# Pediatrics
FOR THE
# Anesthesiologist

# *Pediatrics* FOR THE *Anesthesiologist*

Edited by

**Frederic A. Berry, M.D.**

Professor
Departments of Anesthesiology and Pediatrics
University of Virginia School of Medicine
Charlottesville, Virginia

**David J. Steward, M.B., F.R.C.P.(C.)**

Professor
Department of Anesthesiology
University of Southern California School of Medicine
Director
Department of Anesthesiology
Children's Hospital of Los Angeles
Los Angeles, California

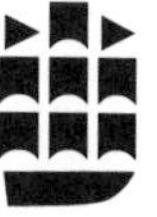

Churchill Livingstone
New York, Edinburgh, London, Madrid, Melbourne, Tokyo

**Library of Congress Cataloging-in-Publication Data**

Pediatrics for the anesthesiologist / edited by Frederic A. Berry, David J. Steward.
p. cm.
Includes bibliographical references and index.
ISBN 0-443-08930-2
1. Pediatric anesthesia. 2. Children—Diseases. I. Berry, Frederic A., Date. II. Steward, David J., Date.
[DNLM: 1. Anesthesia—in infancy & childhood. 2. Drug Therapy—in infancy & childhood. 3. Drug Interactions. WO 440 P3716 1993]
RD139.P44 1993
617.9'6798—dc20
DNLM/DLC
for Library of Congress 93-15587
CIP



Distributed in the United Kingdom by Churchill Livingstone, Robert Stevenson House, 1–3 Baxter's Place, Leith Walk, Edinburgh EH1 3AF, and by associated companies, branches, and representatives throughout the world.

Accurate indications, adverse reactions, and dosage schedules for drugs are provided in this book, but it is possible that they may change. The reader is urged to review the package information data of the manufacturers of the medications mentioned.

The Publishers have made every effort to trace the copyright holders for borrowed material. If they have inadvertently overlooked any, they will be pleased to make the necessary arrangements at the first opportunity.

Copy Editor: *Katharine Leawanna O'Moore*
Production Supervisor: *Patricia McFadden*
Cover Design: *Paul Moran*

Printed in the United States of America

First published in 1993 7 6 5 4 3 2 1

*We dedicate this book to our patients and their parents who have struggled with many years of difficult medical problems and surgical procedures.*

*We also dedicate it to practicing anesthesiologists who, because of the constant technologic and informational advances in medicine, face ever-widening challenges while being harassed by the government and insurance companies with cost-containment measures and voluminous paperwork and by the medicolegal system. It does indeed take dedicated and courageous physicians to practice excellent care under these conditions.*

# Contributors

**Frederic A. Berry, M.D.**
Professor, Departments of Anesthesiology and Pediatrics, University of Virginia School of Medicine, Charlottesville, Virginia

**Charles M. Haberkern, M.D.**
Assistant Professor, Departments of Anesthesiology and Pediatrics, University of Washington School of Medicine; Attending Anesthesiologist, Children's Hospital and Medical Center, Seattle, Washington

**Mark Harris, M.D.**
Associate Professor, Departments of Anesthesiology and Neurosurgery, University of Virginia School of Medicine, Charlottesville, Virginia

**Carol L. Lake, M.D.**
Professor, Department of Anesthesiology, University of Virginia School of Medicine, Charlottesville, Virginia

**John J. Mulroy, Jr.**
Clinical Assistant Professor, University of Utah School of Medicine; Staff Anesthesiologist, Department of Anesthesiology, Primary Children's Medical Center, Salt Lake City, Utah

**Paul C. J. Rogers, M.B., F.R.C.P., F.R.C.P.(C.)**
Senior Consultant, Departments of Hematology and Pediatrics, University of Cape Town, Groote Schuur Hospital, Cape Town, South Africa

**David A. Rosen, M.D.**
Associate Professor, Departments of Anesthesia and Pediatrics, West Virginia University School of Medicine, Morgantown, West Virginia

**Kathleen R. Rosen, M.D.**
Associate Professor, Departments of Anesthesia and Pediatrics, West Virginia University School of Medicine, Morgantown, West Virginia

**Gary M. Scott, M.D., F.A.A.P.**
Clinical Assistant Professor, Department of Anesthesiology, University of Southern California School of Medicine; Attending Anesthesiologist, Department of Anesthesiology, Children's Hospital of Los Angeles, Los Angeles, California

**Michael Seear, M.B., C.H.B., F.R.C.P.(C.)**
Clinical Assistant Professor, Division of Critical Care, University of British Columbia Faculty of Medicine; Attending Staff Member, Pediatric Intensive Care Unit, British Columbia Children's Hospital, Vancouver, British Columbia, Canada

**David J. Steward, M.B., F.R.C.P.(C.)**
Professor, Department of Anesthesiology, University of Southern California School of Medicine; Director, Department of Anesthesiology, Children's Hospital of Los Angeles, Los Angeles, California

**Joseph D. Tobias, M.D.**
Associate Professor, Departments of Anesthesiology and Pediatrics, Vanderbilt University School of Medicine; Associate Director, Division of Pediatric Anesthesiology/Critical Care Medicine, Vanderbilt University Hospital, Nashville, Tennessee

**Louis D. Wadsworth, M.B., F.R.C.P.(C.)**
Clinical Professor, Division of Hematopathology, Department of Pathology and Pediatrics, University of British Columbia Faculty School of Medicine; Program Head, Hematopathology Laboratory, Department of Pathology, British Columbia Children's Hospital; Acting Medical Director, Canadian Red Cross, Vancouver, British Columbia, Canada

**David Wensley, M.B., M.R.C.P., F.R.C.P.(C.)**
Head, Division of Pediatric Critical Care, British Columbia Children's Hospital, Vancouver, British Columbia, Canada

**Andrew M. Woods, M.D.**
Associate Professor, Department of Anesthesiology, University of Virginia School of Medicine; Medical Director, Post-Anesthesia Care Unit and Surgical Admission Suite, University of Virginia Health Sciences Center, Charlottesville, Virginia

**Terrance A. Yemen, M.D.**
Assistant Professor, Division of Pediatrics, Department of Anesthesiology, University of Virginia School of Medicine, Charlottesville, Virginia

# Preface

The anesthesiologist is often faced with a child with a medical disease who needs either some form of diagnostic study or surgery. Until now, there has been no pediatric anesthesia textbook that concisely covered the underlying medical diseases of the pediatric patient. *Pediatrics for the Anesthesiologist* is organized so as to describe, system by system, the medical and infectious diseases encountered in the pediatric patient, and to deal with the special concerns of the pediatric oncology patient.

In several chapters the functions of various body systems are discussed with a view to both proper function and pathophysiology, noting the anesthetic implications of both states. Chapter 8 covers the most common infectious and communicable diseases encountered by the anesthesiologist in the pediatric ward and outpatient facility. Chapter 10 deals with pediatric oncology patients, who often present special challenges since many of the drugs with which they are treated have a cumulative toxicity and have interactions with anesthetic agents that must be taken into consideration by the anesthesiologist.

Finally, in Chapter 11, the needs for pediatric cardiopulmonary resuscitation are approached in a problem-oriented format.

A very helpful feature of this book is the Appendix, which contains comprehensive, easy-to-use tables of the various drugs used to treat pediatric patients, including antibiotics, antihypertensives, and anti-tumor agents. Listed for each drug or agent are the various dosages, as well as the anesthetic interactions and problems that need to be considered by the anesthesiologist. This information—in a quick-reference format—is often not included in pediatric anesthesia books.

This book is not intended to provide the anesthesiologist with a manual on the practice of anesthesia, but rather to assist the anesthesiologist in evaluating the medical problems of the pediatric patient who needs anesthesia.

*Frederic A. Berry, M.D.*
*David J. Steward, M.B., F.R.C.P.(C.)*

# Acknowledgments

We would like to thank Ms. Pat Meté, Ms. Rhonda Taylor, and Mr. Robert Bland for their superb editorial help and assistance.

# Contents

# 1

# Respiratory Diseases

# 1

# Respiratory Diseases

*David Wensley*
*Michael Seear*

## CHANGES IN THE RESPIRATORY SYSTEM AFTER BIRTH

If the preoperative assessment of an adult patient were to read as follows: "high closing volume, significant venous admixture, intracardiac shunting with raised pulmonary arterial pressure, limited exercise tolerance plus abnormally short neck and fat tongue," the average anesthetist would be rather apprehensive. However, even the healthiest newborn fulfills this description, and since surgery in the neonatal period has become a common procedure, it is vital for the anesthetist to have a good working knowledge of the unique physiologic changes that occur after birth.

### Lung Structure

The lung appears as an outgrowth of the foregut at about 3 weeks' gestation (Table 1-1).[1–3] By 16 weeks, the bronchial architecture is complete. Disturbances of growth at this period lead to lung hypoplasia (e.g., diaphragmatic hernia). No further growth of cartilaginous airways is possible. Primitive alveoli (saccules) and surfactant-producing type II cells appear at 24 weeks. By 28 to 30 weeks, the pulmonary capillary bed has developed to the point at which unassisted survival is possible. The muscular layer of the pulmonary artery is thick so that at birth pulmonary and systemic pressures are equal. Pulmonary vascular resistance falls steadily as these arteries remodel over the first 2 to 3 months of extrauterine life. Right-to-left shunting decreases sharply during the first week of life as the pulmonary artery pressure falls and the ductus closes. True alveoli appear at 36 weeks and increase rapidly to a maximum of about 350 million by the age of 6 years. Subsequent lung growth is by increase in alveolar size rather than numbers. The pulmonary capillary bed closely follows the development of these new alveoli.

With development of supporting elastic tissue, lung closing volume falls steadily with age to a minimum around 10 years.

### Lung Volumes

At birth, the child passes from a physiology more suited to the fish to become an air-breathing mammal in about six breaths. The small radius of curvature of the diaphragm allows the child to achieve the high negative pressures ($-70$ cm$H_2O$ or more) necessary to drag the lungs open. A functional residual capacity (FRC) of

**Table 1-1.** Lung Development

| *Gestational Age* | *Lung Development* |
|---|---|
| 4 weeks | Primitive lung buds from foregut |
| 16 weeks | Branching bronchial tree complete down to 28 divisions; no further formation of cartilaginous airways |
| 24 weeks | Primitive alveoli (saccules) and type II cells present; surfactant detectable; survival possible with artificial ventilation |
| 28–30 weeks | Capillary network surrounds saccules; unsupported survival possible |
| 36–40 weeks | True alveoli present, roughly 20 million at birth |
| Birth–3 months | Pulmonary epithelium changes from secretion to net absorption shortly after birth; pulmonary pressure falls below systemic as arterial muscular layer decreases; $PaO_2$ rises as right-to-left mechanical shunts close |
| To 6 years | Rapid increase in alveoli (350 million at 6 years); slow rise in $PaO_2$ as closing volume and consequent venous admixture fall due to development of supporting tissue |

roughly 30 ml/kg is soon established to act as a buffer against changing alveolar gas levels. When related to body weight, static lung volumes are surprisingly close to adult values. However, neonatal alveolar ventilation is over twice as high, reflecting an elevated oxygen consumption. This reduces the buffering capacity of the FRC so changes in inspired gases are rapidly reflected in arterial changes; consequently, gaseous anesthesia induction time is much reduced.

The elastic properties of a neonatal lung are similar to those of a 70-year-old adult (Table 1-2).[3–6] The high closing volume at either end of life may encroach upon FRC, leading to lung collapse and elevated $\dot{V}/\dot{Q}$ mismatch. Closing volume falls during childhood to a minimum at about 10 years. It steadily rises again with age after about 25 years. Small children are particularly at risk from lung collapse and unrecognized hypoxemia during anesthesia. In fact, neonates commonly exhale against a slightly closed glottis, presumably in order to maintain lung volume.

## Lung Mechanics

Although the lungs expand rapidly in the first few breaths, it still takes some days before the interstitial fluid is cleared. This is reflected in the changes in respiratory mechanics. Compliance rises from 1.5 to about 6 ml/cm$H_2O$ during the first week, while resistance falls from 90 cm$H_2O$/L/sec to about 30. When expressed as a ratio of lung volume, respiratory mechanics remain quite constant with growth (Table 1-3).[4–6] Resistance of upper airways is considerable in small children, and since many neonates are obligate nose breathers, any obstruction of the nasal passage (nasogastric tube, mucus) may be clinically significant.

An infant expends about 1 to 2 percent of total energy consumption in quiet breathing. This level is higher in prematures. About 75 percent is elastic work, and the rest is resistive. The highly compliant chest wall combined with horizontal positioning of the ribs makes thoracic ventilation inefficient. Small children rely predominantly on diaphragmatic

**Table 1-2.** Lung Volumes

| *Lung Volume* | *Neonate* | *Adult* |
|---|---|---|
| FVC ml/kg | 35–40 | 50–60 |
| FRC ml/kg | 27–30 | 30–34 |
| RV ml/kg | 20 | 25–30 |
| $V_T$ ml/kg | 6–8 | 5–7 |
| $V_D$ ml/kg | 2–2.5 | 2.2 |
| $V_D/V_T$ | 0.3 | 0.3 |
| $V_A$ ml/min/kg | 100–150 | 60 |
| $V_A$/FRC | 4–5 | 1–2 |
| Closing volume/FRC | ≥1 | <1 but increases again with age |
| Surface area of lung ($m^2$/kg) | 0.9 | 0.9 |

breathing. They have a smaller percentage of slow-twitch, fatigue-resistant muscle fibers in the diaphragm and are predisposed to ventilatory muscle fatigue. They also do not tolerate increases in abdominal pressure.

## Control of Ventilation

Although most measures of respiratory control are normal by 3 to 4 weeks of age, it is likely that the system remains immature for longer than this, especially in preterm infants. Poor respiratory control is probably a major factor in sudden infant death syndrome (SIDS), which is the second commonest cause of infant loss between 3 and 9 months.

Chemoreceptor control is present at birth. Newborns are able to respond to hypercarbia by increasing ventilation, but the slope of the response curve increases with postnatal age. The response to hypoxia is biphasic: there is an initial hyperpnea followed by depression of respiration in about 2 minutes. A fully sustained response does not develop for 2 to 3 weeks. The initial hypoxic response is abolished by hypothermia and very low levels of anesthetic gases. Apart from medullary regulation of ventilation, there are peripheral lung receptors that respond to a variety of stimuli (stretch receptors, irritant receptors, and J-receptors) plus primitive pulmonary reflexes (Head's, Hering-Breuer) that probably help control the depth and frequency of ventilation in this complex system.

Respiratory pauses of about 5 seconds (periodic respiration) are common in infants, especially during rapid eye movement (REM) sleep. They are probably due to immature feedback control and are abolished by administration of oxygen or carbon dioxide or increasing lung volume with positive pressure. Apnea of infancy is defined as respiratory pauses exceeding 20 seconds or those accompanied by bradycardia or cyanosis. Postoperative apneic spells are common in premature infants, and close monitoring is necessary after the most minor procedures. The risk drops rapidly after 45 weeks conceptual age.

**Table 1-3.** Lung Mechanics

| *Lung Mechanics* | *Neonate* | *Adult* |
|---|---|---|
| $C_L$ ml/cm$H_2O$ | 4–6 | 150–200 |
| $C_L$/FRC | 0.04–0.06 | 0.04–0.07 |
| Raw cm $H_2O$/L/sec | 25–40 | 3–5 |
| $f$ | 40–60 | 10–15 |
| Type I fibers (diaphragm %) | 20–30 | 50–60 |

## Oxygen Delivery

Adequate delivery of oxygen to the tissues requires close integration of three components: arterial oxygenation (a final product of pulmonary mechanics, $\dot{V}/\dot{Q}$ mismatch, shunt, and so forth), oxygen carriage (hemoglobin level and oxyhemoglobin dissociation curve), and delivery (cardiac output). Many of the subunits of this complicated system undergo marked changes in the first few weeks of life (Table 1-4),[5,7–14] which makes an assessment of tissue oxygenation difficult. The oxygen consumption index of a newborn is twice as high as an adult, so there is much less margin for error in the delivery system. To some extent, problems with one component can be compensated for by changes in another area; for example, the newborn has a left-shifted dissociation curve[15] plus a high hemoglobin and so delivers a proportionately higher volume of oxygen than the adult, while the reduced hemoglobin level of older children (anemia of childhood) is compensated for by a right shift in the dissociation curve and a higher normal $PaO_2$. Cardiac output is rarely measured in children, so calculations of $\dot{V}O_2$ and $\dot{D}O_2$ are not usually available. Oxygen delivery can only be assessed rather crudely by clinical examination, arterial blood gases (particularly pH and base excess), and serum lactate.

**Table 1-4.** Oxygen Delivery

| *Component* | *Changes with Age* |
|---|---|
| Cardiac output (ml/min/kg) | 400–500 at birth; rapidly falls to 100–150 and remains constant through childhood |
| Hemoglobin (g/100 ml) | 15–20 at birth, falls to 9–13 during early childhood ("physiologic anemia"), then climbs to adult levels 12–15 |
| Oxyhemoglobin dissociation | Curve shifted to left at birth ($P_{50}$ 19 mmHg); shifted to right after 3 months ($P_{50}$ 32 mmHg) probably due to high ATP and 2,3-DPG levels; falls to adult levels coincident with rise in hemoglobin |
| Anatomic shunts | Mechanical shunts (ductus aretriosus and foramen ovale) decrease as pulmonary artery pressure falls during first 2–4 weeks |
| $\dot{V}/\dot{Q}$ mismatch | Mainly due to high closing volume (CV); $\dot{V}/\dot{Q}$ mismatch falls during childhood as CV falls to a minimum around 10 years of age |
| Arterial oxygenation (mmHg) | Rises rapidly as mechanical shunts close, then more slowly as CV drops: 50 on day 1, 70 at week 1, 85 during first year, maximum of 96 around 10-12 years; $Aa\dot{D}O_2$ is 20–25 in neonates and falls to 8–10 in teenagers |

## Practical Points

There are many differences in structure and function between the respiratory systems of older children and infants, especially those born prematurely. Many of these differences have great practical significance for the anesthetist and, just as importantly, for the recovery room staff.

1. Large head, short neck, large tongue, small mouth, anterior larynx, and very compressible upper airway. Intubation and bag and mask ventilation require practice.
2. Horizontal ribs, compliant chest wall, predominantly diaphragmatic breathing. Low percentage of fatigue-resis-

tant muscle fibers; therefore, prone to ventilatory muscle fatigue and also sensitive to raised abdominal pressure.

3. Closing volume may encroach on tidal ventilation. Anesthesia reduces FRC by causing peripheral airway collapse, impaired intercostal activity and diaphragmatic action, and consequently increased $\dot{V}/\dot{Q}$ mismatch. Postoperative hypoxemia is common.[16]
4. Immature respiratory control, particularly before 45 weeks conceptual age. Anesthetic gases accentuate the problem.
5. Unpredictable effects on $\dot{V}/\dot{Q}$ matching and cardiac function in response to positive pressure ventilation. Improved oxygen saturation does not necessarily imply improved oxygen delivery.[17]

## PREOPERATIVE ASSESSMENT OF THE RESPIRATORY SYSTEM

The preoperative workup of a surgical pediatric patient depends, to a large extent, on the planned procedure. Since this can range from tympanostomy tubes in a normal child to a heart-lung transplant in advanced cystic fibrosis, a certain flexibility is required in the initial assessment. There is no end to the tests that can be performed in a tertiary referral center. Each has its own idiosyncrasies and wide range of normal values (that broaden rapidly as age decreases). Occasionally, some of them produce results that, after much discussion, are deemed to be of value. However, as Rufus of Ephesus pointed out nearly 2,000 years ago, there is absolutely no substitute for a complete history and physical examination.

### History

With hospital inpatients, it is probably best to start with a review of the chart. This may reveal the history of the main problem, complications, degree of compromise of the major systems, previous surgery, and response to past anesthetics.

A short talk with the attending physician often makes the task of plowing through a large chart a bit easier. Of course, with day-care patients, this procedure is much simplified, but there is still a core of information that should be obtained from everyone.

Apart from a detailed review of the main complaint and its effects on the respiratory system, it is important to cover the child's past respiratory health, including a careful neonatal and family history (Table 1-5). A review of symptoms can provide a reasonable idea of the functional state of the patient's lungs, and in the young child is probably a better index

**Table 1-5.** History

| | |
|---|---|
| Chart review | Past surgery and anesthetics, test results, history of major problem, etc. |
| Present complaint | Duration, effect on major systems, present drugs, especially bronchodilators, corticosteroids, antibiotics |
| Respiratory problems | Cough, wheeze, cyanosis, stridor, exercise tolerance |
| Past medical health | Asthma, chest infections, previous operations, mechanical ventilation, immunizations, other significant chest problems (e.g., scoliosis, at-home $O_2$) |
| Neonatalogy health | Pregnancy, delivery, gestational age, neonatal illnesses (e.g., hyaline membrane disease, prematurity, prolonged ventilation) |
| Family history | Asthma, allergies, hay fever, eczema, cystic fibrosis |

of operative suitability than any of the available laboratory investigations. Observant parents will have a good idea of the child's exercise tolerance compared with healthy friends and siblings. Symptoms such as wheeze, stridor, respiratory distress, or even cyanosis with exercise will help to quantify the risk of anesthetic.

## Examination

The potential of percussion and auscultation to detect subtle pathology in small children is limited. Most important information comes from careful observations of the calm child, preferably resting on the parent's lap.

Depth and rate of respiration, presence of upper respiratory tract infections, clubbing, cyanosis, alar flare, and respiratory indrawing plus an estimate of the size of face mask and endotracheal tube can all be assessed at without touching the child (Table 1-6).

**Table 1-6.** Examination

| | |
|---|---|
| General | Height, weight, respiratory rate, cyanosis (use oximeter if any doubt), clubbing, alar flare, retractions |
| Head | Size of mask, endotracheal tube, oral airway, laryngoscopy blade; loose teeth |
| Ear/nose/throat | Airway patency, presence of acute upper respiratory tract infection |
| Upper airway | Inspiratory stridor, croupy cough |
| Lower airway | Expiratory wheeze, bronchial breathing, crackles, distribution of air entry |

Although purists might object, it is best to auscultate the chest when a quiet moment occurs and not necessarily to wait until the end of the examination. It is not possible to detect fine wheezes and crackles in a squirming, screaming, or breath-holding child.

Those with a trusting nature will use the height and weight displayed on the chart to calculate drug doses and ventilation settings. Examination should also include mouth, ears, nose, and throat, with a check for loose teeth and the presence of acute upper respiratory tract infections.

## Pulmonary Function Tests in Cooperative Children

Although pulmonary function tests can provide useful information, they are subject to large potential errors. Three main problems should be considered before the results can be taken too seriously:

1. Most tests are effort dependent. Technicians must be specially trained in coaching children and patient enough to obtain maximum cooperation. In general, reliable results will not be obtained in children below about 6 years of age. Test reports must contain a comment or score to indicate degree of cooperation the child displayed.
2. Tests should be performed on well-maintained, calibrated machines capable of measuring small airflows accurately. The American Thoracic Society provides laboratory standardization guidelines.[18]
3. Lung function parameters are usually compared to reference standards based on the patient's age, height, weight, and sex. Prediction equations must be based on a pediatric population and not on wild extrapolations from adult data.

The following tests are commonly performed[19–21] on cooperative children (>6 or 7 years).

### Static Lung Volumes

Inspiratory and expiratory volumes are plotted against time before and during a maximal breath. They are mainly used to measure vital capacity and expired volume at 1 second (Fig. 1-1).

### Flow–Volume Loops

Flow rate can be plotted against its instantaneous integrated value (i.e., volume) to obtain a closed flow–volume loop whose slope is mmHg (time constant). The shape of the curve is diagnostic of some conditions. In addition, various flow rates (peak, mid- and end-expiratory) can be measured and compared with normal values (Fig. 1-2).

### Total Lung Capacity

Residual volume can be calculated by measuring total lung capacity (usually helium dilution from a known volume container) and then subtracting vital capacity.

### Diffusion Capacity

The diffusion capacity of the lung for certain gases can be measured. It provides a broad indication of the efficiency of total gas transfer. The single-breath technique using carbon monoxide is commonly used.

### Bronchial Responsiveness

Various provocative tests (histamine, methacholine, cold air exercise) are available to assess the degree of airway responsiveness. There is a large overlap be-

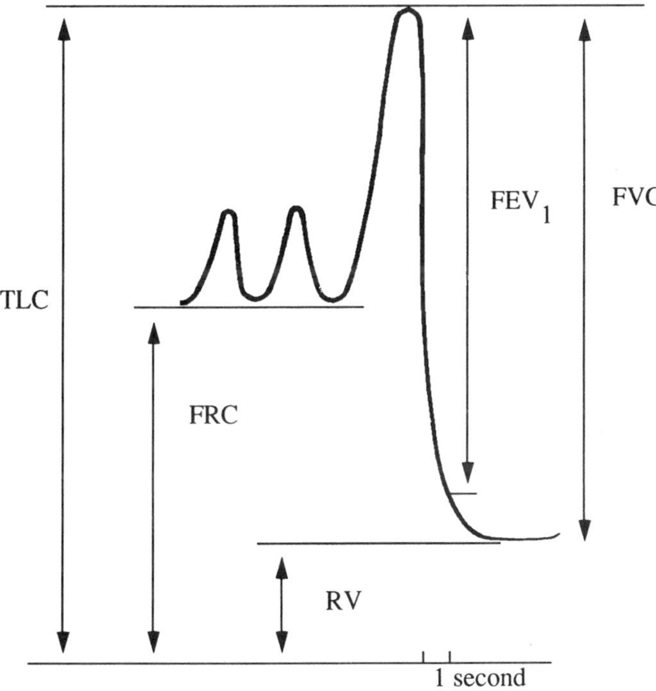


**Fig. 1-1.** Static lung volumes. TLC, total lung capacity; FRC, functional residual capacity; RV, residual volume; $FEV_1$, forced expiratory volume in 1 second; FVC, forced vital capacity.

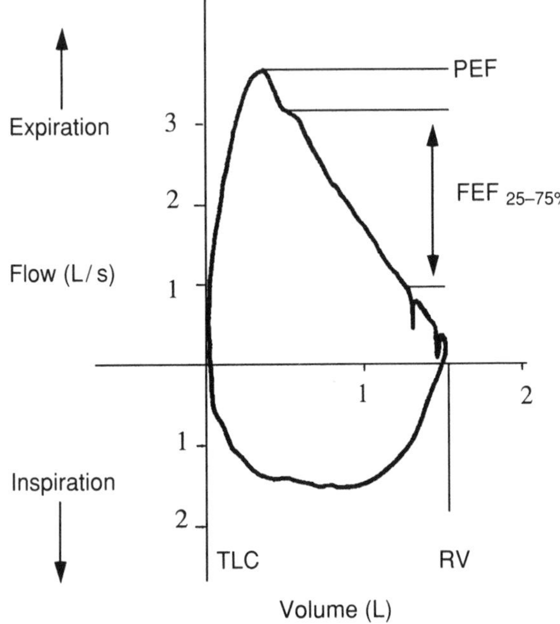


**Fig. 1-2.** Flow–volume loop. PEF, peak expiratory flow; $FEF_{25-75\%}$, expiratory flow between 75 and 25 percent of expired volume.

tween normals and abnormals. Interpretation can be difficult.

### Exercise Testing

Various parameters (oxygen consumption, oximetry, blood pressure, pulse) may be measured during graded exercise and compared with normal values. This can be of value in children down to about 4 years of age.

In general, a well-equipped laboratory can provide useful predictive information in children older than 6 or 7 years. As long as their limitations are remembered, these are useful tests to perform prior to administering an anesthetic.

## Pulmonary Function Tests in Infants

There are several new techniques (including at least two commercially available machines) designed to measure pulmonary mechanics (mainly compliance and resistance) in uncooperative infants. They suffer from common problems:

1. It is difficult to produce reliable and reproducible results when measuring tidal volumes less than 50 ml. Small errors rapidly invalidate the results.
2. Resistance of the upper airway or endotracheal tube is such a large percentage of total resistance that $R_{rs}$ has little predictive power.
3. The tests are time consuming and the child requires sedation.
4. Widely accepted normal values are not available.

The measurement of pulmonary mechanics in intubated children is a relatively straightforward problem. Such patients are easily instrumented, and several techniques exist to measure pulmonary mechanics.[22]

The simplest measurement is peak-inspiratory pressure, although this does not distinguish between elastic and resistive forces. The recent development of hot wire flow meters means that tidal volumes can be measured accurately even on small children. If this volume is divided by end-inspiratory plateau pressure (i.e., no flow, hence no resistance), then static compliance of the respiratory system can be calculated. This provides a simple method of monitoring elastic forces before and during an anesthetic.

Apart from the practical problems of measuring small flows and pressures in infants,[23] the need for sedation and the absence of widely accepted normal values make the measurement of lung mechanics in unintubated infants largely a research tool.[24] It is certainly far from being a routine preoperative test.

The major methods available for unintubated, spontaneously breathing infants are:

#### Esophageal Balloon

Using an esophageal balloon[25] to estimate average pleural pressure, plus face mask and pneumotachograph to measure flow, is a cumbersome means of measuring mechanics in unintubated children. It remains the gold standard but has little practical clinical application for the anesthetist.

#### Multiple Occlusion

Infants usually relax when expiration is occluded (Hering-Breuer reflex). Mouth pressure at this point is assumed to equal alveolar pressure. By performing multiple occlusions and measuring exhaled volume, a pressure volume plot can be constructed. The slope of the graph is lung compliance.[26]

#### Passive Exhalation

A flow–volume plot can be generated from the passive exhaled breath after flow obstruction. The slope of this plot equals time constant (resistance × compliance). Since compliance can also be measured at the same time using occlusion pressure and exhaled volume, it is possible to calculate resistance.[27]

#### Forced Exhalation

Flow–volume curves can be generated in sedated infants by rapidly inflating a close-fitting jacket with air and measuring flow through a tight face mask.[28] Various measurements are made from the curve including flow rate at residual capacity. Although commercial "squeeze" machines are available, the technique has many critics and is the subject of debate.

## COMMON RESPIRATORY DISORDERS

### Upper Respiratory Tract Infections

#### The "Common Cold"

Acute nasopharyngitis is the most frequent childhood infection. The average child contracts five to eight episodes each year. The commonest agents are viral (mainly rhinoviruses and coronaviruses). Group A streptococci and mycoplasma are the most common bacterial causes. The clinical course is usually mild, and side effects are rare. The pediatric anesthetist will frequently be faced with the problem of anesthetizing a child with an active upper respiratory tract infection (URTI). Unfortunately, the information in the literature is sparse and contradictory. Anesthesia in adult patients with upper respiratory tract infection is probably safe,[29] but the pediatric literature has been split between those who feel there is an increased risk of pulmonary side effects[30] and those who feel it is probably safe.[31] The risk of airway incidents is increased in infants of under 1 year, and older children may suffer more complications if anesthetized during an acute URTI.

### Croup

Acute laryngotracheobronchitis[32] is a common childhood problem. Apart from diphtheria the cause is usually viral (parainfluenza). The typical croupy cough and respiratory stridor develop after 2 to 3 days of coryza. The major area of swelling is in the subglottic area. The child usually does not look toxic. Bacterial superinfection may produce an associated tracheitis that is difficult to distinguish from epiglottitis. Mild cases settle without treatment while most others can be controlled with nebulized epinephrine. Rare cases requiring intubation are a management problem because the swelling takes some days to subside and there is a real danger of endotracheal tube blockage by secretions. Occasional cases still require tracheotomy to allow the area to heal without the irritation of an endotracheal tube.

### Epiglottitis

Acute bacterial infection of the epiglottis and surrounding tissues is a potentially lethal disease.[33] It can usually be distinguished from croup without problem. A typical patient has a rapid onset, is febrile, septic, drooling, aphonic, and progresses rapidly toward respiratory obstruction. The most common cause is *Haemophilus influenzae*. Blood cultures are usually positive. The child should be attended continuously by a physician able to maintain an airway. Acute obstruction may be precipitated by examination. Although some units manage less severe cases with antibiotics and observation, most would include intubation under anesthetic in their management for at least 24 hours. The infection is systemic: septic shock and meningitis are potential side effects. Prophylactic rifampin should be given to the family if there is a sibling below 48 months of age. Chloramphenicol or cefotaxime are usually added to ampicillin because of increasing antibiotic resistance.

## Lower Respiratory Tract Infections

### Bronchiolitis

Acute bronchiolitis is a viral disease that causes inflammatory obstruction at the small airway level. The clinical picture of air trapping, wheeze, lung hyperinflation, and areas of atelectasis is identical to asthma.[34] The commonest cause is respiratory syncytial virus (RSV), but adenovirus, parainfluenza 3, and mycoplasma can cause similar clinical pictures. Children with underlying cardiorespiratory disease (congenital heart disease, bronchopulmonary dysplasia, and so forth) are particularly at risk for respiratory failure. A large percentage of these children will subsequently develop reactive airways disease and, in some cases, a picture of chronic lung disease due to obliterative bronchiolitis. Ribavirin given by aerosol early in the disease has been shown to improve outcome when the agent is RSV.[35] The drug is expensive and is usually reserved for the more serious cases.

### Pneumonia

Acute infections of the lung are common. The severity of the illness and the etiologic agent depend largely on the child's age and underlying immune state. Organ transplantation and cancer treatment make unusual organisms, such as pneumocystis and fungi, increasingly common respiratory pathogens in a hospital-based population. Table 1-7 gives the common organisms found at various ages in otherwise healthy children.[36]

Viral diagnosis has become easier with

**Table 1-7.** Common Causes of Pneumonia

| | |
|---|---|
| Newborns | Group B streptococcus, gram negatives, listeria, cytomegalovirus, herpes, chlamydia |
| Under 5 | Respiratory syncytial virus, parainfluenza, influenza adenovirus, pneumococcus, *H. influenza*, *S. aureus* |
| School age | Mycoplasma, pneumococcus, chlamydia (TWAR), group A streptococcus, influenza, adenovirus |

the development of rapid antigen testing, but bacterial diagnosis is difficult. Blood cultures are usually negative, while sputum cultures are of little help. The gold standard is percutaneous needle puncture of the lung, which for obvious reasons is not commonly performed. Treatment consists of antibiotics and good supportive care. Infants are at particular risk of respiratory failure.

## Cystic Fibrosis

Cystic fibrosis is a systemic disease characterized by mucus accumulation and plugging that affects many areas of the body. The major cause of mortality is due to progressive lung disease, probably due to a cycle of obstruction and infection of small airways, with eventual destruction of large parts of the lung. A similar pathology explains pancreatic duct obstruction, malabsorption, focal cirrhosis, and male infertility. The disease is genetic and is transmitted as an autosomal recessive. The major gene responsible for the disease has recently been discovered on the long arm of chromosome 7. The carriage rate for whites is roughly 4 to 5 percent, with a homozygous incidence of 1 in 2,000. Treatment consists of chest physiotherapy, pancreatic enzyme supplementation, and aggressive treatment of lung infections. Median survival is over 30 years in some centers. Males have a better prognosis than females. Preoperative preparation with intensive physiotherapy, antibiotic coverage, and good nutrition is very important prior to any planned anesthetic.[37]

## Foreign Bodies

Aspiration of foreign bodies into the airway is a common problem in young children. The object usually follows the straight course of the right main stem bronchus and lodges in the right lung. After an initial period of coughing and gagging, the child may be surprisingly free from symptoms. Objects causing a check valve effect may present with unilateral wheeze, shift of the trachea, and hyperinflation of the affected lung. (This may be more obvious on inspiratory/expiratory chest films.) Large objects can cause acute respiratory failure and even death. Clinically silent objects may present some time later as asthma, recurrent pneumonia, or hemoptysis. Vegetable matter, especially oily nuts, can cause a chronic local reaction that necessitates lobectomy. Recovery is usually complete after successful removal by bronchoscopy.[38]

## Asthma

Asthma is a poorly defined disease that produces recurrent episodes of cough, wheezing, and breathlessness resulting from variable increases in airway resistance. Airflow obstruction occurs in the small airways as a result of an inflammatory response to a variety of stimuli causing narrowing of the lumen from bronchial muscle constriction, mucosal edema, and increased mucus and debris in the airway.[39,40] Asthmatics appear to have an increased response to the stimuli that cause airway narrowing, and this bronchial hyperactivity varies with time and under a variety of influences. The prevalence varies (depending on the population studied) from less than 1 percent in some developing countries to over 25 percent in New Zealand. In North America, figures vary from 4 to 13 percent.[41] Genetic factors seem important, but the mode of inheritance is unclear. Atopic symptoms, either in the child or family members, are common.

The clinical features vary from a persistent cough, often more marked at night, through episodes of wheezing and breathlessness, to life-threatening episodes of respiratory distress. A number of studies have reported an increase in morbidity in the preschool ages and in mortality in teenage and young adults over the past 15 years.[42] The symptom pattern and triggering factors vary widely, but often the young child develops episodic wheezing and chronic cough associated with respiratory infections, even in infancy, while in the older child, allergens, irritants, and stress and exercise assume greater importance. Some children have persistent symptoms, while in others asthma is episodic or seasonal. Children with milder symptoms (by far the larger group) tend to improve with age and are generally symptom free by late childhood, while the more severely affected will also improve somewhat but often require therapy into adult life.[41] Asthma is diagnosed by exclusion, and although it is the most common cause of recurrent cough and wheezing in childhood, other pathology, such as inhalation injury from large foreign bodies or liquids (reflux and swallowing problems), large airway compression, and cystic fibrosis need to be considered.

Acute episodes often follow shortly after a triggering event and may progress to coughing paroxysms, at times associated with retching and vomiting, tachypnea, retractions and hyperinflation, and wheezing. Progression is heralded by increasing respiratory distress, tachycardia, increasing pulsus paradoxus, anxiety, and eventually somnolence and coma. A few children have severe life-threatening episodes with rapid progression to respiratory failure, sometimes as a result of an identifiable allergic trigger. The airway obstruction results in air trapping, hypoxemia from ventilation–perfusion mismatch, and eventually hypercarbia from ventilatory failure.

Management of the acute episode includes the use of oxygen, guided by pulse oximetry, and early inhaled bronchodilators. A chest radiograph may be helpful in confirming the diagnosis and ruling out foreign body inhalation. It should also be performed if a pneumothorax or pneumomediastinum is suspected. Findings in uncomplicated asthma are generally hyperinflation, peribronchial thickening, perihilar infiltrate, and segmental or lobar atelectasis commonly involving the right middle lobe. The decision to hospitalize a child with a mild asthmatic attack is generally based on previous history, current triggering event, response to inhaled bronchodilators, and ability of the family to manage the situation. Children with moderate or severe asthma and those who do not improve with inhaled bronchodilators should be hospitalized. Despite vomiting and increased respiratory effort, it is rare for children with asthma and bronchiolitis to be significantly dehydrated at presentation. However, they often require IV fluid therapy as oral intake may be reduced. Most inflammatory lung diseases result in retention of fluid and increase in lung water, which may cause increased respiratory difficulty. Maintenance fluid intake is adequate to ensure hydration, and fluid is not replaced unless significant signs of dehydration are present. Blood gases may indicate the severity of asthma in older children. However, they are more difficult to obtain and may be difficult to interpret in infants and young children. With mild distress, the $PCO_2$ is reduced, but with increasing airway obstruction, hypercarbia occurs. This is reached earlier in the course in younger children and clinical assessment is more important in the diagnosis of respiratory failure. Laboratory tests should include an aminophylline level in children on oral therapy. The white blood count is often elevated (>15,000) in response to the asthmatic attack. Spirometry is useful in the older child with mild distress to evaluate the degree of obstruction and response to therapy. Drug therapy is given in Table 1-8. Inhaled $\beta_2$-agonists should be given early, and an effective method of delivery to ensure adequate drug is available in particles in the 1 to 5 μm range is essential.[43–45]

Complications include air leaks and respiratory failure. Pneumothorax is suggested by sudden acute deterioration of respiratory status, occasionally accompanied by chest pain and subcutaneous emphysema. In the nonventilated child with asthma this is a rare complication that requires urgent assessment and management. The lung on the affected side may remain partially inflated and is often slow to expand following insertion of a chest tube. Pneumothoraces occur commonly in ventilated asthmatics. Respiratory failure during asthmatic attacks in children is a clinical diagnosis. The child develops increasing anxiousness and agitation with signs of desaturation, and the breath sounds and wheezing are decreased (silent chest). Pulsus paradoxus and tachycardia may increase. The child becomes less responsive and eventually the respiratory rate is reduced.

Management of respiratory failure is outlined in Table 1-9.

Paralyzing drugs should be used with caution since the intermittent positive pressure ventilation (IPPV) may not be as effective as spontaneous ventilation with marked expiratory obstruction. An endotracheal tube may increase bronchospasm and this should be anticipated. Slow ventilatory rates (<12/min) with low inspiratory pressures (<45 $cmH_2O$) and mild hypercarbia ($CO_2$ 45 to 60 mmHg) minimize barotrauma.[46]

Bronchial hyperactivity persists for some weeks following an asthmatic attack. Bronchodilators and antiinflammatory agents should be continued until symptoms resolve. Chronic management is outlined in Table 1-10.[47]

Inhaled medications can be given to

**Table 1-9.** Management of Respiratory Failure

1. IV $\beta_2$-agonist (salbutamol, isoproterenol)
2. Intubation and ventilation
   Anesthetic agents to treat bronchospasm:
      Halothane[87] (risk of arrhythmias with $\beta$-agonists and theophyllines)
      Ketamine[88]

**Table 1-8.** Management of Acute Exacerbation

1. Inhaled $\beta_2$-agonist
2. Level 1 + oral steroid
3. Level 1 + IV steroid ± inhaled ipratropium bromide
4. Level 3 + IV theophylline (epinephrine s.c.)
5. Management of respiratory failure

**Table 1-10.** Chronic Therapy

1. Inhaled $\beta_2$-agonist as needed ± cromoglycate (before provocation)
2. Level 1 + regular cromoglycate or low-dose inhaled steroid
3. Level 1 + high-dose inhaled steroid ± sustained release theophylline ± inhaled ipratropium bromide
4. Level 3 + oral prednisone

**Table 1-11.** Replacement Corticosteroid Therapy in Adrenosuppressed Patients

| |
|---|
| Basal output: 12–15 mg/m$^2$/d cortisol |
| Minor stress/surgery: basal replacement |
| Moderate–severe stress/surgery: 2–4 times basal output/d |
| Replacement continued while effects of stress/surgery evident |

children from 2 to 3 years old quite effectively using a metered dose inhaler with a spacer device,[48,49] and in older children with breath-activated dry powder devices.

Education of parents and children is crucial to asthma management, since they control chronic therapy in this fluctuating disease. An understanding of the disease and the medications is needed, along with a simple writing strategy for adjusting medications and guidelines for when medical attention should be sought. Avoidance of triggers, allergens, and particularly smoking in the home needs to be stressed.

In children who have had a number of courses of systemic corticosteroids over a few weeks or who are on long-term oral steroids, adrenal suppression should be considered. Assessment of adrenocortical function can be obtained from a morning cortisol level or a stimulation test. Guidelines for replacement therapy are given in Table 1-11.

## Neonatal Lung Disorders

### Respiratory Distress Syndrome (Hyaline Membrane Disease)

Respiratory distress syndrome results from surfactant deficiency and is the most common cause of both respiratory distress in newborns and perinatal mortality. Surfactant is generated in the type II alveolar cells from about 24 weeks, but an amount sufficient for extrauterine survival occurs at lung maturity equivalent to about 35 weeks, which can occur as early as 30 weeks gestational age in some infants or as late as term in infants acutely stressed or born to diabetic mothers. Surfactant deficiency results in atelectasis, reduced compliance, and hypoxemia. The infant may be normal at birth but soon develops signs of increasing work of breathing and hypoxemia. Chest radiographs show a diffuse reticulogranular pattern throughout both lung fields with air bronchograms extending into the periphery and some progress to a "white-out" involving both lungs. Management is supportive, with oxygen, positive end-expiratory pressure, and mechanical ventilation, and some units are evaluating the use of high-frequency ventilation. Avoidance of stress, particularly thermal stress and hypoglycemia, and attention to fluid status without excessive fluid administration are important. Prevention by corticosteroid administration to mothers in premature labor appears to help infants at 30 to 34 weeks' gestation.[50] A number of trials of surfactant replacement therapy are underway, and preliminary results suggest a reduction in mortality and complications, although these are not striking.[51] Differentiation from bacterial pneumonia may be difficult, and antibiotics are commonly given. Complications include air leaks (pulmonary interstitial emphysema, pneumomediastinum, and pneumothorax), disseminated intravascular coagulation, cerebral hemorrhage, secondary infection, and patent ductus arteriosus. Five to 30 percent of these infants go on to develop bronchopulmonary dysplasia.

### Bronchopulmonary Dysplasia

Bronchopulmonary dysplasia is a chronic lung disease characterized by hypoxia and hypercapnia, usually following intensive therapy for respiratory distress, as first described by Northway.[52] It commonly follows hyaline membrane disease, but a similar picture is seen complicating other causes of neonatal respiratory distress. Pathologic changes represent damage and repair with areas of emphysema surrounded by atelectasis, an increase in fibrous tissue and bronchial mucosal, and muscle hyperplasia. Early chest radiograph changes are indistinguishable from hyaline membrane disease, but after 10 days small radiolucent cysts appear in the perihilar areas and extend to the entire lung fields, eventually producing a generalized cystic appearance with areas of hyperlucency and streaky infiltrates. Management is supportive, with oxygen and ventilation. Mortality up to 30 percent has been described, but if these infants can be weaned from the ventilator, after a period of oxygen dependence which may last for months, they often show no clinical respiratory compromise. Pulmonary function abnormalities may persist into late childhood and there appears to be a higher incidence of reactive airways disease in these children. Neurologic and developmental abnormalities are common in this group.[50]

A small group of preterm infants will develop chronic respiratory distress not associated with ventilatory support in the immediate neonatal period. This condition was first described by Wilson and Mikity,[53] and is now termed chronic pulmonary disease of prematurity. The absence of structural change in the pulmonary tissue is striking. Mortality may be high (30 percent) in the early stages, but survivors frequently show complete resolution. Management is similar to that for bronchopulmonary dysplasia.

### Meconium Aspiration Syndrome

Meconium in the amniotic fluid at birth is abnormal and indicates an episode of asphyxia. Aspiration of particulate meconium present at the time of birth can result in severe respiratory distress. In the presence of meconium the hypopharynx should be suctioned when the head has just crowned. If the infant has not commenced vigorous respiration immediately after delivery, endotracheal suctioning, using the endotracheal tube as the aspirator, should be performed two or three times to remove as much particulate meconium as possible.[54] Vigorous resuscitation may be required, and the infant may go on to develop respiratory failure with hypoxemia, hyperinflation, and chest radiograph findings of patchy increased lucency and mottled increased densities throughout the lung fields. Air leaks, persistent pulmonary hypertension with right-to-left shunting, and hypoglycemia commonly complicate the course in severe cases. Mortality is high and neurological sequelae are common.[50]

### Persistent Pulmonary Hypertension of the Newborn

Pulmonary vascular resistance is high in utero to maintain the normal fetal circulation and initially drops with aeration of the lungs and then gradually over the first few days of life. Hypoxemia and acidosis complicating a number of conditions in the newborn period can predispose to persistent pulmonary hypertension of the newborn, but this is also associated with polycythemia, hypoglycemia, and postmaturity, and may occur without obvious underlying cause. Clinically the infants present with marked cyanosis and tachypnea, and the lung fields are clear or reflect the underlying cause. Cardiac evaluation shows the heart to be normal anatomically, but pulmonary hypertension with right-to-left shunting through the foramen ovale and ductus arteriosus is present. This condition is associated with a significant mortality, and pathologic examination in primary cases generally shows increased muscularization of the pulmonary arterioles. Management is supportive and consists of hyperventilation to maintain alkalosis, high oxygen levels ($PO_2 > 100$ mmHg) and pulmonary vasodilators such as tolazoline and prostaglandin.[55,56] Minimal handling and avoidance of stress are important.

### Wet Lung

Some infants present with mild respiratory distress in the first day of life. Chest radiographs show linear densities radiating from the perihilar region. Oxygen may be necessary and occasionally these infants require ventilation, but generally the distress resolves over a few days. It is thought that the syndrome results from delayed clearing of fetal lung water.[57]

### Pulmonary Hemorrhage

Symptomatic massive pulmonary hemorrhage is generally a complication of other disorders such as sepsis, hemolytic disease of the newborn, asphyxia, and kernicterus. It is often a terminal event in these conditions. Rarely it occurs spontaneously without obvious underlying disease, although at autopsy local extravasations of blood into the alveoli is a common incidental finding.

### Apnea

Apnea is common in high-risk neonates and may be a sign of sepsis or other stress. In premature infants from about 30 weeks it can occur spontaneously, probably as a result of immature control of central respiratory drive or control of upper airway tone. Management is aimed at exclusion of underlying causes, minimizing stress (temperature and hypoglycemia), respiratory stimulants (theophylline), and ventilation. With time the infant will develop a regular respiratory drive, and the problem generally resolves.[58]

Stress up to 45 weeks conceptual age may precipitate further episodes of apnea. This is seen particularly in infants with bronchopulmonary dysplasia when they develop a respiratory tract infection, particularly RSV, or following minor surgery such as hernia repair. Infants need monitoring for apnea around these events.[59–61]

## Sudden Infant Death Syndrome

SIDS is defined as the death of any infant or young child that is unsuspected by history, and in which a thorough postmortem examination has failed to demonstrate an adequate cause of death. The incidence is about 2 in 1,000 live births; most occur between 2 weeks and 6 months of age, with the peak between 2 and 3 months. A number of risk factors have been implicated, including low socioeconomic class, low birthweight, smoking and drug abuse in mothers, and siblings who have died of SIDS. Many mechanisms causing the syndrome have been postulated, including cardiac arrhythmias, seizures, hypoglycemia, and central and obstructive apnea.[62,63]

A larger group of infants (up to 2 percent of the population) present with apparent life-threatening events (ALTE). These are episodes of apnea, often with a color change; the observer has suspected the infant is dead. In about half of this group an etiology can be shown, such as gastroesophageal reflux, infection, neurologic problems, and upper airway obstruction. Of the group in whom no cause is suggested, the risk of SIDS may be as high as 10 percent if the episode occurred during sleep.[64] Home monitoring programs have not been shown to reduce the incidence of SIDS.

## Congenital Defects Affecting the Respiratory System

### Esophageal Atresia and Tracheoesophageal Fistula

An abnormal separation of the esophagus from the trachea may occur some time after the 24th day of gestation. Esophageal atresia occurs in 1 in 3,000 to 4,500 live births, of which one-third are premature and one-third have associated anomalies. The most common form consists of an upper blind esophageal pouch and fistula from the trachea to the lower esophagus (87 percent). Esophageal atresia without fistula is the next most common (8 percent), with H-type fistula (without atresia) occurring in 4 percent of cases.[65] Esophageal atresia is associated with polyhydramnios and may be noted on prenatal ultrasound. It should be suspected in mucous infants or if choking occurs on feeding. In the common form, aspiration can occur when pharyngeal or gastric secretions cause respiratory distress. Positive pressure ventilation is difficult in the presence of a fistula, and if ventilatory support is required, consideration should be given to urgent ligation of the fistula. Emergency gastrostomy may be lifesaving in the infant with gastric distension and ventilatory failure. Other congenital defects should be suspected, particularly involving the following areas: vertebrae, anus, cardiac, tracheoesophageal, renal and limb (to make up the VACTERL syndrome). H-type tracheoesophageal fistula presents with recurrent aspiration and is often diagnosed later in infancy or childhood.

Pulmonary complications following repair are common and consist of recurrent bronchitis, pneumonia, and wheezing, particularly in early childhood. Esophageal motility is abnormal, and recurrent aspiration accounts for some of these symptoms. Tracheomalacia is common, resulting in a characteristic harsh cough. Some infants have life-threatening airway obstruction. By late childhood only a small number continue to have significant respiratory symptoms.[66]

### Diaphragmatic Hernia

Congenital diaphragmatic hernia generally results from passage of the bowel through a defect in the posterolateral part of the diaphragm, the foramen of Bochdalek, usually on the left side. It occurs in 1 in 4,000 births and infants usually present soon after birth with respiratory distress.[67] Infants diagnosed by ultrasound early in pregnancy appear to have a higher mortality than the 50 percent overall mortality generally reported.[68] The lung on the ipsilateral side is very small, but that on the contralateral side is also abnormal, with reduced airway generation and increased muscularization of the pulmonary arterioles,[69] resulting in the clinical picture of increased pulmonary resistance. The severely affected infant needs resuscitation at birth. Management consists of paralysis, hyperventilation and maintenance of $PaO_2$ above 100 mmHg to minimize episodes of pulmonary hypertension.[70] Minimal handling and avoidance of stress are important. Other congenital defects (cardiac or chromosomal abnormalities) need to be excluded. Surgical correction of the defect is required, but in recent years this has been delayed for a number of days until the infant is stable.[71] Following the stress of surgery the infant may deteriorate, but once stability is maintained, ventilatory support is gradually discontinued. Newer promising methods of support include high-frequency and extracorporeal membrane oxygenation (ECMO).[72]

A few patients present out of the newborn period. Symptoms include mild respiratory distress, failure to thrive, vomiting, bowel sounds in the chest on routine physical examination, or an incidental finding on chest radiograph. Rarely, strangulation of the hernia can occur in the chest, presenting a confusing picture with a high fatality.[73]

Late bowel obstruction may occur as a result of the malrotation, but long-term respiratory compromise is rare in survivors.[74]

## Congenital Lobar Emphysema

Congenital lobar emphysema is a rare abnormality that generally causes respiratory distress in the newborn period, although it may present later and occasionally is an incidental finding on a chest radiograph obtained for other reasons. Frequently the left upper lobe is involved and hyperinflation of the affected area results in compression of normal ipsilateral lung and shift of the mediastinum to the opposite side. The radiographic appearance may be confused with a pneumothorax, but lung markings are usually visible in the hyperlucent area. A chest radiograph obtained in the first day of life may demonstrate delayed clearance of lung water in the affected lobe. Urgent excision of the affected lobe may be necessary and is generally curative. Pathologic examination of the tissue is often surprisingly normal, and various etiologies have been considered, including extrinsic obstruction of the bronchial supply to the area, abnormalities of cartilage development in the bronchus, and abnormal alveolar elasticity.[75]

## Lung Cysts

The pathologic classification of lung cysts is imprecise and depends on the site, association, airway and vascular connections, and microscopic features.[76–78] Extrapulmonary cysts in close association with the trachea or major bronchi are termed bronchogenic cysts. They generally occur near the carina and occasionally communicate with the airway. Differential diagnosis includes lymph node enlargement, neurogenic tumors, and teratomas. The most common presenting features result from large airway compression (cough, wheezing, and respiratory distress), occasionally in the newborn period.

Intrapulmonary cysts may be single or multiple and pathologically appear similar to bronchogenic cysts, with walls composed of connective tissue, smooth muscle, and cartilage, lined by epithelium, and containing mucus. The cysts may communicate with the airway, sometimes expanding due to a check valve and resulting in respiratory distress from displacement of normal lung tissue. The cyst may occur as a result of infection, and it may be difficult to differentiate between a congenital cyst that became infected and one acquired as a result of staphylococcal disease. Occasionally simple cysts may rupture, resulting in pneumothorax. Spontaneous pneumothorax is rare in children and an underlying cause should always be suspected.

Congenital cystadenomatous malformation of the lung is a rare dysplastic or harmartomatous lesion containing disorganized terminal bronchi and alveoli, and at times tissues not normally present in the lung. Frequently the lesion is limited to one lobe, although the whole lung is rarely involved. The cysts may expand as a result of air trapping, causing respiratory distress, or occasionally rupture, causing a pneumothorax. Rhabdomyosarcomas are very occasionally associated with these lesions.[79]

Pulmonary sequestration is an area of lung supplied from systemic arteries, generally associated with the left lower lobe. Most extralobar sequestrations do not produce symptoms since the tissue is generally isolated from the airway. Intralobar sequestrations present in childhood with recurrent infection.[80] Occasionally sequestration causes respiratory distress in infancy from left-to-right shunting through the abnormal lung.[81] Pathologic examination demonstrates disorganized bronchial and alveolar elements with systemic arterial supply.

Occasionally lung cysts demonstrate pathologic features of more than one of the categories above, suggesting a spectrum of abnormalities. Frequently lesions in all the above groups do not cause symptoms and are incidental findings on chest radiograph or autopsy. Investigations to delineate the abnormality may include computed tomography, angiography, and bronchoscopy. Surgical excision is generally recommended to treat presenting symptoms or minimize later complications of infection or pneumothorax.[41]

## Lung Diseases Associated with Immune Deficiency

The approach to pulmonary disease in the immune-compromised host differs from that in the normal host, since clinical features and radiologic findings are nonspecific in these patients, the organisms encountered differ, and the diseases and their therapy may produce lung damage.

### Organisms

Viruses and bacteria implicated in lung disease in normal hosts tend to cause more severe disease in immunocompromised hosts. Gram-negative bacteria probably occur more commonly. Tuberculosis and nontuberculous mycobacterial diseases are being seen more commonly, particularly in patients with acquired immunodeficiency syndrome (AIDS); the latter are particularly difficult to control.

*Pneumocystis carinii*, a ubiquitous protozoan of low virulence, is one of the more common unusual organisms seen. It produces an acute illness characterized by cough, respiratory distress, fever, and a diffuse generalized pulmonary infiltrate on chest radiograph (although this may be normal). Prophylaxis with oral cotrimoxazole or inhaled pentamidine is given to high-risk groups, particularly patients undergoing treatment for lymphoproliferative disorders, and those with AIDS. Very occasionally it has been found in otherwise normal infants. Diagnosis is established by bronchioalveolar lavage or lung biopsy and the disease treated with high-dose systemic cotrimoxazole or pentamidine. Corticosteroids are also helpful.[82]

Viruses that cause relatively trivial disease in normal hosts may cause severe pulmonary problems in immunocompromised hosts. Giant cell pneumonia is frequently caused by measles, although other viruses have been implicated. Respiratory failure progresses over days to weeks, and survivors are few. Hyperimmune globulin may be useful. Cytomegalovirus (CMV) is often cultured from airway secretions in immunocompromised children without clinical disease, but it also causes a fatal inclusion pneumonitis in some children. Disseminated varicella zoster is associated with a pneumonitis, and treatment with acyclovir has been successful. Immunocompromised patients coming into contact with people with varicella or zoster should be given zoster immune globulin within 72 hours to prevent infection. Herpes simplex may produce a tracheobronchitis or pneumonia that can be treated with acyclovir if the diagnosis is established by demonstration of virus in lesions in the upper airway or lung tissue.

Fungi, particularly candida and aspergillus, cause invasive disease in immunocompromised patients. The course is typically a slow progressive deterioration despite broad-spectrum antibiotics. Diagnosis is difficult since colonization with fungi is common and biopsy is essential to show invasive disease. The effects of antifungal agents have been disappointing once the infection is established.

### Immune Disorders

The primary immune disorders usually associated with lung disease are those that result in immunoglobulin deficiency and in chronic granulomatous disease. Chronic suppurative lung disease resulting in bronchiectasis is common in sex-linked agammaglobulinemia and ataxis telangiectasia. Treatment with immunoglobulin replacement appears to prevent the bronchiectasis. Chronic granulomatous disease results from the failure of phagocytic cells to kill certain ingested organisms due to enzyme defects in pathways that produce hydrogen peroxide. Diagnosis is established by failure of patients' phagocytes to oxidize nitroblue tetrazolium. Recurrent or chronic bacterial lung infections are common and progress to abscess formation. Fungal infection is also common. Extrapulmonary involvement is common. Treatment consists of long term cotrimoxazole and specific antibiotic therapy for established infections. Occasionally surgery is necessary for identification of the infecting organism and drainage of abscesses.[75,83]

AIDS in children is usually acquired perinatally, although blood products (hemophilia), infected needles, or sexual contact have been implicated. Opportunistic pulmonary infections, particularly pneumocystis, CMV, and mycobacterium infections are common in these children. "Noninfectious" pulmonary lymphoid hyperplasia (lymphocytic interstitial pneumonitis) is common in young children with AIDS. This is an insidious process with gradually increasing cough, hypoxemia, and respiratory distress. Chest radiographs show a bilateral diffuse reticulonodular interstitial infiltrate that is worse in the lower lung fields. Diagnosis is established by lung biopsy. Hypoxemia can be reversed and chest radiographic findings improved with corticosteroids.[84]

Therapy of malignant disorders, particularly the lymphoproliferative processes, results in an immune-deficient state with attendant risks for the opportunistic pulmonary infections described above. Pulmonary involvement may also occur with the disease and therapy. Some solid tumors, particularly the sarcomas, metastasize to the lung. Pulmonary fibrosis results from radiotherapy to the thorax and from a number of chemotherapeutic agents, including bleomycin, carmustine (BCNU), methotrexate, and occasionally cyclosphosphamide. The presenting features are fever, dyspnea, cough, and hypoxemia. Reduced diffusing capacity of the lung for carbon monoxide (DLCO) and a restrictive pattern are seen on pulmonary function testing. This is occasionally reversible on discontinuation of the drug. Hypersensitivity reactions also occur.[41] Graft versus host disease following bone marrow transplant can result in progressive obstruction, and necrotizing bronchiolitis has been described.[85,86]

## Miscellaneous Lung Diseases

A number of lung diseases more commonly seen in adults occasionally present in children. These are listed in Table 1-12; the reader is referred to more extensive texts for details.[41,75] These disorders usually present with cough, gradually increasing respiratory distress, and cyanosis. The vasculitides may present with hemoptysis. Often lung biopsy is required to establish the diagnosis, although in some conditions it may be hazardous, precipitating an exacerbation of the underlying condition. Some of the conditions

**Table 1-12.** Miscellaneous Lung Diseases

| |
|---|
| Interstitial pneumonitis |
|   Fibrosing alveolitis (classical interstitial pneumonia) |
|   Bronchiolitis obliterans |
|   Desquamative, lymphoid, and giant cell interstitial pneumonias |
| Hypersensitivity pneumonitis |
| Pulmonary eosinophilic syndromes |
| Pulmonary vasculitides and granulomatous diseases |
|   Pulmonary hemosiderosis |
|   Collagen vascular diseases |
|     Goodpasture syndrome, systemic lupus erythematosus, others |
|   Wegener's granulomatosis |
|   Bronchocentric granulomatosis |
| Sarcoid |
| Alveolar diseases |
|   Pulmonary alveolar microlithiasis |
|   Pulmonary alveolar proteinosis |

are responsive to antiinflammatory therapy.

## REFERENCES


1. Murray JF: Prenatal growth and development of the lung. p. 1. In: The Normal Lung. WB Saunders, Philadelphia, 1986
2. Polgar G, Weng TR: Functional development of the respiratory system. Am Rev Respir Dis 120:625, 1979
3. Inselman L, Mellins R: Growth and development of the lung. J Pediatr 98:1, 1981
4. Nelson NM: Neonatal pulmonary function. Pediatr Clin North Am 13:769, 1966
5. Scarpelli E, Auld P: Pulmonary Physiology of the Fetus, Newborn and Child. Lea & Febiger, Philadelphia, 1975
6. Respiration and Circulation (Biological Handbooks). Federation of American Societies for Experimental Biology, Bethesda, 1971
7. Mansell A, Bryan C, Levison H: Airway closure in children. J Appl Physiol 33:711, 1972
8. Sorbini C, Grassi V, Solinas E, Muiesan G: Arterial oxygen tension in relation to age in healthy subjects. Respiration 25:3, 1968
9. Pang L, Mellins R: Neonatal cardiorespiratory physiology. Anesthesiology 43: 171, 1975
10. Rudolph AM: Changes in the circulation after birth. In: Congenital Disease of the Heart. Year Book Medical Publishers, Chicago, 1974
11. Motoyama E, Zigas C, Troll G: Functional basis of childhood anemia. Abstr Am Soc Anesth 283, 1974
12. Bryan A, Bryan M: Control of respiration in the newborn. Clin Perinatol 5:269, 1978
13. Gerhardt T, Bancalari E: Apnea of prematurity. I. Lung function and regulation of breathing. Pediatrics 74:58, 1984
14. Gerhardt T, Bancalari E: Apnea of prematurity. II. Respiratory reflexes. Pediatrics 74:63, 1984
15. Delivoria-Papadopoulous M, Rancevic N, Oski F: Postnatal changes in oxygen transport of term, premature and sick infants. Pediatr Res 5:235, 1971
16. Glazener C, Motoyama E: Hypoxemia in children following general anesthesia. Anesthesiology 61:416, 1984
17. Finch C, L'Enfant C: Oxygen transport in man. N Engl J Med 286:407, 1972
18. American Thoracic Society: Standardization of spirometry, 1987 update. Am Rev Respir Dis 136:1285, 1987
19. Motoyama E: Airway function tests in children. Int Anesth Clin 26:6, 1988
20. Sly P, Robertson C: Testing children for pulmonary function. Aust Fam Phys 18: 810, 1989
21. Eisenberg J, Wall M: Pulmonary function testing in children. Clin Chest Med 8:661, 1987
22. Sly P, Brown K, Bates J et al: Non-invasive determination of respiratory mechanics during mechanical ventilation of neonates. Pediatr Pulmonol 4:39, 1988
23. Stocks J, Beardsmore C, Helms P: Infant lung function: measurement conditions and equipment. Eur Resp J 2:123, 1989
24. England S: Current techniques for assessing pulmonary function in the new-

born and infant. Pediatr Pulmonol 4:48, 1988
25. Beardsmore C, Helms P, Stocks J et al: Improved esophageal balloon technique for use in infants. J Appl Physiol 49:735, 1980
26. Olinsky A, Bryan AC, Bryan MH: A simple method of measuring total respiratory system compliance in newborn infants. S Afr Med J 50:128, 1976
27. Le Souef P, England S, Bryan A: Passive respiratory mechanics in newborns and children. Am Rev Respir Dis 129:552, 1984
28. Taussig L, Landau L, Godfrey S, Arad I: Determinants of forced expiratory flows in newborn infants. J Appl Physiol 32: 1220, 1982
29. Fennelly M, Hall G: Anesthesia and upper respiratory tract infections—a nonexistent hazard? Br J Anesth 64:535, 1990
30. Tait A, Knight P: Intraoperative respiratory complications in patients with upper respiratory tract infections. Can J Anaesth 34:300, 1987
31. Hinkle AJ: What wisdom is there in administering elective general anesthesia to children with active upper respiratory tract infection? Anesth Anal 68:413, 1989
32. Denny F, Murphy T, Clyde W: Croup: an 11 year study in a pediatric practice. Pediatrics 71:871, 1984
33. Battaglia J, Lockhart C: Management of acute epiglottitis by nasotracheal intubation. Am J Dis Child 120:334, 1975
34. Henderson F, Clyde W, Collier A: The etiological and epidemiologic spectrum of bronchiolitis in pediatric practice. J Pediatr 95:183, 1979
35. Hall C, McBride J, Walsh E: Aerosolized ribavirin treatment of infants with respiratory syncytial viral infection: a randomized double blind study. N Engl J Med 308:1443, 1983
36. Peter G: The child with pneumonia: diagnostic and therapeutic considerations. Pediatr Infect Dis J 7:453, 1988
37. Lamberty J, Rubkin B: The management of anesthesia for patients with cystic fibrosis. Anesthesia 40:448, 1985
38. Blazer S, Naveh Y, Friedman A: Foreign body in the airway: a review of 200 cases. Am Rev Dis Child 134:68, 1980
39. Konig P: Asthma: a pediatric pulmonary disease and a changing concept. Pediatr Pulmonol 3:264, 1987
40. Abraham WM, Wanner A: Inflammatory mediators of asthma. Pediatr Pulmonol 4: 237, 1988
41. Phelan PD, Landau LI, Olinsky A: Respiratory Illness in Children. 3rd Ed. Blackwell Scientific Publications, Oxford, 1990
42. Mao Y, Semencin R, Morrison H et al: Increased rates of illness and death from asthma in Canada. Can Med Assoc J 258: 349, 1987
43. Clay M, Pavia D, Newman SP et al: Assessment of jet nebulizers for lung aerosol therapy. Lancet 2:592, 1983.
44. Wood JA, Wilson RS, Bray C: Changes in salbutamol concentration in the reservoir solution of a jet nebulizer. Br J Dis Chest 80:164, 1986
45. Mallol J, Robertson C, Olinsky A: Aerosol penetrance and deposition in infants with cystic fibrosis. p. 105. 10th International Cystic Fibrosis Congress, Sydney, Australia, March 5–10, 1988
46. Cox RG, Barker GA, Bohn DJ: Efficacy, results and complications of mechanical ventilation in children with status asthmaticus. Pediatr Pulmonol 11:120, 1991
47. Hargreave F, Dolovich J, Newhouse M: The assessment and treatment of asthma: a conference report. J Allergy Clin Immun 85:1098, 1990
48. Pool JB, Greenough A, Gleeson JGA, Price JF: Inhaled bronchodilator treatment via the nebuhaler in young asthmatic patients. Arch Dis Child 63:288, 1988
49. Kernig P, Gayer D, Kantak A: A trial of metaproterenol by metered-dose inhaler and two spacers in preschool asthmatics. Pediatr Pulmonol 5:247, 1988
50. Stahlman MT: Acute respiratory disorders in the newborn. p. 418. In Avery GB (ed): Neonatology, Pathophysiology and Management of the Newborn. 3rd Ed. JB Lippincott, Philadelphia, 1987
51. Yee WF, Scarpelli EM: Surfactant replacement therapy. Pediatr Pulmonol 11: 65, 1991
52. Northway WH, Rosan RC, Porter DY: Pul-

monary disease following respiratory therapy of hyaline membrane disease. N Engl J Med 276:357, 1967
53. Wilson MG, Mikity VG: A new form of respiratory disease in premature infants. Am J Dis Child 99:489, 1960
54. Eisner P: Suctioning meconium from the trachea: a new solution to an old problem. Pediatrics 78:713, 1986
55. Sandor GS, Macnab AJ, Rastogi RB: Persistant Foetal Circulation: Etiology, Clinical Aspects and Therapy. Futura Press, New York, 1984
56. Drummond WH, Gregory GA, Herman MA, Phibbs RA: The independent effects of hyperventilation, tolazoline and dopamine on infants with PPHN. J Pediatr 98: 603, 1981
57. Avery ME, Garewood OB, Brumley G: Transient tachypnea of the newborn. Am J Dis Child 3:380, 1966
58. Marshal F, Bairam A, Vert P: Neonatal apnoea and aponea syndromes. Clin Perinatol 14:509, 1987
59. Steward DJ: Manual of Pediatric Anesthesia. 3rd Ed. Churchill Livingstone, New York, 1990
60. Mayhew JF, Bourke DL, Guinee WS: Evaluation of the premature at risk for postoperative complications. Can J Anaesth 34:627, 1987
61. Hall CB, Kopelman AE, Douglas RG et al: Neonatal respiratory syncytial virus infection. N Engl J Med 300:393, 1979
62. Krous HF: Pathological considerations of SIDS. Pediatrician 15:231, 1988
63. Southall DP: Can we predict or prevent sudden unexpected deaths during infancy? Pediatrician 15:183, 1988
64. Oren J, Kelly DH, Shannon DC: Identification of a high risk group for SIDS among infants who were resuscitated for sleep apnea. Pediatrics 77:495, 1986
65. Behrman RE, Vaughan VC: Nelson Textbook of Pediatrics. 13th Ed. WB Saunders, Philadelphia, 1987
66. Chetcuti P, Meyers NA, Phelan PD, Beasley SW: Adults who survived repair of oesophageal atresia and tracheo-oesophageal fistula. Br Med J 297:344, 1988
67. Cullen ML, Klein MD, Philippart AI: Congenital diaphragmatic hernia. Surg Clin North Am 65:1115, 1985
68. Adzick NS, Vacanti JP, Lillehei CW et al: Fetal diaphragmatic hernia: ultrasound diagnosis and clinical outcome in 38 cases. J Pediatr Surg 24:654, 1989
69. Thurlbeck WM, Kida K, Langston C et al: Postnatal lung growth after repair of congenital diaphragmatic hernia. Thorax 34: 338, 1979
70. Bohn D, Tamura M, Perrin D et al: Ventilatory predictors of pulmonary hypoplasia in congenital diaphragmatic hernia, confirmed by morphologic assessment. J Pediatr 111:423, 1987
71. Breaux CW, Rouse TM, Cain WS, Georgeson KE: Improvement in survival of patients with congenital diaphragmatic hernia utilizing a strategy of delayed repair after medical and/or extracorporeal membrane oxygenation stabilization. J Pediatr Surg 26:333, 1991
72. O'Rourke PP, Lillehei CW, Crone RK, Vacanti JP: The effect of extracorporeal membrane oxygenation on the survival of neonates with high-risk congenital diaphragmatic hernia: 45 cases from a single institution. J Pediatr Surg 26:147, 1991
73. Booker PD, Meerstadt PWD, Bush GH: Congenital diaphragmatic hernia in the older child. Arch Dis Child 56:253, 1981
74. Freyschuss U, Lannergren K, Freckner B: Lung function after repair of congenital diaphragmatic hernia. Acta Pediatr Scand 73:589, 1984
75. Chernick V, Kendig EL: Kendig's Disorders of the Respiratory Tract in Children. 5th Ed. WB Saunders, Philadelphia, 1990
76. Stocker JT, Drake RM, Madwell JE: Cystic and congenital lung disease in the newborn period. Perspec Pediatr Pathol 4:93, 1974
77. Wesley JR, Heidelberg KP, DiPietro MA, et al: Diagnosis and management of congenital cystic disease of the lung in children. J Pediatr Surg 21:202, 1986
78. Clements BS, Warner JO: Pulmonary sequestration and related congenital bronchopulmonary vascular malformations: nomenclature and classification based on anatomical and embryological considerations. Thorax 42:401, 1987
79. Krous HF, Sexauer CL: Embryonal rhabdomyosarcoma arising within a congenital

bronchogenic cyst in a child. J Pediatr Surg 16:506, 1981

80. Savic B, Birtel FJ, Tholen W et al: Lung sequestration: report of seven cases and review of 540 published cases. Thorax 34: 96, 1979
81. Wensley DF, Robertson CF, Goh TH et al: Management of pulmonary sequestration and scimitar syndrome presenting in infancy. Pediatr Surg Int [in press]
82. Consensus statement on the use of corticosteroids as adjunctive therapy for pneumocystis pneumonia in the acquired immunodeficiency syndrome. N Engl J Med 323:1500, 1990
83. Sotomayor JL, Douglas SD, Wilmott RW: Pulmonary manifestations of immune deficiency diseases. Pediatr Pulmonol 6: 275, 1989
84. Rubenstein A, Bernstein LJ, Charytan M et al: Corticosteroid treatment for pulmonary lymphoid hyperplasia in children with the acquired immune deficiency syndrome. Pediatr Pulmonol 4:13, 1988
85. Johnson LF, Stokes DC, Ruggiero M et al: Chronic obstructive airways disease after bone marrow transplantation. J Pediatr 105:370, 1984
86. Edwards JR, Matthay KK: Hematologic disorders affecting the lungs. Clin Chest Med 10:723, 1989
87. O'Pourke P, Crone RK: Halothane in status asthmaticus. Crit Care Med 10:341, 1982
88. Rock MJ, De La Rocha S, L'Hommedieu CS, Truemper E: Use of ketamine in asthmatic children to treat respiratory failure refractory to conventional therapy. Crit Care Med 14:514, 1986

# 2
# Cardiovascular Diseases

# 2

# Cardiovascular Diseases

*Carol L. Lake*

Cardiac disease in the pediatric population is usually congenital, although a few acquired diseases resulting from metabolic deficiencies, infectious processes, and even atherosclerotic vascular occlusion are seen. Congenital heart disease is present in 6 to 8/1,000 live births. The eight lesions seen in Table 2-1 comprise 80 percent of the congenital cardiac lesions, with ventricular septal defect being the most common (20 percent incidence). The approach to these lesions may be anatomic (valvular, septal, atrial, ventricular, conduction system) or pathophysiologic (shunting leading to excessive pulmonary blood flow, cyanosis from inadequate pulmonary blood flow, outflow track obstruction, heart failure, and arrhythmias), as presented in Table 2-2. Obstruction can be either fixed or dynamic. Increased pulmonary blood flow may impair pulmonary function (secondary to distended pulmonary vessels obstructing large/small airways and increasing the work of breathing, increased pulmonary venous return distending the left atrium and causing left mainstem bronchial obstruction, and increased left atrial pressure and pulmonary blood flow increasing pulmonary venous congestion and interstitial/alveolar lung water), may lead to pulmonary vascular obstructive disease, or may cause congestive heart failure. Finally, abnormalities of the cardiac conduction system causing complete atrioventricular block may be congenital or secondary to structural cardiac anomalies.

The anatomic and pathophysiologic approaches may be combined by creating a diagram of the lesions using the helpful atlas by Mullins and Mayer.[1] Once the anatomy is clearly indicated, the pathophysiology can be appreciated. Specific segments of the lesion may be affected differently by alterations in preload, afterload, heart rate, or contractility, as described by Moore (Table 2-3). Hemodynamically significant aspects of proposed diagnostic or operative procedure should be added to the effects of preload, afterload, and other cardiovascular variables. An example of this approach is shown in

**Table 2-1.** Classification of Congenital Heart Disease[a]

| |
|---|
| Ventricular septal defect |
| Pulmonic stenosis |
| Patent ductus arteriosus |
| Ventricular septal defect with pulmonic stenosis (including tetralogy of Fallot) |
| Atrial septal defect |
| Aortic stenosis |
| Coarctation of the aorta |
| Transposition of the great arteries |

[a] In decreasing order of incidence.

**Table 2-2.** Pathophysiologic Approaches to Congenital Heart Disease

- Left-to-right shunting, increased pulmonary blood flow
  - Ventricular septal defect
  - Atrial septal defect
  - Anomalous left coronary artery
  - Endocardial cushion defect
  - Patent ductus arteriosus
  - Partial anomalous pulmonary venous drainage
- Ventricular outflow track obstruction
  - Aortic stenosis
  - Coarctation of the aorta
  - Pulmonic stenosis
- Right-to-left shunting
  - Increased pulmonary blood flow
    - Transposition of the great arteries
    - Double outlet right ventricle
    - Truncus arteriosus
    - Partial anomalous pulmonary venous drainage
    - Hypoplastic left heart syndrome and similar lesions
  - Decreased pulmonary blood flow
    - Tetralogy of Fallot
    - Pulmonic stenosis, pulmonary atresia with ventricular septal defect
    - Tricuspid atresia

**Table 2-3.** Desirable Hemodynamic Changes in Congenital Heart Diseases

| | *Preload* | *Pulmonary Vascular Resistance* | *Systemic Vascular Resistance* | *Heart Rate* | *Contractility* |
|---|---|---|---|---|---|
| Atrial septal defect (L to R shunt) | ↑ | ↑ | ↓ | N | N |
| Ventricular septal defect | | | | | |
| R to L shunt | N | ↓ | ↑ | N | N |
| L to R shunt | ↑ | ↑ | ↓ | N | N |
| Idiopathic hypertrophic subaortic stenosis | ↑ | N | N-↑ | ↓[a] | ↓[a] |
| Patent ductus arteriosus | ↑ | ↑ | ↓ | N | N |
| Coarctation | ↑ | N | ↓ | N | N |
| Pulmonic stenosis | | | | | |
| Valvular | ↑ | ↓ | N | ↓ | ↑ |
| Infundibular | ↑ | ↓ | N | ↓ | ↓[a] |
| Aortic stenosis | ↑ | N | ↑[a] | ↓[a] | N-↑ |
| Mitral stenosis | ↑ | N-↓ | N | ↓[a] | N-↑ |
| Aortic regurgitation | ↑ | N | ↓ | N-↑ | N-↑ |
| Mitral regurgitation | ↑ | N-↓ | ↓ | N-↑ | N-↑ |
| Tetralogy of Fallot | ↑ | N-↓ | ↑ | ↓ | ↓[a] |

[a] An overriding consideration.
(Adapted from Moore,[2] with permission.)

A 4 1/2-year-old 12 kg cyanotic female with TGA, (A) pulmonary (D) and tricuspid (B) atresia (hypoplastic right ventricle; (C) functionally a single ventricle), also small ASD (F) VSD, (E) Down's syndrome, and radiologic evidence of cervical spine hypermobility needs extensive dental restorative surgery. She has a functioning systemic to pulmonary shunt (G) performed at age 5 days. Hematocrit 55%. Child has history of congestive heart failure.

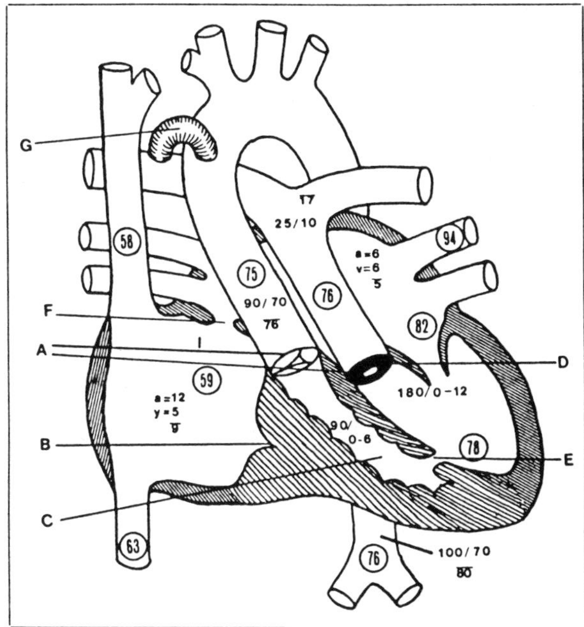


PATHOPHYSIOLOGIC IMPORTANCE TO ANESTHESIA*

| | Preload | PVR | SVR | HR | Contractility |
|---|---|---|---|---|---|
| ASD/VSD | N | ↓ | ↑ | N | N |
| P→S Shunt | → | ↓ | ↑ | ↑ | ↑ |
| TGA | N | ↓ | N-↑ | N | N |

*Other issues include avoidance of intravascular air and control of cervical spine.

**Fig. 2-1.** Combination of the anatomic and physiologic approach to a child with congenital heart disease. At top is a verbal description of the child and her lesions, followed by an anatomic view of the lesions, with the pressures indicated in the various cardiac chambers. The oxygen saturations (circles) are indicated in the cardiac chambers and vessels. At bottom is pathophysiologic importance of the lesions to anesthetic management. The problem of atlantoaxial subluxation and cervical cord compression is discussed in detail in Moore et al.[120] (Modified from Mullins and Mayer[1], with permission.)

Figure 2-1. The final step in management is to assess the known pharmacologic effects of anesthetic drugs and to design a rational anesthetic plan, taking account of their effects on the lesion.

## GROWTH AND DEVELOPMENT OF THE CARDIOVASCULAR SYSTEM

### Cardiac Embryology

Although knowledge of the embryonic development of cardiac structure is helpful for understanding the congenital cardiac anomalies, a detailed discussion of cardiac embryology is beyond the scope of this chapter. Embryologic development of the human heart occurs between 3 and 8 weeks' gestation. The heart begins as angioblastic cells in the embryonic splanchnic mesoderm arrange themselves into myoepicardial and endocardial tubes. The tubes fuse ventral to the foregut and differentiate into bulbar, middle ventricular, and caudal atrial portions. The heart tube forms a loop when it undergoes unequal growth on its right and ventricular portions. It begins beating at this stage. Development of septa between the atria and ventricles and endocardial cushions dividing atria from ventricles occurs after cardiac loop formation.

The main outlet from the developing heart is the truncus arteriosus, which is septated into the aorta and pulmonary artery by the truncoconal septum. The remaining portions of the aorta, pulmonary arteries, and other great vessels develop from the six pairs of branchial arches that run between the two embryonic dorsal and single ventral aortas. Branch pulmonary arteries develop from the sixth branchial arch at 5 to 7 weeks' gestation. The right pulmonary artery develops from the proximal portion of the right sixth arch while the left pulmonary artery develops from a portion of the left sixth arch. Peripheral pulmonary arteries develop within the lung buds. Pulmonary vein development begins at 4 weeks' gestation from an evagination of the left atrium termed the primitive pulmonary vein. The primitive pulmonary vein joins the capillary plexus in the lung buds and becomes the common pulmonary vein opening into the primitive left atrium. As the atrium expands, the common pulmonary vein and its branches are incorporated into the atrial wall, resulting in the four separate pulmonary vein openings into the left atrium. For additional details, the reader is referred to the appropriate chapter in Lake.[3]

In embryologic development, the importance of neural crest abnormalities in the development of cardiac outflow track must be appreciated.[4] Truncus arteriosus results from removal of cardiac cells, or their replacement with cranial neural crest cells, in developing chick embryos.[4] Less complete ablation of the cardiac neural crest results in double outlet right ventricle, Eisenmenger's complex, and tetralogy of Fallot.[4] Embryologic defects of the bulbus cordis (the upper portion is the truncus arteriosus), pulmonic valve, or tricuspid valve are responsible for most complex congenital cardiac anomalies.

### Fetal Circulation

In the developing fetus, umbilical venous blood from the placenta enters the liver to join the portal vein. This blood is relatively well oxygenated, with a $PO_2$ of 30 to 35 mmHg (saturation of 80 percent).[5] The ductus venosus unites the umbilical and portal veins with a physiologic constrictor at its origin diverting 40 to 60 percent of umbilical venous blood away from the liver.[6] The ductus venosus connects to the inferior vena cava at the junction of the hepatic veins. The $PO_2$ of the blood in the inferior vena cava is only 28 to 30 mmHg due to mixing with the splanchnic circulation. As blood from the inferior vena cava enters the heart, about one-third is diverted by the crista dividends through the foramen ovale to the left atrium, while the remainder enters the right ventricle. Only 2 to 3 percent of superior vena caval blood crosses the foramen ovale and the majority enters the right ventricle. Although the theory of right ventricular dominance in utero has been questioned,[7–9] the fetal right ventricle has a relative volume overload, as demonstrated by greater tricuspid than mitral flow velocities.[10] The right ventricle pumps about 66 percent of the combined ventricular output. Blood leaving the right ventricle is primarily shunted through the ductus arteriosus into the systemic circulation, with only 7 to 20 percent reaching the pulmonary circulation. Fetal pulmonary vascular resistance is high. Pressures in the pulmonary circulation, right and left ventricles, are similar in the fetus. Thus, the lower body is supplied with more desaturated blood ($PO_2$ 26 to 28 mmHg, saturation 55 to 60 percent) from the ductus arteriosus, while the left ventricle ejects better oxygenated blood to the cerebral and coronary circulation. Left ventricular output is only 33 percent of the combined ventricular output. Systemic resistance is low due to the placenta. The ductus arteriosus remains open due to the low $PO_2$ and endogenous prostaglandin $E_2$ concentrations.[11]

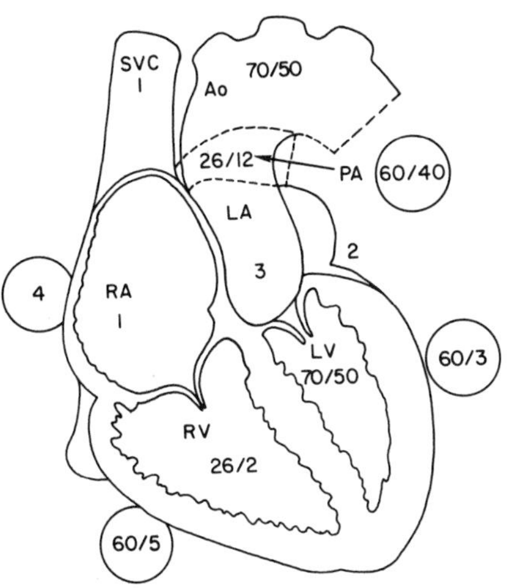


**Fig. 2-2.** Differences in intracardiac pressures in the fetal and neonatal heart. The pressures in circles outside the chambers are those found in the fetus while those within the chambers are typical of the neonatal circulation. (From Lake,[3] with permission.)

## Transitional Circulation

After birth, the circulation is in a transition between the fetal and adult states until the foramen ovale, ductus venosus, and ductus arteriosus close. The differences in pressures between these two states are shown in Figure 2-2. Systemic vascular resistance increases due to loss of the placenta. Pulmonary blood flow increases 450 percent as pulmonary vascular resistance decreases with lung expansion and the onset of respiration. Increased arterial oxygenation relaxes pulmonary vascular smooth muscle, producing dilatation of muscular pulmonary arteries. However, other factors including leukotrienes or prostaglandins may also be involved. Right ventricular and pulmonary artery pressures rapidly decrease in the first 24 hours of life. As the thickness of media of the pulmonary artery decreases and the size and number of pulmonary arteries increase, pulmonary pressures continue to decrease toward adult values. Pulmonary artery wall thickness is comparable to adult values in infants at 4 months of age. Although the right and left ventricle are similar in thickness at birth, the left ventricle increases rapidly in weight and thickness in the first few weeks of life due to its increased workload. Left ventricular mass increases through hyperplasia and an increase in number of cells, rather than hypertrophy.

Closure of the normal human ductus arteriosus occurs in two steps: functional closure caused by constriction of the medial muscle layers, which occurs soon after birth, and anatomic closure, occurring by 3 weeks of age. However, flow in the ductus continues during the first 24 hours of life, as indicated by retrograde systolic aortic velocities and retrograde diastolic pulmonary artery velocities in 91 percent of infants.[12] In the majority of normal infants, the ductus is closed by the second day of life. Physiologic closure of the foramen ovale also occurs shortly after birth, but some left-to-right shunting may be present for the first year of life. Tricuspid insufficiency may also be present in normal infants in the first 24 hours of life.[12] Umbilical arteries rapidly close after birth by contraction of their intrinsic musculature. Complete obliteration by fibrous proliferation occurs within 2 to 3 months. Umbilical veins close shortly after the umbilical arteries, eventually becoming the ligamentum teres. Closure of the ductus venosus forms the ligamentum venosum.

The normal neonatal changes in pulmonary resistance affect the flow through nonrestrictive septal defects. In the neonate, there may be only a small left-to-right shunt, but as pulmonary vascular resistance decreases with growth, the left-to-right shunt increases and eventually will produce pulmonary hypertension and heart failure. The pulmonary vasculature reacts to the increased flow caused by left-to-right shunts or other lesions by increased pulmonary artery pressures, vascular resistance, and reactivity, as described below.

## PERSISTENT PULMONARY HYPERTENSION

Persistence of the transitional circulation beyond the time framework detailed above may occur in full-term infants, premature infants with respiratory distress syndrome, or infants with congenital heart defects. Transient right-to-left shunting at the atrial level may occur in normal infants during coughing, "bucking," or straining during anesthetic induction or emergence.[13] Acute or chronic hypoxia occurring either pre- or postnatally may affect the normal reduction in pulmonary resistance. The state of development of the pulmonary vasculature also determines its response to hypoxia.

Symptoms and signs of persistent pulmonary hypertension include severe hypoxia, tachypnea, and acidosis. A systolic murmur, loud second heart sound, and parasternal heave are present on physical examination. The chest radiograph shows diminished vascular flow without parenchymal disease. Confirmatory evidence is provided by the presence of a higher $PO_2$ in the radial (R) rather than in the umbilical artery. Contrast echocardiography via an upper extremity vein or Doppler studies reveals right-to-left shunting at the atrial level.

## PEDIATRIC CARDIAC PHYSIOLOGY

The important differences between the heart of the infant or small child and the adult heart are given in Table 2-4. They

**Table 2-4.** Differences between Infant and Adult Heart

| |
|---|
| Heart rate |
| Contractility |
| Compliance |
| Afterload mismatch susceptibility |
| Ventricular interdependence |
| Response to catecholamines |

include rate, contractility, compliance, afterload mismatch susceptibility, ventricular interdependence, and response to catecholamines. Cardiac output in the neonate is rate dependent; heart rates less than 90 bpm are associated with hypotension or inadequate tissue perfusion. The infant increases cardiac output by increasing heart rate rather than stroke volume.[14] However, in certain circumstances such as patent ductus arteriosus (increased preload and decreased afterload), stroke volume may be increased substantially.[15] During the first 6 weeks of life, cardiac output increases markedly, and continues to increase until 7 to 24 months of age.[16]

Myocardial length–tension relationships are reduced compared with adults (Fig. 2-3).[17] The immature myocyte also shortens less rapidly than the adult.[18] As development progresses, the myocardial cell changes from a short, round form to a long, rodlike form. As maturation proceeds, intracellular myofibrils become oriented to the long axis of the cell in a subsarcolemmal shell.[18] The volume of the cell occupied by the myofibrils also increases with development.

Reduced contractility in newborns may

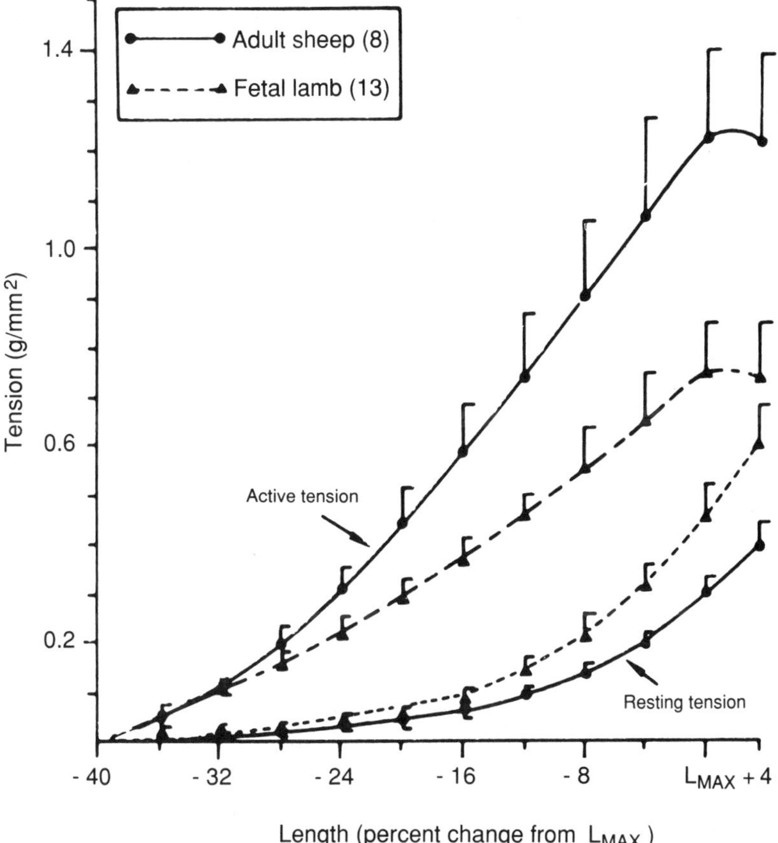


**Fig. 2-3.** Length–tension relationships in sheep and fetal myocardium are similar to those of human adult and infant myocardium. The adult sheep (solid line) shows a lower resting tension and greater active tension development. Fetal myocardium has a higher resting tension and less active tension development. (From Friedman,[17] with permission.)

be partly due to lower cytosolic calcium concentrations.[17] The immature heart is also more dependent upon transarcolemmal calcium fluxes to regulate beat-to-beat contractility. In the immature myocardium, the source of activator calcium is primarily extracellular. Extensive maturational changes occur in the sarcoplasmic reticulum and in its relationship to the sarcolemma. The transverse tubular system of the sarcolemma develops as the myocardial cell increases in volume. Thus, maturational changes in the structure and organization of the myofilaments, membrane systems controlling cytosolic calcium concentration, and contractile proteins controlling the sensitivity of myofilaments to calcium result in a gradual maturational increase in contractility.[18]

Immature ventricles are less compliant, so that increasing preload does not increase stroke volume as it does in the adult. Although the immature ventricle obeys Starling's law, the ascending limb of the Starling curve is short, steep, and plateaus at 5 to 7 mmHg. In younger infants, the plateau occurs at lower filling pressures (Fig. 2-4).[19] Left ventricular regional wall motion is altered during the first few days of life. Due to systolic right ventricular hypertension, the interventricular septum is flattened and the left ventricle is distorted in systole. Responses to exogenous catecholamines are also reduced in the neonate due to reduced receptor responsiveness and incomplete development of myocardial sympathetic receptors (Fig. 2-5).[17] Measurement of the ventricular shortening fraction by M-mode echocardiography is unreliable before 4 to 5 days of age because of variance in contractility among different ventricular segments.[20] Global left ventricular function in neonates is best assessed by measuring the ejection fraction.[20]

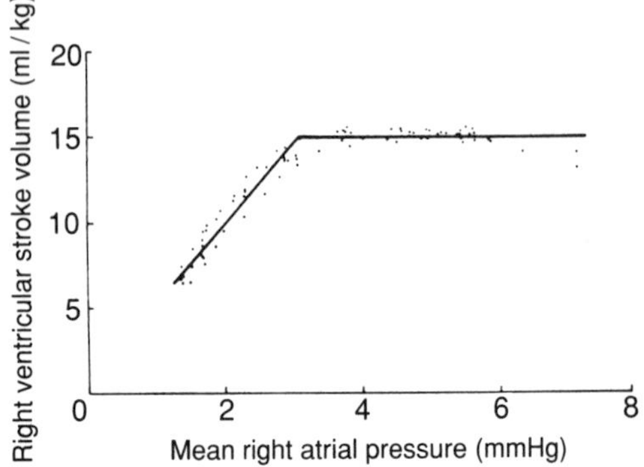


**Fig. 2-4.** The Starling curve of the right ventricle in a fetal lamb is similar to that of the human neonate. The ascending limb is short and the plateau occurs at filling pressures of 5 to 7 mmHg. The left ventricle responds in a similar fashion. (From Thornburg and Morton,[19] with permission.)

Although studies of myocardial metabolism in neonates have recently appeared, it is controversial whether the neonatal heart is more sensitive or more resistant to hypoxia/ischemia. Normally, the immature heart uses lactate as its primary substrate and glucose only under hypoxic conditions. Increased susceptibility to hypoxia/ischemia may also result from alterations in cardiac metabolism secondary to congenital cardiac lesions. Resilience of the neonatal heart has been attributed to increased concentrations of glycogen substrate with enhanced energy production through the glycolytic pathway, greater resistance to acidosis due to increased buffer capacity, and the reduced contractile function of the immature ventricle described earlier. However, acidosis depresses cardiac contractility and increases coronary blood flow in the immature heart.

Changes in myocardial metabolism occur within hours of birth. Mitochondrial enzymatic activity increases, particularly lipolytic and gluconeogenic activity.[21] The neonatal myocardium has converted completely to fatty acid oxi-

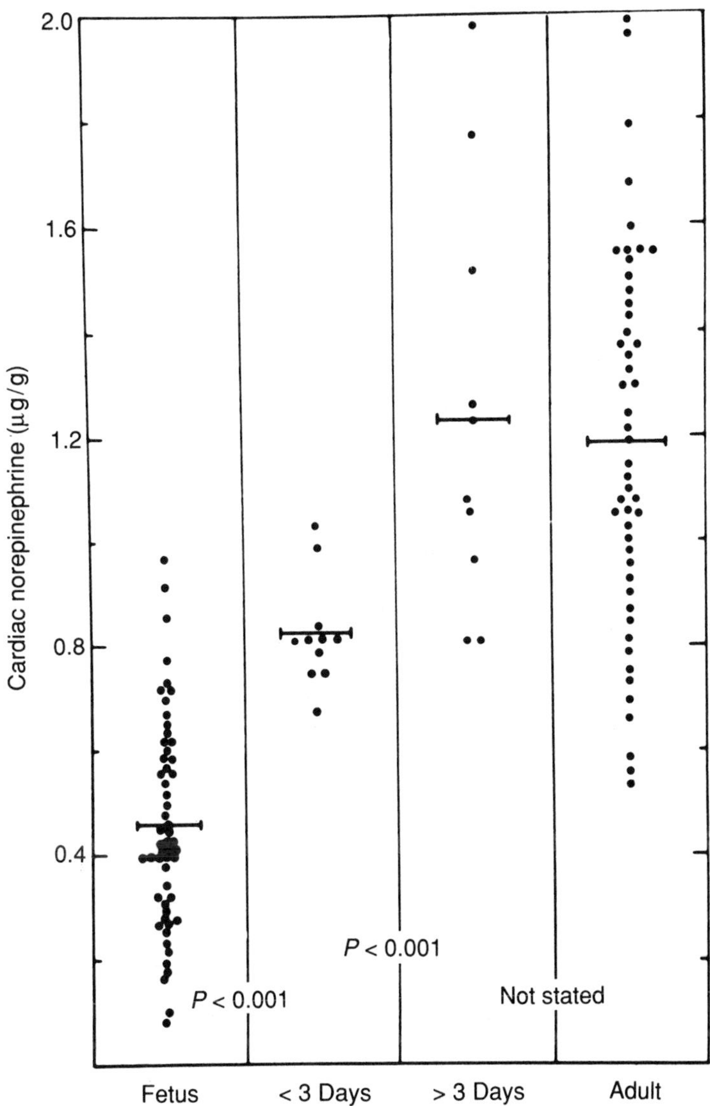


**Fig. 2-5.** Myocardial norepinephrine content in fetal and adult sheep. Myocardial sympathetic receptors are incompletely developed in the fetus and their response to endogenous or exogenous catecholamines is reduced. (From Friedman,[17] with permission.)

dation by 1 to 2 years of age. However, the oxidation of fatty acids is impaired by hypoxia, leading to reduced myocardial contractility and arrhythmias. During hypoxia, myocardial glucose metabolism produces more energy without the deleterious effects of unmetabolized lipids.[21]

## DIAGNOSTIC EVALUATION OF THE CHILD'S HEART

### History and Physical Examination

The important historical questions include whether the child has frequent respiratory infections, is ever visibly cyanotic, keeps up with peers, suffers from easy fatigability, or requires pharmacologic therapy to maintain acceptable cardiovascular function. On physical examination, retardation of growth and delayed developmental milestones frequently accompany the heart failure associated with congenital heart disease. Other notable signs of heart failure in infants and children are respiratory distress, wheezing, hepatosplenomegaly, diaphoresis, cardiomegaly, and reduced peripheral perfusion. Prior cardiac surgical procedures (such as subclavian flap angioplasty for coarctation or subclavian to pulmonary artery shunts) may affect the availability of sites for monitoring blood pressures, requiring planning for alternate sites.

### Chest Radiography

The chest radiograph should be evaluated prior to more expensive or invasive procedures for heart size, cardiac position (malpositioned in asplenia, polyspenia, and situs inversus), heart shape (boot-shaped in tetralogy of Fallot, egg-shaped in transposition, or figure-of-eight shape in total anomalous pulmonary venous return), pulmonary vascularity (increased with left-to-right shunts), and contours of aorta and pulmonary artery. Cardiomegaly indicates either failure or volume overload resulting from recirculation via shunts or valvular regurgitation. Other important chest radiograph findings to be noted prior to surgical procedures are atelectasis, acute respiratory infections, and elevated hemidiaphragms. More sophisticated radiographic techniques such as magnetic resonance imaging are reserved for uncommon anomalies such as vascular rings or slings, pulmonary venous obstruction, and complex cardiac defects.[22] Prior to surgical or diagnostic procedures, minimal laboratory evaluation should include hematocrit, electrolytes, and arterial blood gases if not previously obtained during catheterization.

### Electrocardiography

Pediatric electrocardiograms differ substantially from those of the adult because of the gradual evolution of the transitional anatomy and physiology to the adult form. Decreased pulmonary and increased systemic resistance cause gradual reductions in right ventricular muscularity. The "normal" right ventricular hypertrophy of the infant regresses as the patient ages. Detailed criteria for the components of the electrocardiogram at different ages are listed in Table 2-5. Ventricular hypertrophy is indicated by the lack of normal R/S progression across the precordium. Except in cyanotic children, ischemic ST-T wave changes are infrequent. Conduction disturbances such as right bundle branch block are common in many congenital cardiac anomalies.

## Table 2-5. Summary of Normal ECG Values in Children[a]

| Age Group | Heart Rate (bpm) | Frontal Plane QRS Vector (degrees) | PR Interval (sec) | Q III (mm) | Q $V_6$ (mm) | $RV_1$ (mm) | $SV_1$ (mm) | R/S $V_1$ | $RV_6$ (mm) | $SV_6$ (mm) | R/S $V_6$ | $SV_1 + RV_6$ (mm) | R + S $V_4$ (mm) |
|---|---|---|---|---|---|---|---|---|---|---|---|---|---|
| Less than 1 day | 93–154 (123) | +59 to −163 (137) | 0.08–0.16 (0.11) | 4.5 | 2 | 5–26 (14) | 0–23 (8) | 0.1–U (2.2) | 0–11 (4) | 0–9.5 (3) | 0.1–U (2.0) | 28 | 52.5 |
| 1–2 days | 91–159 (123) | +64 to −161 (134) | 0.08–0.14 (0.11) | 6.5 | 2.5 | 5–27 (14) | 0–21 (9) | 0.1–U (2.0) | 0–12 (4.5) | 0–9.5 (3) | 0.1–U (2.5) | 29 | 52 |
| 3–6 days | 91–166 (129) | +77 to −163 (132) | 0.07–0.14 (0.10) | 5.5 | 3 | 3–24 (13) | 0–17 (7) | 0.2–U (2.7) | 0.5–12 (5) | 0–10 (3.5) | 0.1–U (2.2) | 24.5 | 49 |
| 1–3 weeks | 107–182 (148) | +65 to +161 (110) | 0.07–0.14 (0.10) | 6 | 3 | 3–21 (11) | 0–11 (4) | 1.0–U (2.9) | 2.5–16.5 (7.5) | 0–10 (3.5) | 0.1–U (3.3) | 21 | 49 |
| 1–2 months | 121–179 (149) | +31 to +113 (74) | 0.07–0.13 (0.10) | 7.5 | 3 | 3–18 (10) | 0–12 (5) | 0.3–U (2.3) | 5–21.5 (11.5) | 0–6.5 (3) | 0.2–U (4.8) | 29 | 53.5 |
| 3–5 months | 106–186 (141) | +7 to +104 (60) | 0.07–0.15 (0.11) | 6.5 | 3 | 3–20 (10) | 0–17 (6) | 0.1–U (2.3) | 6.5–22.5 (13) | 0–10 (3) | 0.2–U (6.2) | 32 | 61.5 |
| 6–11 months | 109–169 (134) | +6 to +99 (56) | 0.07–0.16 (0.11) | 8.5 | 3 | 1.5–20 (9.5) | 0.5–18 (4) | 0.1–3.9 (1.6) | 6–22.5 (12.5) | 0–7 (2) | 0.2–U (7.6) | 32 | 53 |
| 1–2 years | 89–151 (119) | +7 to +101 (55) | 0.08–0.15 (0.11) | 6 | 3 | 2.5–17 (9) | 0.5–21 (8) | 0.05–4.3 (1.4) | 6–22.5 (13) | 0–6.5 (2) | 0.3–U (9.3) | 39 | 49.5 |
| 3–4 years | 73–137 (108) | +6 to +104 (55) | 0.09–0.16 (0.12) | 5 | 3.5 | 1–18 (8) | 0.2–21 (10) | 0.03–2.8 (0.9) | 8–24.5 (15) | 0–5 (1.5) | 0.6–U (10.8) | 42 | 53.5 |
| 5–7 years | 65–133 (100) | +11 to +143 (65) | 0.09–0.16 (0.12) | 4 | 4.5 | 0.5–14 (7) | 0.3–24 (12) | 0.02–2.0 (0.7) | 8.5–26.5 (16) | 0–4 (1) | 0.9–U (11.5) | 47 | 54 |
| 8–11 years | 62–130 (91) | +9 to +114 (61) | 0.09–0.17 (0.13) | 3 | 3 | 0–12 (5.5) | 0.3–25 (12) | 0–1.8 (0.5) | 9–25.5 (16) | 0–4 (1) | 1.5–U (14.3) | 45.5 | 53 |
| 12–15 years | 60–119 (85) | +11 to +130 (59) | 0.09–0.18 (0.14) | 3 | 3 | 0–10 (4) | 0.3–21 (11) | 0–1.7 (0.5) | 6.5–23 (14) | 0–4 (1) | 1.4–U (14.7) | 41 | 50 |

[a] Values are limits of normal, with means in parentheses. U, undefined.
(From Garson,[118] with permission.)

## Exercise Testing

Exercise tolerance is a good indicator of functional cardiac status. Most infants or children with congenital cardiac disease limit their activities to their physical capacities. Data from exercise testing in children with specific cardiac defects indicate that exertional endurance is commonly reduced, but is adequate for normal childhood activities. However, children with cyanosis or severe defects have greater limitations. In children with pulmonic stenoses, increased right ventricular end-diastolic pressure during exercise occurred only when pulmonic valve area was less than 0.5 $cm^2/m^2$.[23] However, even with severe pulmonic stenosis, cardiac index increases during exercise.

Cardiac and functional reserve after surgery can be easily determined by exercise testing. Usually tests using a combination of bicycle ergometry or treadmill, radionuclide angiography, and respiratory gas exchange measurements are employed. The radionuclide angiography assesses ventricular function, while respiratory gas exchange globally assesses work capacity.[24] However, this technique is applicable only to children old enough to perform such exercise (5 to 6 years). An alternative method for younger children is afterload stress testing in which the response of ventricular ejection to increased systemic pressure induced by peripheral vasoconstrictor drugs is noted.

Exercise testing may also be useful in the detection of arrhythmias.[25] However, in 58 percent of children, ventricular ectopy decreased and atrioventricular block was suppressed during exercise.[25] Successful suppression of arrhythmias by pharmacologic or surgical therapy can be documented by exercise testing.

## Imaging Techniques

In addition to roentgenography (described earlier) and cineangiography (which will be described later), imaging techniques useful for diagnosing congenital heart disease include fluoroscopy, digital subtraction angiography, nuclear cardiology, computed tomography, positron emission tomography, and nuclear magnetic resonance imaging. A detailed discussion of all these modalities is beyond the scope of this chapter; the reader is referred to Wiles.[26]

Echocardiography is the most commonly used imaging technique for diagnosis of congenital cardiac anomalies. Complete echocardiographic examination provides essential details of the anatomy and pathophysiology to complement the history and physical examination and avoid the risk of cardiac catheterization in ill neonates. Many cardiac lesions (patent ductus arteriosus, ventricular septal defect, atrial septal defect, atrioventricular canal, aortic stenosis, tetralogy of Fallot, and transposition of the great vessels) can be diagnosed and treated based only upon echocardiographic findings.[27–29] In certain instances, the information obtained on echocardiography may be unique or may change the clinical diagnosis from that determined from catheterization.[27,28]

Two-dimensional, M-mode, and Doppler echocardiography are commonly used in the pediatric population. Doppler echocardiography is used to measure flow velocities, permitting estimation of pulmonary to systemic flow ratios, pressure gradients, and intracardiac pressures.[30] Fetal echocardiography identifies structural abnormalities while altered flow velocities indicate abnormal flow patterns in utero in congenital heart lesions.[31] Contrast echocardiography identifies cardiac structures, intracardiac shunts, and valvular lesions.[32,33]

**Table 2-6.** Normal Oxygen Saturations and Intracardiac Pressures

| *Location* | *Oxygen Saturation (%)* | *Intracardiac Pressure (mmHg)* | |
|---|---|---|---|
| | | *Neonate* | *Child* |
| Right atrium | 75 ± 5 | 0–5 | 2–6 |
| Right ventricle | 75 ± 5 | 60/0–5 | 20/5 |
| Pulmonary artery | 75 ± 5 | 60/30 | 20/12 |
| Left atrium | 95 ± 1 | 4–5 | 5–10 |
| Left ventricle | 95 ± 1 | 70/0–5 | 90–110/7–9 |
| Aorta | 95 ± 1 | 70/45 | 90–110/65–75 |

Echocardiographic delineation of atrial septal defects is obtained from right parasternal, apical, or subxiphoid four-chamber views. The diagnosis is confirmed by echocardiographic dropout and pulsed color flow Doppler imaging in the area of the interatrial septum from the right parasternal view, with the ultrasound perpendicular to the atrial septum. Ventricular septal defects are similarly defined from a parasternal long or short axis view. Patency of the ductus arteriosus is often difficult to demonstrate by echocardiography, although the great vessels, pulmonary veins, and systemic veins can be imaged from the suprasternal notch. Endocardial cushion defects with their accompanying valvular anomalies are imaged on the apical four-chamber view. Valvular abnormalities are visualized with two-dimensional and color flow Doppler imaging. Measurement of the left ventricular outflow volume (from the left ventricular ejection flow velocity and left ventricular outflow track diameter) and left ventricular inflow volume (from transmitral flow velocity and mitral valve motion) permits noninvasive assessment of pulmonary to systemic flow ratios (Qp/Qs).[30] Quantitation of ventricular function is performed by measurement of the shortening fraction, the fractional shortening of the short axis of the left ventricle. Normal values are 30 to 40 percent.

## Catheterization and Angiography

Indications for cardiac catheterization include identification of specific congenital lesions, demonstration of their functional significance, continued follow-up of the pathophysiology, and evaluation after surgical therapy. Catheterization is usually required for accurate measurement of the pulmonary artery pressures and assessment of the responsiveness of the pulmonary circulation to vasodilators.[34] Pressures and oxygen saturation are measured in each cardiac chamber (Table 2-6). Cardiac output is determined using the Fick principle with measured

**Table 2-7.** Calculation of Hemodynamic Variables

| *Variable* | *Calculation* |
|---|---|
| Cardiac index | Cardiac output/body surface area |
| Systemic vascular resistance | MAP − CVP/CO × 79.9 |
| Pulmonary vascular resistance | PAP − PWP/CO × 79.9 |
| Valve area | $\frac{Q}{K \sqrt{\Delta P}}$ |

*Abbreviations:* MAP, mean arterial pressure; CVP, mean central venous pressure; PAP, mean pulmonary artery pressure; PWP, pulmonary wedge pressure; Q and CO, cardiac output; K, 44.5 for aortic valve and 31.5 for the mitral valve; P, mean transvalvular pressure gradient.

or estimated oxygen consumption. Systemic or pulmonary vascular resistance and gradients across valves are then calculated from this data using the equations in Table 2-7.

In addition to diagnosis, interventional cardiac catheterization provides either palliation or therapy in some lesions.[35] Examples include atrial septostomy, embolization, umbrella occlusion, and balloon dilatation angioplasty. Atrial septostomy is usually performed in the neonatal period when the foramen ovale is thin and membranous. The procedure im-

**Table 2-8.** Features of Cyanotic

| *Lesion* | *Anatomy* | *History* | *Physical Findings* | *ECG* |
|---|---|---|---|---|
| Tetralogy of Fallot | VSD<br>Right ventricular hypertrophy<br>Pulmonic stenosis/atresia<br>Overriding aorta | Cyanosis<br>Clubbing<br>Growth retardation | Systolic ejection murmur at LSB<br>Systolic thrill at LSB<br>Absent pulmonic component of $S_2$ | Right axis deviation<br>Right ventricular hypertrophy |
| Transposition of great vessels | Systemic venous return to RA → RV → aorta<br>Pulmonary venous return to LA → LV → pulmonary artery | Cyanosis<br>Dyspnea<br>Developmental delay<br>Frequent URI | Left parasternal prominence<br>Enlarged anterior ventricle | Right axis deviation<br>Right ventricular hypertrophy |
| Tricuspid atresia | Absent tricuspid valve<br>RV hypoplastic<br>Often ASD/VSD/PDA present | Cyanosis<br>Dyspnea<br>Retarded growth<br>Clubbing<br>Fatigue | Single $S_1$<br>Systolic murmur<br>Hepatomegaly<br>Presystolic liver pulsation<br>Giant "A" waves on CVP | ↑ LV voltage<br>Left axis deviation<br>P pulmonale |
| Total anomalous pulmonary venous drainage | Supracardiac connection (left or right IVC)<br>Cardiac connection (coronary sinus or RA)<br>Intracardiac (portal vein or IVC) | Cyanosis<br>Heart failure<br>Exercise intolerance | Hyperkinetic RV<br>Widely split $S_2$<br>Systolic ejection murmur | RV dominance |
| Hypoplastic left heart syndrome | Hypoplastic aortic arch<br>Mitral/aortic valve atresia<br>LV atresia and/or hypoplasia | Cyanosis<br>Tachypnea<br>↓ Systemic perfusion as ductus closes | Dominant RV impulse<br>Nonspecifric systolic murmur<br>Diminished peripheral pulses | RA enlargement<br>RVH |

*Abbreviations:* ASD, atrial septal defect; CVP, central venous pressure; ECG, electrocardiography; IVC, fraction; PA, pulmonary artery; PDA, patent ductus arteriosus; P, P wave; PVR, pulmonary vascular resistricular outflow track; SVC, superior vena cava; SVR, systemic vascular resistance; URI, upper respiratory

proves oxygenation in patients with transposition, tricuspid atresia, pulmonary atresia with intact ventricular septum, mitral atresia, and other anomalies. Embolization of bronchial collateral vessels or pulmonary atriovenous malformations is performed to reduce left ventricular volume overload, protect the pulmonary circulation from excess flow, and reduce collateral flow. Umbrella occlusion of atrial septal defects and balloon closure of patent ductus arteriosus currently are being introduced with some success. Balloon dilatation angioplasty has been used suc-

Congenital Heart Disease

| *Echocardiography* | *Chest Radiograph* | *Catheterization* | *Pathophysiology* |
|---|---|---|---|
| Subaortic VSD<br>Anterior deviation of infundibular septum | "Boot-shaped" heart with concave PA segment and dominant RV | ↑ RV pressure<br>Gradient across RVOT<br>Normal PA pressures<br>Step-up in oxygen saturation at ventricular level | RVOT obstruction<br>Left-to-right shunting ("pink" tetralogy of Fallot)<br>Right-to-left shunting<br>↓ Pulmonary blood flow |
| RV to aorta and LV to PA connection | Egg-shaped enlarged heart due to RA enlargement and dominant RV | Communication between venous ventricle and aorta<br>Oxygen saturations reveal left-to-right shunts through ductus, atrial, or ventricular septa | Pulmonary blood flow determined by PVR; systemic oxygenation determined by intracardiac/extracardiac mixing and pulmonary blood flow |
| Absence of tricuspid valve<br>↓ RV size | No pathognomic features | ↑ PA pressure<br>↓ PA oxygen saturation<br>RV inaccessible with catheter | Absent RV inflow |
| Normal RVEF<br>↑ RV EDV<br>↓ LVEF | Figure-of-8 or "snowman" of right and left SVC and heart | ↑ RA pressure<br>↑ RV pressure<br>↑ PVR<br>↓ LVEF | Decreased arterial saturation coupled with pulmonary arterial or venous hypertension |
| Aortic atresia<br>Hypoplastic ascending aorta<br>Mitral atresia<br>Small or absent LV<br>Primum ASD | Moderate cardiomegaly<br>Increased pulmonary vascularity<br>R heart enlargement | Confirms echocardiography findings | Flow to head and upper body via ductus arteriosus (retrograde)<br>Flow to lower body via descending aorta (antegrade)<br>Flow distribution between pulmonary and systemic circulations depends on PVR/SVR ratio |

inferior vena cava; LA, left atrium; LSB, left sternal border; LV, left ventricle; LVEF, left ventricle ejection tance; RA, right atrium; RV, right ventricle; RVEF, right ventricular ejection fraction; RVOT, right ven- infections; VSD, ventricular septal defect.

Table 2-9. Features of Acyanotic

| *Lesion* | *Anatomy* | *History* | *Physical Findings* | *ECG* |
|---|---|---|---|---|
| Atrial septal defect | Ostium primum<br>Ostium secundum<br>Sinus venosus | Fatigue<br>Dypnea<br>Arrhythmias/heart failure (4th–5th decade of life) | Fixed splitting $S_2$<br>Systolic murmur LSB<br>Hyperdynamic RV lift | rsR′ pattern over right precordum |
| Ventricular septal defect | Membranous<br>Muscular | Frequent URI<br>↓ Growth | Systolic thrill LSB<br>Holosystolic murmur | Rightward QRS<br>Biventricular hypertrophy |
| Patent ductus arteriosus | Small, moderate, or large duct between aorta and pulmonary artery | Asymptomatic or heart failure<br>Respiratory distress | Systolic thrill at sternal notch<br>Continuous machinery murmur at LSB | Left atrial hypertrophy<br>Left ventricular hypertrophy |
| Coarctation of aorta | Preductal<br>Juxtaductal<br>Postductal | Dyspnea<br>Feeding problems<br>Decreased growth<br>Lower extremity claudication in older children | Gradient between upper extremity and lower extremity blood pressures | Left ventricular hypertrophy<br>Nonspecific ST-T wave changes |
| Pulmonic stenosis | Valvular<br>Infundibular<br>Peripheral | Dyspnea<br>Exercise intolerance<br>Respiratory infections | Systolic ejection murmur at LSB<br>Widely split $S_2$ | RVH<br>Tall, peaked P waves in II |
| Aortic stenosis | Valvular<br>Subvalvular<br>Supravalvular | Dyspnea<br>Syncope<br>Chest pain<br>Heart failure | Systolic ejection murmur right second ISC<br>LV lift and/or thrill | LVH/strain |

*Abbreviations:* CFD, color flow doppler; ECG, electrocardiography; ISC, intercostal space; L → R, left LVH, left ventricular hypertrophy; PA, pulmonary artery; PVR, pulmonary vascular resistance; RA, right URI, upper respiratory infection; $V_{cf}$, velocity circumferential fiber.

cessfully in recurrent coarctation, pulmonic stenosis, stenotic Blalock-Taussig shunts, aortic valvular stenosis, and obstructed intra-atrial baffles.

## PREOPERATIVE ASSESSMENT

The specific diagnostic features of several common congenital cardiac defects are given in Tables 2-8 and 2-9. The anesthetic and/or surgical risk of a given cardiac lesion is often difficult to assess. It depends upon patient age, type of correction of the cardiac lesion (palliative or definitive), presence of other congenital defects or diseases, and status of the pulmonary circulation, as discussed later. However, children with Down syndrome appear to be at increased risk.[36] According to the American Heart Association guidelines, prophylactic antibiotics are mandatory for patients with congenital heart disease undergoing surgical or diagnostic procedures in which bacteremia may occur (Table 2-10). Desirable he-

Congenital Heart Disease

| *Echocardiography* | *Chest Radiograph* | *Catheterization* | *Pathophysiology* |
|---|---|---|---|
| ↑ RA/RV size<br>Paradoxical septal motion<br>Septal defect on 2D, CFD, contrast echocardiography | Mild/moderate cardiac enlargement<br>Prominent main PA | Step-up oxygen saturation at atrial level<br>Slight ↑ RV, PA pressures | L → R shunting |
| Septal defect on 2D, CFD | ↑ Pulmonary blood flow<br>Mild/moderate cardiac enlargement | Step-up in oxygen saturation at ventricular level<br>Normal to ↑ RV/PA pressure | L → R shunting<br>Bidirectional shunting |
| Left atrial enlargement<br>↑ LVEDD<br>↑ $V_{cf}$ shortening<br>Ductus not usually visualized | Enlarged aorta and PA<br>Enlarged LV | Step-up in oxygen saturation at PA<br>Catheter passage from PA to aorta | L → R shunting<br>(R → L shunting if PVR increased) |
| Associate anomalies such as bicuspid aortic value seen, but coarctation not usually visualized | Left ventricular hypertrophy<br>Notching of ribs due to enlarged intercostal arteries | Pressure gradient across coarctation | Upper extremity hypertension<br>Decreased pressures in lower extremities<br>↑ LV afterload |
| RV hypertropthy<br>Valvular/infundibular stenosis | Normal heart size<br>Convex main PA<br>Prominent RA and RV | ↑ RV pressure<br>Gradient across pulmonic valve<br>Postobstruction pulmonary artery dilution | RV outflow obstruction |
| Valvular stenosis<br>Subvalvular membrane or hypertrophied muscle<br>LV hypertrophy | Usually normal | ↑ LV pressure<br>Gradient between left ventricle and aorta | LV outflow obstruction |

to right; LSB, left sternal border; LV, left ventricle; LVEDD, left ventricular end-diastolic dimensions; atrium; R → L, right to left; RV, right ventricle; RVH, right ventricular hypertrophy; 2D, two-dimensional;

modynamic changes in common congenital cardiac disease are shown in Table 2-3.

## PATHOPHYSIOLOGIC EFFECTS OF CONGENITAL HEART DISEASE

Untreated congenital heart disease carries a significant risk of complications secondary to the pathophysiologic alterations. These complications include pulmonary vascular changes, shunting, congestive heart failure, arrhythmias, bacterial endocarditis, syncope, brain abscesses, and cerebrovascular accidents.

### Effects on Growth

Growth retardation is common in children with severe cardiac malformations, particularly those associated with cyanosis or heart failure. Height and weight measurements are often below the third percentile for age. Heart failure usually

**Table 2-10.** Prophylactic Antibiotic Therapy

| *Drug* | *Dose* |
|---|---|
| | *Dental, Oral, or Upper Respiratory Tract Procedures* |
| Standard regimen | |
| Amoxicillin | 3.0 g orally 1 hour before procedure; then 1.5 g 6 hours after initial dose |
| Amoxicillin/penicillin-allergic patients | |
| Erythromycin | Erythromycin ethylsuccinate, 800 mg, or erythromycin stearate, 1.0 g orally 2 hours before procedure; then half the dose 6 hours after initial dose |
| Or clindamycin | 300 mg orally 1 hour before procedure and 150 mg 6 hours after initial dose |
| Pediatric | Amoxicillin, 50 mg/kg; erythromycin ethylsuccinate or erythromycin stearate, 20 mg/kg; and clindamycin, 10 mg/kg. Follow-up dose should be one-half the initial dose. Total pediatric dose should not exceed total adult dose. The following weight ranges may also be used for the initial pediatric dose of amoxicillin; < 15 kg, 750 mg; 15–30 kg, 1,500 mg; and > 30 kg, 3,000 mg (full adult dose) |
| | *Alternative Prophylactic Regimens for Dental, Oral, or Upper Respiratory Tract Procedures* |
| Patients unable to take oral medications | |
| Ampicillin | Intravenous or intramuscular administration of ampicillin, 2.0 g 30 minutes before procedure; then intravenous or intramuscular administration of ampicillin, 1.0 g, or oral administration of amoxicillin, 1.5 g, 6 hours after initial dose |
| Ampicillin/amoxicillin/penicillin-allergic patients unable to take oral medications | |
| Clindamycin | Intravenous administration of clindamycin, 300 mg, 30 minutes before procedure and intravenous or oral administration of 150 mg 6 hours after initial dose |
| Pediatric | Ampicillin, 50 mg/kg; clindamycin, 10 mg/kg; gentamicin, 2.0 mg/kg; and vancomycin, 20 mg/kg. Follow-up dose should be one-half the initial dose. Total pediatric dose should not exceed total adult dose. |
| | *Regimens for Genitourinary/Gastrointestinal Procedures* |
| Standard regimen | |
| Ampicillin, gentamicin, and amoxicillin | Intravenous or intramuscular administration of ampicillin, 2.0 g, plus gentamicin, 1.5 mg/kg (not to exceed 80 mg), 30 minutes before procedure; followed by amoxicillin, 1.5 g orally 6 hours after initial dose; alternatively, the parenteral regimen may be repeated once, 8 hours after initial dose |
| Ampicillin/amoxicillin/penicillin-allergic patients | |
| Vancomycin and gentamicin | Intravenous administration of vancomycin, 1.0 g, over 1 hour plus intravenous or intramuscular administration of gentamicin, 1.5 mg/kg (not to exceed 80 mg), 1 hour before procedure; may be repeated once, 8 hours after initial dose |
| Pediatric | Initial pediatric doses are as follows: ampicillin, 50 mg/kg; amoxicillin, 50 mg/kg; gentamicin, 2.0 mg/kg; and vancomycin, 20 mg/kg. Follow-up dose should be one-half the initial dose. Total pediatric dose should not exceed total adult dose |

(Modified from Dajani AS et al.[119])

retards growth in weight rather than height. Cyanosis reduces growth in both weight and height. Skeletal growth retardation is usually associated with weight or height retardation and is monitored by bone age. Factors associated with the cardiac disease also affect growth. These include insufficient caloric intake, frequent infections, dyspnea, subnormal birth weight, intrauterine growth retardation, or extracardiac anomalies.

## Effects of Cyanosis

Cyanosis, which depends upon the presence of 5 g percent deoxyhemoglobin, produces multiple pathophysiologic changes. Detection of cyanosis depends upon the hemoglobin concentration, oxygen saturation, and cutaneous perfusion. Greater arterial desaturation is required to produce visible cyanosis when fetal hemoglobin is present. Oxygen transport is maximized by alveolar hyperventilation, polycythemia, and increased blood volume.

Global ventricular function is impaired by cyanosis. Cardiac output is reduced and redistributed to the brain and heart at the expense of splanchnic organs, muscle, bone, and skin.[37] Renal dysfunction is also common in patients with cyanotic congenital heart disease. The incidence of renal abnormalities increases with both degree and duration of cyanosis.[38] Both structural and functional renal abnormalities are present, including decreased renal plasma flow and glomerular filtration rate as well as glomerular enlargement, glomerular capillary congestion, segmental sclerosis, and mesangial hypercellularity.[38]

## Hematologic Effects

The hematologic effects of cyanotic congenital heart disease include erythrocytosis, thrombocytopenia, shortened platelet survival, and coagulopathy. Such abnormalities are found in about 19 percent of patients.[39] Decreased vitamin K-dependent factors have been reported in patients with congenital heart disease.[39] Platelet function is abnormal with defective aggregation due to failure of release of adenosine diphosphate from platelets.[40] Bleeding time may be prolonged. The severity of the hematologic defects seems to correlate with the degree of hypoxia and polycythemia.[39,40] Laboratory results of coagulation tests may also be in error if adjustments of the amount of anticoagulant in collection tubes are not made when the hematocrit is greater than 55 percent.

Tissue hypoxia causes production of erythropoietin from specialized renal cells. In turn, erythropoietin induces proliferation and differentiation of erythrocyte precursors in bone marrow spacing. An increased number of erythrocytes are released into the circulation to increase erythrocyte mass. Erythrocytosis can be either compensated (stable hematocrit and no symptoms of hyperviscosity) or uncompensated (unstable, increasing hematocrit and symptoms of impaired tissue perfusion). Common symptoms of hyperviscosity due to erythrocytosis are fatigue, dizziness, headache, paresthesia, myalgia, decreased mentation, anorexia, and irritability.[41] Polycythemia may also lead to cerebral or renal thrombosis. Systemic vascular resistance is increased at hematocrits over 65 percent.

Children with hematocrits over 55 to 60 percent should be subjected to hemodilution or erythrophoresis to decrease their hematocrits to less than 50 percent before a surgical procedure. However, it is essential to differentiate increased blood viscosity due to iron-deficient microspherocytes from that due to decompensated erythrocytosis.[41] The symptoms of hyperviscosity listed above are similar to those of iron deficiency. Inappropriate phlebotomy may cause iron deficiency. In the perioperative period, adequate hydration and antipyretic therapy are mandatory in children with polycythemia.

## Pulmonary Vascular Obstructive Disease

Pulmonary vascular obstructive disease (PVOD) develops in patients with congenital heart diseases in which pulmonary blood flow is increased, pulmonary venous pressure is increased, or pulmonary blood flow is decreased and hypoxia is present. In the neonatal period, persistence of the transitional circulation (persistent pulmonary hypertension) may accompany congenital heart disease. Pulmonary vascular obstruction also progresses more rapidly in children with nonrestrictive ventricular septal defect, Down syndrome, truncus arteriosus, and partial or complete atrioventricular canal defects.[36,42]

### Clinical Signs

Clinical signs of pulmonary hypertension include accentuation and splitting of the pulmonic second heart sound and softening or shortening of heart murmurs. The main pulmonary artery is enlarged and tortuous, with "pruning" of the intrapulmonary arteries on chest radiograph. In advanced stages the electrocardiogram (ECG) shows right ventricular hypertrophy. However, right heart catheterization is the only method that accurately assesses pulmonary artery pressures and vascular resistance (PVR). Pulmonary vascular resistances of 8 to 10 Wood units/m$^2$ are borderline, while resistances greater than 10 suggest irreversible pulmonary hypertension. Reversibility may be present if vasodilators such as oxygen, tolazoline, or isoproterenol reduce resistance to below 6 Wood units. Other diagnostic information regarding the pulmonary vasculature can be obtained from a pulmonary wedge angiogram or lung biopsy, as described by Rabinovitch et al.[43,44] However, since lung biopsy carries a 20 percent mortality risk and carefully measured pulmonary vascular resistance and pulmonary to systemic resistance ratios reliably indicate the condition of the pulmonary vasculature, lung biopsy is performed infrequently.[45]

**Table 2-11.** Heath-Edwards Classification of Pulmonary Vascular Obstructive Disease

| *Grade* | *Morphology* | *Status* |
|---|---|---|
| 1 | Medial hypertrophy | Reversible |
| 2 | Medial hypertrophy with cellular intimal proliferation | Reversible |
| 3 | Grades 1 and 2 changes plus luminal occlusion by fibroelastic tissue | Variably reversible |
| 4 | Grades 1, 2, and 3 plus luminal occlusion by fiborous tissue with arterial dilatation | Irreversible |
| 5 | Angiomatoid formation | Irreversible |
| 6 | Fibrinoid necrosis | Irreversible |

(From Heath and Edwards,[46] with permission.)

The vascular changes of pulmonary vascular occlusive disease were classified by Heath and Edwards[46] into six grades of increasing severity (Table 2-11). In addition, Rabinovitch[47] has further stratified the changes into grades A, B, and C. Grade A has abnormal extension of muscle into normally nonmuscular, peripheral pulmonary arteries and is associated with increased pulmonary blood flow. Grade B has abnormal muscular extension and mild medial hypertrophy in the proximal pulmonary arteries associated with mildly increased pulmonary artery pressure and increasing pulmonary blood flow. Later developments in grade B include severe medial hypertrophy and abrupt tapering of arteries with moderate to severely increased pulmonary artery pressure and mildly increased pulmonary vascular resistance. Grade C has all the findings of grade B plus reduced numbers and sizes of arteries, abrupt tapering of vessels on pulmonary wedge angiogram, and moderate to severely increased pulmonary vascular resistance. There is probably failure of arterial development to maintain pace with alveolar proliferation in grade C.[47] An increase in β-adrenergic receptor density in the lungs of patients with pulmonary hypertension secondary to congenital heart disease has been recently reported using radioligand binding techniques.[48] The increased density of β-receptors correlates well with mean pulmonary arterial pressure and may result from adaptive changes.[48]

## Effects on Pulmonary Function

PVOD affects lung mechanics. Dilated pulmonary arteries obstruct large bronchi while increased pulmonary blood flow obstructs the peripheral airways. Decreased pulmonary compliance and increased airway resistance result from these pathologic changes. Even the alveolar ducts and respiratory bronchioles may be narrowed. Ventilation–perfusion imbalance is often present.[49] The increased pulmonary blood flow resulting from left-to-right shunts may be abnormally distributed, while the associated pulmonary congestion reduces alveolar ventilation. The normal gravitational effects on ventilation/perfusion mismatch are accentuated in patients with right-to-left shunts. Increased physiologic dead space requires greater minute ventilation and work of breathing to eliminate carbon dioxide.[49] The slope of phase III (the "alveolar plateau") of carbon dioxide expiration is increased by right-to-left shunting.[50] In addition to these secondary changes, some children with congenital heart disease have abnormal lung parenchyma, which also increases the gradient between arterial and expired carbon dioxide.[50]

## Management

In the perioperative period, hypocarbia, alkalosis (pH controls pulmonary vascular tone), oxygen, and ventilation at a normal functional residual capacity (avoidance of positive end-expiratory pressure and lung hyperinflation) are used to maintain low pulmonary vascular resistance. Lung retraction or abdominal distention increase PVR and should be avoided or performed cautiously. Various pharmacologic and mechanical modalities have been used in attempts to control persistent pulmonary hypertension, including prostaglandins, high-frequency oscillation,[51] and extracorporeal membrane oxygenation.[52]

Because excessive pulmonary blood flow often intensifies the vascular changes in the pulmonary circulation, banding of the pulmonary artery is performed in some children to allow growth prior to definitive surgery. Children with pulmonary artery bands should have arterial oxygen saturations between 87 and 92 percent, with lower values indicating inadequate pulmonary blood flow.[53,54]

# Shunting

Children with septal defects, patency of the ductus arteriosus, or truncus arteriosus may have shunting of blood from the pulmonary to systemic circulation (right to left), systemic to pulmonary circulation (left to right), or bidirectionally. The direction and flow through the shunt depend upon the size of the defect and the ratio of pulmonary to systemic resistance. A shunt-producing defect is nonrestrictive if there is no pressure gradient across the defect. If a defect is restrictive, there is significant resistance across it and a pressure gradient develops between the two chambers connected by the defect. The amount of shunt through a restrictive defect is fixed by the size of the defect, rather than the ratio of systemic/pulmonary resistance. The obvious sequelae of intracardiac shunts include arterial desaturation (right to left), paradoxical embolization, pulmonary circulatory overload with the associated vascular changes (left to right), volume overload of the right ventricle, and ventilatory changes. The end stage of pulmonary vascular obstructive disease caused by left-to-right shunting is shunt reversal and Eisenmenger's syndrome.

Left-to-right shunts causing pulmonary overperfusion increase airway resistance and work of breathing while decreasing physiologic dead space/tidal volume ratio at unchanged lung compliance.[55] Right-to-left shunts, by mixing desaturated blood with arterial blood and reducing pulmonary blood flow, cause hypoxia. Blunted ventilatory responses to hypoxemia are present in cyanotic patients with shunts.[56] Ventilatory requirements for a given metabolic rate are increased, while the ventilatory responses to hypoxemia are reduced, increasing the vulnerability of these children to postoperative respiratory depression. Sietsema et al.[57] report decreased end-tidal carbon dioxide and oxygen saturation, increased minute ventilation, and unchanged arterial pH and $PCO_2$ in patients with right-to-left shunts.

The presence of intracardiac shunts theoretically affects the uptake of volatile anesthetics.[58] With a left-to-right shunt, which augments pulmonary blood flow, speed of induction should be increased with a volatile agent and slowed with an intravenous agent. With a right-to-left shunt, blood that leaves the lungs with a certain concentration of volatile anesthetic has that concentration diluted by blood that has bypassed the lungs, slowing induction. Intravenous induction is rapid in patients with right-to-left shunts. In adequately premedicated children, the effects of shunt on the speed of anesthetic induction is minimal. However, the cardiovascular effects of the volatile anesthetics may also alter the direction or magnitude of the shunt. Hensley and colleagues[59] noted that oxygen saturation improved substantially in a series of children with tetralogy of Fallot during halothane induction. Although halothane decreases systemic vascular resistance, the relaxation of infundibular stenosis and the decrease in total body oxygen consumption were the more important effects in these children. Conversely, shunt reversal can occur during surgery, as demonstrated by Greeley and coworkers[60] using echocardiography in a patient with tetralogy of Fallot. In patients with tetralogy of Fallot whose primary lesions are right ventricular outflow track obstruction and shunting at the ventricular level, increased systemic vascular resistance to enhance left-to-right shunting and decreased right ventricular contractility to reduce outflow obstruction are important to maintain systemic oxygenation and flow. Obstruction of the right ventricular outflow track increases with decreased venous return, sympathetic stimulation, infundibular spasm, and reduced systemic vascular resistance. Perioperative hypercyanotic episodes are treated by acute volume administration, leg flexion, peripheral vasoconstrictors such as phenylephrine, and morphine or β-blockers during noncardiac surgery.

In addition to naturally occurring shunts, palliative shunts are created to enhance pulmonary blood flow and arterial oxygenation when pulmonary flow is limited by congenital lesions. Such shunts permit recirculation of blood through the lungs as long as normal systemic arterial pressures are maintained. Adequate systemic oxygenation requires shunt flow to be several times that of systemic flow. Maneuvers that increase pulmonary vascular resistance substantially reduce flow through these shunts, causing desaturation.

## Heart Failure

In the first few hours of life, neonates with ventricular volume overload (as from severe valvular regurgitation) may demonstrate heart failure. Other causes of early heart failure include myocarditis, supraventricular tachycardia, complete heart block, or endocardial fibroelastosis. Heart failure in the first week of life is due to obstruction to systemic flow (coarctation, aortic stenosis, interrupted aortic arch, aortic atresia). Lesions causing heart failure later in neonatal life are ventricular septal defects, truncus arteriosus, transposition, complete atrioventricular canal, and patent ductus arteriosus.

The presenting symptoms of heart failure in infants are different from those in adults. Rapid (greater than 60 bpm), grunting, gasping respiration is the most common symptom. Dyspnea is recognized by nasal flaring and subcostal or intercostal retractions. Rales or wheezing may be heard on auscultation. Feeding difficulties are common because the infant cannot feed as rapidly or vigorously as the normal baby. Weight gain is poor, with growth retardation affecting weight more than length. Other common symptoms are tachycardia, diaphoresis due to increased sympathetic tone, cool or moist skin, and hepatomegaly. Frequent upper respiratory infections occur. Peripheral edema is uncommon. Chest radiographs reveal cardiomegaly.

## Arrhythmias

Arrhythmias are uncommon in normal children. Possible developmental changes in the cardiac conduction system are presently under investigation. However, it is known that the resting membrane potentials in Purkinje fibers, atrial cells, and ventricular cells are less negative than later in life, due to a lower intracellular potassium activity.[61] Uncorrected cardiac defects are often associated with arrhythmias. Both bradyarrhythmias and tachyarrhythmias may occur in children. Atrial arrhythmias including flutter, fibrillation, or tachycardia are present in adults with atrial septal defects. Atrial flutter is infrequent in infants under 1 year of age. Flutter rates of 250 to 350/min occur in children with abnormal hearts over the age of 1 year. Atrial flutter is a serious arrhythmia in children because of sudden death, which may occur secondary to 1:1 conduction of rates over 300/min, progressive conduction block, or sudden spontaneous cessation of flutter with asystole.

Supraventricular tachycardias have rates of 120 to 350/min in children. Types of supraventricular tachycardia include atrial ectopic, junctional ectopic, and junctional reciprocating, but specifically exclude atrial flutter and fibrillation. In addition to narrow QRS complexes, supraventricular tachycardias may have no visible P waves but a greater than normal ventricular rate, visible P waves and normal P-wave axis but AV dissociation, visible P waves with abnormal P-wave axis, or visible P waves at a rate over 230/min or greater than normal for age.[62] Paroxysmal tachycardia is most commonly due to Wolff-Parkinson-White syndrome. Aberration with supraventricular tachycardia is rare in children; ventricular tachycardia is usually present if the QRS complex differs from that seen in sinus rhythm. Ventricular tachycardias usually indicate a cardiac abnormality such as congestive cardiomyopathy, prolonged QT interval syndrome, ventricular tumor, or arrhythmogenic right ventricular dysplasia. Ventricular arrhythmias are also frequent in patients after ventriculotomy to repair tetralogy of Fallot or the aortic valve.

## MANAGEMENT OF CONGENITAL HEART DISEASE

### Medical Therapy

#### Heart Failure

Although its therapeutic efficacy is sometimes questioned, digoxin remains the therapy of choice for infants and children with heart failure. Digoxin improves left ventricular contractile indices in neonates and infants with heart failure.[63] Digoxin is also effective in the treatment of supraventricular tachycardia other than those caused by an accessory pathway. However, in heart failure, heart rate is often slowed by digoxin therapy. Absorption, protein binding, and metabolism of digoxin are similar in infants and adults. However, infants between 2 months and 2 years of age have a larger volume of distribution and increased excretion. Higher serum concentrations of digoxin are often found in infants and children, but a therapeutic need for these increased concentrations has not been established by pharmacokinetic studies. Except when rapid treatment is needed, as for arrhythmias, digoxin can be initiated at oral maintenance doses without a loading dose (see Appendix). As in adults, its effects on the ECG include slowing of the heart rate, shortening of the Q-T interval, and downsloping/sagging ST segments.

Digitalis toxicity, although infrequent, may occur in children, usually within the first week of therapy. Signs include marked sinus arrhythmia, prolonged P-R interval (first degree atrioventricular block), atrial or junctional premature beats, anorexia, and nausea.

Digoxin is usually combined with diuretics such as furosemide, ethacrynic acid, spironolactone, chlorthiazide, or metolazone. These drugs are given orally unless severe congestion requires intravenous administration. The diuretic action of furosemide may be enhanced by combination with metolazone. A longer acting diuretic is chlorothiazide. Spironolactone, an aldosterone antagonist, can be given to enhance diuresis and minimize the hypokalemia associated with thiazide or loop diuretics. Careful monitoring of fluid balance and serum potassium and chloride are essential with high-dose or combination diuretic therapy.

Vasodilator therapy with hydralazine or prazosin is useful in heart failure or hypertension not caused by left-to-right shunts. Captopril and enalapril, angiotensin-converting enzyme inhibitors (ACEI) that block the conversion of angiotensin I to the pressor angiotensin II, are also useful for chronic vasodilator therapy of either hypertension or heart failure in children. Captopril actually decreases pulmonary blood flow in patients with ventricular septal defects.[64] In patients with heart failure, ACEI reduce systemic vascular resistance and left ventricular filling pressures while increasing cardiac output without a change in heart rate. However, captopril actually has a direct negative inotropic effect.[64] The efficacy of ACEI can be monitored by measurement of the plasma renin activity, angiotensin I or II, and aldosterone levels. A therapeutic effect is indicated by a reduction in plasma angiotensin II and aldosterone levels and increased plasma renin activity and angiotensin I concentrations.[64] Several second-generation ACEI (lisinopril, cilazapril, and ramipril) are effective in adults but no data have been reported for their use in children.

## Arrhythmias

Bradyarrhythmia therapy is usually permanent electrical pacing. Tachyarrhythmias are often amenable to pharmacologic therapy to minimize the lifestyle disruption, chest pain, dyspnea, lethargy, syncope, or more serious cardiovascular decompensation associated with tachycardia.[61] Atrial tachyarrhythmias are poorly tolerated in children. Therapy is directed at elimination of episodes rather than control of ventricular response. Digoxin is the usual treatment. Pacemakers are also recommended in patients with sinus bradycardia who require drugs other than digitalis, such as quinidine, β-blockers, or amiodarone, to control atrial flutter.

Therapy for supraventricular tachycardia is similar to that in adults. Carotid sinus massage and Valsalva maneuver are effective in older children, and the diving reflex is effective at all ages. Cardioversion or overdrive pacing may be effective in tachycardias resistant to physiologic maneuvers. Digoxin is usually a safe therapy for atrial tachyarrhythmias, but is hazardous in patients with Wolff-Parkinson-White syndrome, in which it decreases the refractory period in the accessory pathway. Verapamil therapy for supraventricular tachycardia should be avoided in neonates due to its side effects of negative inotropism, hypotension, electromechanical dissociation, and shock. However, verapamil is the drug of choice for termination of sinus node reentry, AV nodal reentry, and circus movement tachycardias associated with Wolff-Parkinson-White syndrome in older children.

Effective drugs for ventricular tachycardia include intravenous lidocaine for short-term control and oral phenytoin, mexiletine, tocainide, and propranolol for long-term therapy. Quinidine, procainamide, and amiodarone are used to control both atrial and ventricular tachyarrhythmias. However, these drugs have significant side effects. Side effects of quinidine include "quinidine syncope" (due to polymorphic ventricular tachycardia or torsade de pointes), increased brain concentrations of digoxin (when given concurrently), gastrointestinal disturbances, and cinchonism. Procainamide therapy is associated with lupus erythematosus, hypotension, bradycardia, agranulocytosis, and gastrointestinal disturbances. Amiodarone produces pulmonary toxicity, neurologic symptoms, bluish skin, hypothyroidism, hypotension, and bradycardia. The side effects of mexiletine are hypotension, bradycardia, ventricular fibrillation, and neurologic symptoms.

**Pacemakers.** The indications for pacemakers in children are similar to those recommended for adults by the Joint Task Force of the American College of Cardiology and the American Heart Association.[66] However, Kugler and Danford[66] point out several circumstances in which pacemaker insertion is appropriate in children in addition to those listed by the Task Force. Bradycardia is age dependent; sinus rates should be greater than 40/min in teenagers, greater than 50/min in children, and over 70/min in infants. Congenital complete atrioventricular (AV) block that results in heart rates less than 50 bpm is treated with a pacemaker. Infants with congenital heart disease and heart rates less than 70 to 80 bpm usually also require pacemakers. Other children with faster ventricular rates may require pacemakers if their symptoms suggest cardiac insufficiency (reduced exercise tolerance). The presence of long QT interval syndrome with or without congenital complete AV block may require cardiac pacing in addition to beta blockade to minimize the possibility of sudden-death episodes secondary to sinus node dysfunction or torsade de pointes.[66] However, not all children with bradycardia-tachycardia syndrome require pacemakers, as adults do.[66]

Children should always have physiologic, rate-responsive pacemakers. Both transvenous and epicardial leads are used, but transvenous leads are advantageous because of easier placement and lower pacing thresholds. Bipolar leads are most frequently used because of the need for selective sensing with dual-chamber pacemakers. Pulse generators are usually placed in the abdomen for cosmetic reasons. Pacemaker followup protocols are similar to those for adults and are detailed by Kugler and Danford.[66]

## Surgical Therapy

Interventional cardiac catheterization and palliative or definitive surgery are possible for nearly all types of congenital cardiac defects.

Specific surgical procedures provide anatomic and physiologic improvement for most of the common congenital defects (Table 2-12). Cardiac surgical procedures can be classified as palliative, anatomic, or physiologic corrections. Palliative procedures are performed to mitigate the hemodynamic consequences of the lesion, alleviate symptoms, and enhance growth or development. However, the primary cardiac defect remains unchanged. Examples of palliative proce-

**Table 2-12.** Surgical Therapy for Congenital Heart Disease

| *Lesion* | *Procedure* |
|---|---|
| Atrial septal defect | Suture, pericardial, prosthetic patch closure |
| Ventricular septal defect | *Palliative*—pulmonary artery banding<br>*Definitive*—suture, pericardial, prosthetic patch closure |
| Patent ductus arteriosus | Direct ligation and division |
| Tetralogy of Fallot | *Definitive*—patch closure ventricular septal defect, pulmonary valvulotomy, right ventricular outflow track enlargement<br>*Palliative*—Brock blind pulmonary valvulotomy, Blalock-Taussig subclavian-to-pulmonary artery shunt, Waterston ascending aorta-to-right pulmonary artery shunt, Potts left pulmonary artery-to-descending thoracic aorta shunt |
| Transposition of great vessels | *Palliative*—Rashkind balloon atrial septostomy<br>*Definitive*—arterial switch, atrial correction (Mustard or Senning procedures), Rastelli (with ventricular septal defect) |
| Anomalous pulmonary venous return | Atrial patch repair |
| Atrioventricular canal (endocardial cushion defects) | Patch repair atrial and ventricular septal defects, mitral/tricuspid valvuloplasty |
| Coarctation of aorta | Subclavian flap angioplasty, resection/end-to-end anastomosis, patch angioplasty |
| Valvular stenosis (aortic, pulmonic, mitral) | Open valvulotomy, valve replacement |
| Valvular insufficiency (aortic, pulmonic, mitral) | Valvuloplasty, valve replacement |
| Tricuspid atresia | Balloon atrial septostomy, Fontan procedure, Glenn shunt |
| Pulmonic atresia | Balloon atrial septostomy, Blalock-Taussig shunt, central shunt |
| Hypoplastic left heart syndrome | Norwood procedure, Sade modification, transplantation |

dures are pulmonary artery banding to reduce pulmonary blood flow, systemic-to-pulmonary anastomoses or central shunts to increase pulmonary blood flow, and atrial septectomy to increase intracardiac mixing. In some circumstances, palliative procedures precede definitive operations, while for complex defects, only palliation may be possible. Some complex defects may be amenable only to palliative procedures. Physiologic repairs correct hemodynamically significant cardiac defects. However, cardiac physiology is not normalized. Examples include Mustard, Senning, Glenn, and Fontan procedures. Anatomic corrections include closures of septal defects, arterial switching for transposition of great arteries, and repair of the pulmonary outflow track in tetralogy. Indications for pulmonary valvulotomy include peak right ventricular to pulmonary artery pressure gradients greater than 60 mmHg, ECG evidence of right ventricular hypertrophy, and right ventricular pressures of 70 percent or greater of the systemic systolic pressure. Aortic valvulotomy for congenital aortic stenosis is indicated when heart failure, syncope, angina, peak systolic gradient on echocardiography of 75 mmHg, or calculated valve area of 0.5 $cm^2/m^2$ or less are present.

Pulmonary regurgitation is usually well tolerated. Indications for aortic valvuloplasty or replacement are increasing left ventricular dilatation, chest pain, heart failure, or complicating infective endocarditis. For lesions such as hypoplastic left heart syndrome, tricuspid atresia, and complex congenital lesions, cardiac transplantation is a useful, although not readily available, alternative. The timing of transplantation in children is important. Addonizio and coworkers[67] noted that pediatric patients with pulmonary hypertension or hemodynamic decompensation had significant increased mortality compared with 100 percent survival for children without these risk factors.

## CONGENITAL HEART DISEASE AFTER CARDIAC SURGERY

The anesthesiologist who cares for a patient after anatomically corrective cardiac surgery must appreciate the fact that the cardiac anatomy may have been repaired but the patient's heart is not completely normal. Stark[68] has defined corrective cardiac operations as those that (1) achieve and maintain normal function; (2) result in normal life expectancy; and (3) required no additional medical or surgical therapy. True total correction or complete cure is limited to division of an uncomplicated patent ductus arteriosus in a patient without pulmonary hypertension and, perhaps, closure of simple ostium secundum atrial septal defects.[69] Rarely, however, recanalization of the ductus does occur. Common residual abnormalities include residual shunts, outflow obstructions, heart block or other arrhythmias, and complications from specific defects (mitral regurgitation after endocardial cushion defects, systemic venous obstruction after Mustard repair of transposition, among others). Prosthetic materials are always at risk for thrombus formation and infective endocarditis. Conduits with or without valves are subject to development of thickening of the lining and bioprosthetic valves are prone to calcification and/or degeneration. Right, left, or biventricular dysfunction secondary to chronic volume or pressure overload, myocardial oxygen supply–demand imbalances, ventriculotomy scars, or altered coronary blood flow may adversely affect postoperative cardiac function in many lesions. Complications from the cardiac surgical procedure, such as diaphragmatic paralysis or neurologic deficits, also affect general functional capacity.

## Neurologic Injuries

One of the most devastating sequelae of congenital cardiac repairs is neurologic dysfunction, occurring in 2 to 25 percent of cases.[70] Both permanent sequelae (seizures, motor disorders) and higher cortical dysfunction (learning disability, mental retardation) have been described.[70] While most children with acyanotic congenital heart disease have normal preoperative neurologic function, those with cyanotic lesions are often neurologically impaired. Correction of cyanotic congenital heart disease at later ages is associated with impaired cognitive performance.[71] This finding suggests that prolonged hypoxia is detrimental to perceptual, intellectual, and motor function.

Although the exact etiology of the postoperative neurologic sequelae is unclear, pathogenetic factors may include preoperative cerebral anomalies, low flow-low pressure bypass, hypothermic circulatory arrest, postoperative low cardiac output syndrome, and emboli. There is a frequent association of cerebral anomalies (microencephaly, altered cortical development) in hypoplastic left heart syndrome that may affect postoperative neurologic sequelae.[72,73] McConnell et al.[74] describe ventriculomegaly and dilatation of the subarachnoid space in one-third of children undergoing repairs for cyanotic or acyanotic disease using moderate hypothermic nonpulsatile membrane bypass. Four of their 15 patients developed clinically insignificant but magnetic resonance imaging-demonstrable subdural hematomas. Glauser et al.[72] noted that 45 percent of infants with hypoplastic left heart syndrome had intracranial hemorrhages or hypoxic-ischemic lesions. The principal factor associated with these lesions was a prolonged period of circulatory arrest (more than 40 minutes) during palliative surgery, although other associated factors were diastolic hypotension and hyperglycemia.

## Septal Defects

Patients whose atrial septal defects were corrected before age 25 have actuarial survival rates similar to controls.[75] However, residual shunts secondary to patch dehiscence or uncorrected defects, right ventricular dysfunction (particularly after ventriculotomy), damage to the cardiac conduction system (sinus or atrioventricular nodes, bundle branch block, premature ventricular contractions (in 17 percent of patients after repair of ventricular septal defect), pulmonary hypertension, and atrioventricular valvular regurgitation may be present.[76] Electrophysiologic dysfunction is particularly common after repair of atrioventricular canal defects. Thirty-eight percent of patients have new electrophysiologic abnormalities involving the sinus node in 19 percent and the AV node in 25 percent after surgical repair.[77] First-degree AV block and right bundle branch block are frequent postoperative abnormalities.[77] In adult patients undergoing repair of atrial septal defect, the incidence of atrial fibrillation/flutter increases with age at repair.[75] Aortic regurgitation or obstruction may occur after repair of subaortic ventricular septal defects and subaortic obstruction may follow patch closures of ventricular septal defects.

Shunt reversal must be avoided in patients with residual defects by preventing factors known to increase PVR (hypoxia, acidosis, hypercarbia) or decrease systemic resistance. Even with apparent left-to-right shunts, arterial air embolism is possible. Perioperative mortality is about 15 percent in patients with Eisenmenger's syndrome, but numerous case reports indicate successful outcomes with careful maintenance of myocardial contractility and systemic vascular resistance.

## Aortic Valve Disease

Bicuspid aortic valve is a common congenital malformation. It may remain functionally normal throughout a normal lifespan but more commonly develops either regurgitation or stenosis. Regurgitation secondary to the bicuspid valve may be mild or gradually increase in severity, eventually requiring replacement. Valvular stenosis develops from calcification and fibrosis of the abnormal valve. Residual or recurrent stenosis occurs after valvulotomy of congenitally stenotic aortic valves.

## Pulmonary Valve Disease

Valvular pulmonic stenosis that is noncritical is usually well tolerated throughout childhood, as the orifice size increases with growth. However, valvular calcification or secondary hypertrophic subpulmonic stenosis may augment the obstruction with aging. In contrast, exercise testing reveals that patients with pulmonic atresia and ventricular septal defect have significantly reduced total work, maximal power achieved, exercise time, and maximal oxygen uptake prior to surgery. If the lesion is incompletely corrected (placement of conduit between ventricle and pulmonary artery without closure of the defect), exercise performance improves but not to normal levels. Complete correction achieves near normal arterial oxygen saturation and ventilatory function, but exercise performance remains subnormal.[78]

## Tetralogy of Fallot

Surgical therapy, usually definitive, rather than palliative, is indicated for severe hypoxia, documented hypercyanotic episodes, and suprasystemic right ventricular pressure in patients with tetralogy of Fallot. Residual defects after repair include pulmonary hypertension, ventricular septal defect, tricuspid regurgitation occurring in 65 percent of patients, aortic regurgitation, pulmonic insufficiency occurring in 78 percent of patients with the severity correlating with right ventricular cavity area, right ventricular dysfunction, right ventricular outflow track obstruction, right bundle branch block, and arrhythmia including ventricular tachycardia and premature ventricular contractions in 16 percent of patients.[79] In Sunakawa's series,[80] preoperative hypoxia, severe pulmonary regurgitation, and pulmonic stenosis were the major factors contributing to right ventricular dysfunction. The severity of the tricuspid regurgitation is unrelated to the degree of pulmonic stenosis or pulmonic regurgitation.[79] However, both tricuspid and pulmonic regurgitation increase ventricular volume and pressure, contributing to ventricular dysfunction.

In a large series of patients undergoing correction of tetralogy of Fallot at a mean age of 7 months, 24/203 were found to have right ventricular outflow track obstruction in excess of 40 mmHg, but only 3 had residual ventricular septal defect and only 2 had ventricular ectopy.[81] The most common outflow track obstruction is subvalvular pulmonic stenosis, but annular or main pulmonary artery stenosis may also be present.[82] Although the right/left ventricular pressure ratio is usually highest immediately postoperatively, additional outflow repair should be performed if the ratio is greater than 0.65. Gradients across the pulmonic outflow track often increase with exercise even when normal at rest. In the series of Kirklin and colleagues,[83] the long-term probability of death was inversely related to pulmonary artery size. Early, intermediate, and long-term survival was worse in patients with pulmonary atresia compared with those who had pulmonic stenosis.[83]

Postoperative arrhythmias may be due to ventricular scar surrounded by cells with increased automaticity that serve as a site for reentry for ventricular tachycardia. Right bundle branch block is present in almost all patients after repair of tetralogy of Fallot.[84] In Chandar et al.'s series,[85] spontaneous premature ventricular contractions were found in 48 percent of patients after tetralogy repair. Inducible ventricular tachycardia was noted in 17 percent of patients. Residual outflow obstruction with right ventricular systolic hypertension, older age at time of repair, longer follow-up time, pulmonic insufficiency, and biventricular dysfunction (particularly right ventricular enlargement and low left ventricular ejection fraction) have been suggested as causes of postoperative arrhythmias after repair of tetralogy, leading to late sudden death in 5 percent of patients.[86,87] However, Vaksman and coworkers[88] reported no increased mortality in a group of untreated patients with ventricular arrhythmias after tetralogy repair. Vaksman's[88] patients had a very low incidence (9 percent) of poor hemodynamic results. Ambulatory ECG monitoring for 24 hours should be performed in all patients after repair of tetralogy. Exercise testing may detect arrhythmias not present on resting ECG. Electrophysiologic studies should be performed in patients with frequent premature ventricular contractions or complex ventricular arrhythmias and abnormal right ventricular function (increased right ventricular systolic pressure and dilatation).[89]

Respiratory function is often abnormal in patients after repair of tetralogy of Fallot. Rowe and colleagues[90] demonstrated statistically significant decreases in vital capacity to less than 80 percent of predicted on long-term follow-up. Breathing reserve, defined as $1 - (Vmax/MVV) \times 100$, where Vmax is maximal ventilation and MVV is maximal voluntary ventilation, is decreased. The respiratory rate at peak exercise is reduced compared with control subjects (Fig. 2-6).

Perrault and coworkers[91] compared patients 12 to 19 years of age who had undergone repair of a ventricular septal defect or tetralogy of Fallot before the age of 5 years with age-matched controls. Maximal exercise tolerance was normal in all subjects. Although there were no significant differences in oxygen consumption among the groups, maximum heart rate was reduced in all postcardiac patients.[91] Cardiac index was also subnormal in the patient group, resulting from the chronotropic limitation. The inadequate chronotropic response may result from impaired reflex control of heart rate or autonomic dysfunction, although the etiology is unclear. The reduction in cardiac output/stroke volume response to exercise is due to right ventricular dysfunction secondary to endocardial fibroelastosis, exercise-induced ectopy, increased right ventricular outflow track obstruction on exercise, and increased right ventricular area from pulmonic regurgitation.

## Transposition of the Great Arteries

Without palliation, transposition is nearly always fatal in the first year of life. Balloon atrial septostomy is performed during diagnostic cardiac catheterization to increase arterial oxygen saturation in the early neonatal period. Transposition is repaired at the atrial level by the Mustard or Senning procedures, at the arterial level by the arterial switch or Jatene procedure, and at the ventricular level with a valved conduit or Rastelli procedure

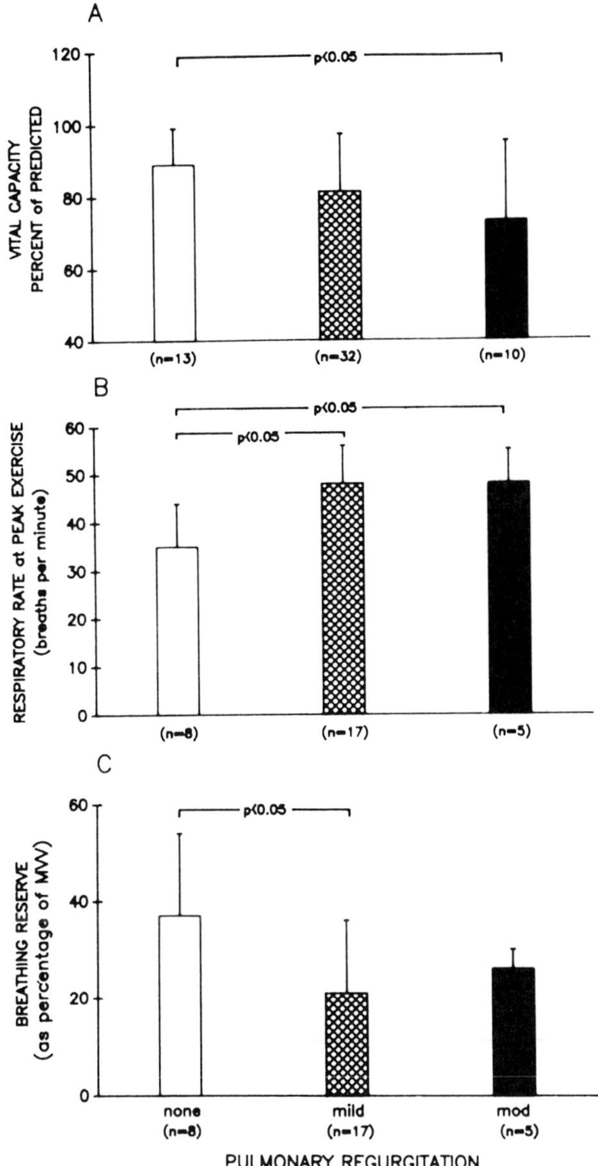


**Fig. 2-6.** Ventilatory function is reduced after repair of tetralogy of Fallot. (**A**) The reduction of vital capacity associated with increasing pulmonic regurgitation. (**B**) Respiratory rate fails to increase during peak exercise as the amount of pulmonary regurgitation increases. (**C**) Breathing reserve is reduced as pulmonic regurgitation increases. Breathing reserve is 1 − (Vmax/MVV) × 100, where Vmax is maximal ventilation and MVV is maximal voluntary ventilation. The amount of pulmonic regurgitation was estimated by Doppler. (From Rowe et al,[90] with permission.)

when a ventricular septal defect is present.

## Atrial Correction

The Mustard and Senning operations are clearly not corrective, although excellent results have been reported in some series.[92] After atrial repairs, both right and left, but particularly systemic (right) ventricular dysfunction has been reported during rest and with exercise.[93] The ventricular contractile pattern is abnormal in infants with Senning repairs. The greatest inward motion of the endocardium occurs in the free wall and infundibulum in normal infants, but septal motion is greatest after Senning procedures.[94] Although the end-diastolic and end-systolic areas of the ventricle are greater than normal in patients after Senning procedures, the area change fraction is nearly normal.[94] Causes of dysfunction include preoperative hypoxia, limited capacity of the right ventricle to function as a systemic ventricle, and adhesion of the right ventricular free wall to the sternum and anterior chest wall, restricting right ventricular free wall contraction.[95] Downward movement of the tricuspid valve ring, an important component of right ventricular function, is also reduced by adhesions.[95] Dilatation and poor function of the right (systemic) ventricle probably also contribute to the 33 percent incidence of tricuspid regurgitation noted after atrial correction.[96] In patients studied 15 years after the Mustard repair, Wong et al.[97] found that ventricular function, although reduced, remained stable over a 5-year period.

Even in asymptomatic patients after Mustard repairs, maximum aerobic exercise capacity (duration of exercise, work capacity, and oxygen consumption compared with controls) is reduced, although cardiac output increases normally.[98] During exercise, heart rate increases less in patients after Mustard repair than in controls. The normal increase in stroke volume during exercise is also blunted by Mustard repairs. However, the normal ejection variables of a systemic right ventricle are unclear.

Constriction of the intra-atrial baffle may partially occlude either pulmonary or systemic venous return. Superior vena caval obstruction occurs in 5 to 10 percent of patients after the Mustard procedure and is less common after the Senning repair. Inferior vena caval obstruction occurs in 1 to 2 percent after either Mustard or Senning repairs. Pulmonary venous obstruction occurs in 2 to 3 percent of patients after atrial repair.

Eight to 10 years after atrial repair, 10 percent of patients experience sudden death, possibly from arrhythmias or hemodynamic complications. Between 10 and 80 percent of patients are free of rhythm disturbances in the late postoperative period.[92] Arrhythmias after atrial repairs are due to preexisting arrhythmias associated with transposition, septostomy/septectomy with excision of internodal pathways, or damage to sinus or AV node or their blood supply.[99] The most common arrhythmia is atrial flutter, which is treated with digoxin or quinidine. Pacemakers must be inserted into any patient after an atrial repair who requires antiarrhythmic drugs that suppress the sinus node. Other options for patients with resistant atrial flutter are antitachycardia pacemakers, AV node ablation, or antiflutter surgery.

Rastelli procedures are curative for varying periods of time. However, the homograft conduit eventually develops stenosis or obstruction and requires replacement.

## Arterial Correction

Long-term studies of children after arterial correction of transposition are still incomplete. Operative mortality rates are similar with either atrial or arterial correction. On a long-term basis, survival is better with arterial than with atrial correction. However, short-term studies demonstrate supravalvular pulmonic stenosis, supravalvular aortic stenosis, aortic regurgitation, arrhythmias, and ventricular dysfunction in some patients.[93]

After neonatal arterial correction of transposition of the great arteries, flow velocities across the tricuspid valve are greater than in normal children.[100] Some degree of pulmonic stenosis (about a 34-mmHg gradient) at the anastomotic site is frequently present.[100] However, flow velocities across the mitral valve and in the ascending aorta are comparable to those in normal children.[100] Supravalvular aortic stenosis has been reported by Martin et al.[93] in 14 percent of patients. Aortic regurgitation, seen in about one-half of patients, is more frequent after the two-stage anatomic repair in which a pulmonary artery band is initially placed to maintain anatomic left ventricular contractility.[93,101] The aortic root diameter is increased compared with normal for age and weight, enhancing the possibility of later aortic regurgitation.

Arrhythmias are less frequent after arterial than after atrial correction. The majority of patients have no significant arrhythmias.[99] Occasional premature ventricular contractions are present, in less than one-third of patients.

On short-term followup, ventricular function is normal after arterial switching.[96,102] Although symptomatic dysfunction has been reported primarily in children with interatrial repairs, it occasionally occurs after arterial (anatomic) correction.[93,95] Ventricular function may be reduced if other defects, aortic regurgitation, or pulmonary hypertension are present. It is also reduced when arterial correction is performed at an older age. Echocardiographic assessment of regional wall motion identifies children with myocardial ischemia after arterial switch procedures.[103] Long-term studies of aortocoronary anastomoses and myocardial perfusion are still incomplete.

## Aortic Coarctation

Patients with uncorrected coarctation rarely present for other surgical procedures, since the lesion is usually diagnosed and repaired at a young age. Upper extremity hypertension with diminished lower extremity pulses should alert the anesthesiologist to the possibility of coarctation in an otherwise healthy patient presenting for noncardiac surgery. Cerebral hemorrhage, bacterial endocarditis, pericoarctation aortic aneurysm, or congestive heart failure generally preclude survival beyond middle age with an uncorrected coarctation.

After surgical repair of coarctation of the aorta, survival is 95 percent when the lesion is repaired at less than 20 years of age. However, postoperative survival declines with older age at repair.[104]

Only 20 percent of patients whose coarctations were repaired after 1 year of age were free from cardiovascular disease 25 years later.[68] Associated anomalies such as a bicuspid aortic valve may become stenotic or insufficient as the patient ages. Other potential problems are aneurysmal aortic dilatation or recurrence of stenosis at the site of the coarctation. Recurrent stenosis is more likely with repair at a young age, but occurs with either end-to-end anastomosis or subclavian flap angioplasty.[105] The type of surgical repair affects the long-term results. Aortic isthmoplasty with resection of the posterior fibrous ridge predisposes to late development of pericoarctation aneurysm, which has an incidence of 1 to 25 percent depending upon the surgical series.[106] A recent evaluation by Parikh et al.[107] demonstrated aneurysm formation in 5 percent of patients after Dacron patch repair of coarctation but not after subclavian flap angioplasty or end-to-end anastomoses. These investigators also noted that preductile bulges were present in 23 percent of patients with coarctation prior to surgery.[107] Subclavian flap angioplasty decreases blood flow velocities in the left brachial artery, potentially causing ischemia during exercise.[108] The extremity is in a permanent state of maximal or submaximal vasodilatation. In contrast, blood flow velocity after resection with end-to-end anastomosis is comparable to control values.[108] Perioperative management of the postcoarctectomy patient is determined by the presence of hypertension and the condition of the aortic valve or other cardiac lesions.

Almost 80 percent of patients with repaired coarctation have normal or only slightly increased blood pressures, but the remainder are hypertensive.[105] The incidence of hypertension varies from 6 to 50 percent (6 percent of patients with surgery performed between 1 and 5 years of age, 30 percent of patients with surgery performed between 6 and 18 years of age, 47 percent of patients with surgery performed between 19 and 40 years of age, ad 50 percent of patients with operation performed over age 40 years.[104,109,110] Postoperative hypertension is increased by older age at correction and reduces long-term survival.[104]

## Hypoplastic Left Heart Syndrome

In the hypoplastic left heart syndrome, the left ventricle, aortic arch, aortic valve, and mitral valve are hypoplastic, stenotic, or atretic. Without surgery (Norwood procedure) or transplantation, the lesion is fatal in the first year of life. Components of the Norwood procedure are atrial septectomy, pulmonary homograft augmentation of the ascending aorta and aortic arch, and anastomosis of the transected proximal pulmonary artery to the augmented aorta via a 4-mm polytetrafluoroethylene shunt. After the Norwood repair, which offers up to an 84 percent survival in some centers, significant tricuspid regurgitation predicts poor outcomes from the subsequent Fontan procedure. Additional potential problems to be evaluated in such patients in between the Norwood and Fontan procedures are restrictive interatrial communications, aortic outflow gradients (arch obstruction), pulmonary hypertension (pulmonary branch stenosis), aortic regurgitation, inadequate shunt, and reduced right ventricular function.[111,112]

## Fontan Procedure

Tricuspid atresia, hypoplastic left heart syndrome after Norwood stage I procedures, and other right heart anomalies are palliated by the Fontan procedure. Arrhythmias, including bradyarrhythmias, atrial tachyarrhythmias, bradycardia-tachycardia syndrome, and supraventricular ectopy occur in about 45 percent of patients after these right ventricular exclusion procedures. Although the other arrhythmias are generally well tolerated, atrial tachyarrhythmias are associated with hemodynamic decompensation. These arrhythmias are significantly associated with morbidity and increase with long-term survival.[113]

After Fontan procedures, many patients have abnormal ejection fractions at rest and are unable to increase cardiac output during exercise to a normal degree. Abnormal left ventricular function after Fontan procedures is related to preoperative ventricular volume overload and hypoxia. The cardiac output is highly rate dependent.[24] The right atrium probably does not function as a pulmonary pump after the Fontan procedure, as pulmonary flow is more dependent upon respiratory changes in intrathoracic pressure than on atrial contraction.[24] Anastomotic obstructions may be unmasked during exercise.

## The Child with a Transplanted Heart

The success of adult cardiac transplantation has increased interest in the use of transplantation for lesions such as hypoplastic left heart syndrome, tricuspid atresia, or other complex cardiac malformations not amenable to surgical repair. However, the major indications are dilated cardiomyopathy and palliated congenital heart defects with irreversible myocardial dysfunction.[114] Although the reported perioperative mortality and rejection rates are high (about 15 percent) in pediatric cardiac transplantation,[115,116] the need for other procedures, such as myocardial biopsy or cholecystectomy, may necessitate anesthetic intervention after successful pediatric cardiac transplantation.

In such children, the presence of rejection must be identified. Rejection occurs most commonly within the first 6 months. Noncompliance with medical therapy is one of the most common causes of cardiac rejection.[117] Shortening of the isovolumetric relaxation time and the pressure half-time of the maximal velocity of blood flow across the mitral valve noninvasively indicate rejection.[115] Radionuclide scans to determine left ventricular ejection fraction are also performed regularly, since a 5 percent decrease is another good predictor of rejection. Atrial or ventricular arrhythmias are also associated with rejection episodes, although they occur in the first 6 months after transplantation in nonrejecting patients. Serial cardiac biopsies to detect myocyte necrosis are confirmatory. However, a 5-year survival of 70 percent is expected.[115]

In survivors of cardiac transplantation, initial growth is maintained and weight increases markedly. Long-term corticosteroid therapy eventually produces retardation of growth and osteoporosis. Coronary vascular disease, renal dysfunction, and hypertension secondary to cyclosporine are serious long-term problems after both pediatric and adult cardiac transplantation.[116] Despite renal dysfunction, progression to chronic renal failure is uncommon. Monitoring of renal function is most easily accomplished in children using serum creatinine rather than creatinine clearance. Multiple-drug antihypertensive therapy may be necessary to control blood pressure, and these drugs should be continued in the perioperative period. Transplant atherosclerosis, probably on an immunologic basis (indicative of chronic rejection), has been a major cause of mortality in Fricker et al's series.[114] A group at particular perioperative risk comprises patients with congenital heart disease who undergo transplantation because their associated pulmonary vascular disease has caused right ventricular failure even in the transplanted heart. Finally, the need for strict asepsis in immunocompromised patients is mandatory in the perioperative period.

The transplanted heart is essentially normal except for the absence of innervation; therefore, no specific anesthetic technique is mandated. Resting heart rate is determined by the donor sinoatrial node. Heart rate is unresponsive to drugs or physiologic compensatory mechanisms (no response to pancuronium, fentanyl, carotid sinus massage, etc.). The Frank-Starling mechanism remains intact. During exercise, cardiac output initially increases due to increased venous return and subsequently due to increased circulating catecholamines. Coronary autoregulation is also intact in the transplanted heart.

Management of these children requires maintenance of venous return and use of direct-acting chronotropic and inotropic agents such as isoproterenol, dopamine, and epinephrine. Regional techniques (spinal or epidural), which reduce venous return, should be used cautiously. Strict asepsis should be maintained and invasive procedures with infection potential (nasotracheal intubation, prolonged intubation, intra-arterial or pulmonary artery catheters) performed only when necessary.

## REFERENCES


1. Mullins CE, Mayer DC: Congenital Heart Disease. A Diagrammatic Atlas. Alan R Liss, New York, 1988
2. Moore RA: Anesthesia for the pediatric congenital heart patient for noncardiac surgery. Anesth Rev 8:23, 1981
3. Lake CL: Pediatric Cardiac Anesthesia. 2nd Ed. Appleton & Lange, East Norwalk, CT, 1993
4. Kirby ML, Waldo KL: Role of neural crest in congenital heart disease. Circulation 82:332, 1990
5. Rudolph AM: The changes in the circulation after birth. Circulation 41:343, 1970
6. Rudolph AM: Hepatic and ductus venosus blood flows during fetal life. Hepatology 3:254, 1983
7. St. John Sutton MG, Gewitz MH, Shah B et al: Quantitative assessment of growth and function: a prospective longitudinal echocardiographic study. Circulation 69:645, 1984
8. St. John Sutton MG, Raichlen JS, Reicheck N, Huff DS: Quantitative assessment of right and left ventricular growth in the human fetal heart: a pathoanatomic study. Circulation 70:935, 1984
9. DeVore GR, Siassi B, Platt LD: Fetal echocardiography IV: M-mode assessment of ventricular size and contractility during the second and third trimesters of pregnancy in the normal fetus. Am J Obstet Gynecol 150:35, 1981
10. Reed KL, Sahn DJ, Scagnelli S et al: Doppler echocardiographic studies of diastolic function in the human fetal heart: changes during gestation. J Am Coll Cardiol 8:391, 1986
11. Barst RJ, Gersony WM: The pharmacological treatment of patent ductus arteriosus. Drugs 38:249, 1989
12. Mahoney LT, Coryell KG, Lauer RM: The newborn transitional circulation: a two dimensional Doppler echocardiographic study. J Am Coll Cardiol 6:623, 1985
13. Moorthy SS, Dierdorf SF, Krishna G et al: Transient hypoxemia from a transient right-to-left shunt in child during emergence from anesthesia. Anesthesiology 66:234, 1987
14. Rudolph AM: Circulatory changes during the perinatal period. Pediatr Cardiol 4(suppl. II):17, 1983
15. Mellander M, Larsson LE: Effects of left-to-right ductus shunting on left ventricular output and cerebral blood flow velocity in 3-day-old preterm infants with and without severe lung disease. J Pediatr 113:101, 1988
16. Scholler GF, Celermajer JM, Whight CM, Bauman AE: Echo doppler assessment of cardiac output and its relation to growth in normal infants. Am J Cardiol 60:1112, 1987
17. Friedman WF: The intrinsic physiologic properties of the developing heart. Prog Cardiovasc Dis 15:87, 1972
18. Anderson PAW: Maturation and cardiac contractility. Cardiol Clin 7:209, 1989
19. Thornberg KL, Morton MJ: Filling and arterial pressures as determinants of RV stroke volume in the sheep fetus. Am J Physiol 244:H656, 1983
20. Rein AJJT, Sanders SP, Colan SD et al: Left ventricular mechanics in the normal newborn. Circulation 76:1029, 1987
21. Tripp ME: Developmental cardiac metabolism in health and disease. Pediatr Cardiol 10:150, 1989
22. Bisset GS: Magnetic resonance imaging of congenital heart disease in the pediatric patient. Radiol Clin North Am 29:279, 1991

23. Krabill KA, Wang Y, Einzig S et al: Rest and exercise hemodynamics in pulmonary stenosis: comparison of children and adults. Am J Cardiol 56:360, 1985
24. Moreau GA, Graham TP: Clinical assessment of ventricular function after surgical treatment of congenital heart defects. Cardiol Clin 7:439, 1989
25. Weigel TJ, Porter CJ, Mottram CD, Driscoll DJ: Detecting arrhythmias by exercise electrocardiography in pediatric patients: assessment of sensitivity and influence on clinical management. Mayo Clin Proc 66:379, 1991
26. Wiles HB: Imaging congenital heart disease. Pediatr Clin North Am 37:115, 1990
27. Lipshultz SE, Sanders SP, Mayer JE et al: Are routine preoperative cardiac catheterization and angiography necessary before repair of ostium primum atrial septal defect? J Am Coll Cardiol 11:373, 1988
28. Alboliras ET, Seward JB, Hagler DJ et al: Impact of two-dimensional and Doppler echocardiography on care of children aged two years and younger. Am J Cardiol 61:166, 1988
29. Krabill KA, Ring WS, Foker JE et al: Echocardiographic versus cardiac catheterization diagnosis of infants with congenital heart disease requiring cardiac surgery. Am J Cardiol 60:351, 1987
30. Kurokawa S, Takahashi M, Katoh Y et al: Noninvasive evaluation of the ratio of pulmonary to systemic flow in ventricular septal defect by means of Doppler two-dimensional echocardiography. Am Heart J 116:1033, 1988
31. Shenker L, Reed KL, Marx GR et al: Fetal cardiac Doppler flow studies in prenatal diagnosis of heart disease. Am J Obstet Gynecol 158:1267, 1988
32. Valdez-Cruz LM, Pieroni DR, Roland JMA et al: Recognition of residual postoperative shunts by contrast echocardiographic techniques. Circulation 55:148, 1977
33. Fraker TD, Harris PJ, Behar VS, Kisslo JA: Detection and exclusion of interatrial shunts by two-dimensional echocardiography and peripheral venous injection. Circulation 59:379, 1979
34. Cooper MJ, Tyndall M, Silverman NH: Evaluation of the responsiveness of elevated pulmonary vascular resistance in children by Doppler echocardiography. J Am Coll Cardiol 12:470, 1988
35. Mullins CE: Pediatric and congenital therapeutic cardiac catheterization. Circulation 79:1153, 1989
36. Morray JP, MacGillivray R, Duker G: Increased perioperative risk following repair of congenital heart disease in Down's syndrome. Anesthesiology 65: 221, 1986
37. Stork RL, Bredle DL, Chapler CK, Cain SM: Regional hemodynamic responses to hypoxia in polycythemic dogs. J Appl Physiol 65:2069, 1988
38. Flanagan MF, Hourihan M, Keane JF: Incidence of renal dysfunction in adults with cyanotic congenital heart disease. Am J Cardiol 68:403, 1991
39. Colon-Otero G, Gilchrist GS, Holcomb GR et al: Preoperative evaluation of hemostasis in patients with congenital heart disease. Mayo Clin Proc 62:379, 1987
40. Ekert H, Sheers M: Preoperative and postoperative platelet function in cyanotic congenital heart disease. J Thorac Cardiovasc Surg 67:184, 1974
41. Territo MC, Rosove MH: Cyanotic congenital heart disease: hematologic management. J Am Coll Cardiol 18:320, 1991
42. Clapp SK, Perry BL, Farooki ZQ et al: Down's syndrome, complete atrioventricular canal and pulmonary vascular obstructive disease. J Thorac Cardiovasc Surg 100:115, 1990
43. Rabinovitch M, Keane JK, Fellows KE et al: Quantitative analysis of the pulmonary wedge angiogram in congenital heart defects. Correlation with hemodynamic data and morphometric findings in lung biopsy tissue. Circulation 63:152, 1981
44. Rabinovitch M, Haworth SG, Castaneda AR et al: Lung biopsy in congenital heart disease: a morphometric approach to pulmonary vascular disease. Circulation 58:1107, 1978
45. Wilson NJ, Seear MD, Taylor GP et al: The clinical value and risks of lung bi-

opsy in children with congenital heart disease. J Thorac Cardiovasc Surg 99: 460, 1990
46. Heath D, Edwards JE: The pathology of hypertensive pulmonary vascular disease. Circulation 18:533, 1958
47. Rabinovitch M: Structure and function of the pulmonary vascular bed: an update. Cardiol Clin 7:227, 1989
48. Lopes AAB, Liberato MH, Brentani MM et al: Lung beta-adrenoceptors in pulmonary hypertension. Chest 99:637, 1991
49. Banclari E, Jessie MJ, Gelband H et al: Lung mechanics in congenital heart disease with increase and decrease of pulmonary blood flow. J Pediatr 90:192, 1977
50. Fletcher R: Invasive and noninvasive measurement of the respiratory deadspace in anesthetized children with cardiac disease. Anesth Analg 67:442, 1988
51. Kohelet D, Perlman M, Kirplani H et al: High-frequency oscillation in the rescue of infants with persistent pulmonary hypertension. Crit Care Med 16:510, 1988
52. Martin GR, Short BL: Doppler echocardiographic evaluation of cardiac performance in infants on prolonged extracorporeal membrane oxygenation. Am J Cardiol 62:929, 1988
53. Casthely PA, Redko V, Dluzneski J et al: Pulse oximetry during pulmonary artery banding. J Cardiothorac Anesth 1:297, 1987
54. Friesen RH: Pulse oximetry during pulmonary artery surgery. Anesth Analg 64: 376, 1985
55. Yates AP, Lindahl SGE, Hatch DJ: Pulmonary ventilation and gas exchange before and after correction of congenital cardiac malformations. Br J Anaesth 59: 170, 1987
56. Edelman NH, Lahiri S, Braudo L et al: Blunted ventilatory response to hypoxia in cyanotic congenital heart disease. N Engl J Med 282:405, 1970
57. Sietsema KE, Cooper DM, Perloff JK et al: Control of ventilation during exercise in patients with central venous-to-systemic arterial shunts. J Appl Physiol 64: 234, 1988
58. Tanner GE, Angers DG, Barash PG et al: Effect of left-to-right, mixed left-to-right, and right-to-left shunts on inhalational anesthetic induction in children: a computer model. Anesth Analg 64:101, 1985
59. Hensley FA, Larach DR, Martin DE et al: The effect of halothane/nitrous oxide/oxygen mask induction on arterial hemoglobin saturation in cyanotic heart disease. J Cardiothorac Anesth 1:289, 1987
60. Greeley WJ, Stanley TE, Ungerleider RM, Kisslo JA: Intraoperative hypoxemic spells in tetralogy of Fallot. Anesth Analg 68:815, 1989
61. Klitzner TS, Friedman WF: Cardiac arrhythmias: the role of pharmacologic intervention. Cardiol Clin 7:299, 1989
62. Perry JC, Garson A: Diagnosis and treatment of arrhythmias. Adv Pediatr 36:177, 1989
63. Redington ABN, Carvalho JS, Shinebourne EA: Does digoxin have a place in the treatment of the child with congenital heart disease? Cardiovasc Drug Ther 3:21, 1989
64. Schneeweis A: Cardiovascular drugs in children. II. Angiotensin-converting enzyme inhibitors in pediatric patients. Pediatr Cardiol 11:199, 1990
65. Driefuss LS, Fisch C, Griffen JC et al: ACC/AHA guidelines for implantation of cardiac pacemakers and antiarrhythmia devices. Circulation 84:455, 1991
66. Kugler JD, Danford DA: Pacemakers in children: an update. Am Heart J 117:665, 1989
67. Addonizio LJ, Hsu DT, Fuzesi L et al: Optimal timing of pediatric heart transplantation. Circulation 80(suppl. 3):III-84, 1989
68. Stark J: Do we really correct congenital heart defects? J Thorac Cardiovasc Surg 97:1, 1989
69. Perloff JK: Adults with surgically treated congenital heart disease. JAMA 250: 2033, 1983
70. Ferry PC: Neurologic sequelae of open-heart surgery in children. An "irritating question." Am J Dis Child 144:369, 1990
71. Newburger JW, Silbert AR, Buckley LP, Fyler DC: Cognitive function and age at

repair of transposition of the great arteries in children. N Engl J Med 310:1495, 1984

72. Glauser TA, Rorke LB, Weinberg PM, Clancy RR: Acquired neuropathologic lesions associated with the hypoplastic left heart syndrome. Pediatrics 85:991, 1990
73. Glauser TA, Rorke LB, Weinberg PM, Clancy RR: Congenital brain anomalies associated with the hypoplastic left heart syndrome. Pediatrics 85:984, 1990
74. McConnell JR, Fleming WH, Chu WK et al: Magnetic resonance imaging of the brain in infants and children before and after cardiac surgery. A prospective study. Am J Dis Child 144:374, 1990
75. Murphy JG, Gersh BJ, McGoon MD et al: Long-term outcome after surgical repair of isolated atrial septal defect. N Engl J Med 323:1645, 1990
76. Kaplan S: Natural adult survival patterns. J Am Coll Cardiol 18:319, 1991
77. Fournier A, Young M-L, Garcia OL et al: Electrophysiologic cardiac function before and after surgery in children with atrioventricular canal. Am J Cardiol 57: 1137, 1986
78. Barber G, Danielson GK, Puga FJ et al: Pulmonary atresia with ventricular septal defect: preoperative and postoperative responses to exercise. J Am Coll Cardiol 7:630, 1986
79. Zahka KG, Horneffer PJ, Rose SA et al: Long-term valvular function after total repair of tetralogy of Fallot. Relation to ventricular arrhythmias. Circulation 78: III-14, 1988
80. Sunakawa A, Shirotani H, Yokoyama T, Oku H: Factors affecting biventricular function following surgical repair of tetralogy of Fallot. Jpn Circ J 52:401, 1988
81. Walsh EP, Rockenmacher S, Keane JF et al: Late results in patients with tetralogy of Fallot repaired during infancy. Circulation 77:1062, 1988
82. Chang AC, Vetter JM, Gill SE et al: Accuracy of prospective two-dimensional/ Doppler echocardiography in the assessment of reparative surgery. J Am Coll Cardiol 16:903, 1990
83. Kirklin JW, Blackstone EH, Shimazaki Y et al: Survival, functional status, and reoperations after repair of tetralogy of Fallot with pulmonary atresia. J Thorac Cardiovasc Surg 96:102, 1988
84. Krongrad E: Postoperative arrhythmias in patients with congenital heart disease. Chest 85:107, 1984
85. Chandar JS, Wolff GS, Garson A et al: Ventricular arrhythmias in postoperative tetralogy of Fallot. Am J Cardiol 65:655, 1990
86. Kavey REW, Thomas FD, Byrum CJ et al: Ventricular arrhythmias and biventricular dysfunction after repair of tetralogy of Fallot. J Am Coll Cardiol 4: 126, 1984
87. Kawashima Y, Matsuda H, Hirose H et al: Ninety consecutive corrective operations for tetralogy of Fallot with and without minimal right ventriculotomy. J Thorac Cardiovasc Surg 90:856, 1985
88. Vaksman G, Fournier A, Davignon A: Frequency and prognosis of arrhythmias after operative correction of tetralogy of Fallot. Am J Cardiol 66:346, 1990
89. Garson A: The emerging adult with arrhythmias after congenital heart disease: management and financial health care policy. Pace 13:951, 1990
90. Rowe SA, Zahka KG, Manolio TA et al: Lung function and pulmonary regurgitation limit exercise capacity in postoperative tetralogy of Fallot. J Am Coll Cardiol 17:461, 1991
91. Perrault H, Drblik SP, Montigny M et al: Comparison of cardiovascular adjustments to exercise in adolescents 8 to 15 years of age after correction of tetralogy of Fallot, ventricular septal defect or atrial septal defect. Am J Cardiol 64:213, 1989
92. Turley K, Hanley FL, Verrier ED et al: The Mustard procedure in infants (less than 100 days of age). J Thorac Cardiovasc Surg 96:849, 1988
93. Martin RP, Qureshi SA, Ettedgui JA et al: An evaluation of right and left ventricular function after anatomical correction and intra-atrial repair operations for complete transposition of the great arteries. Circulation 82:808, 1990
94. Trowitzsch E, Colan SD, Sanders SP:

Global and regional right ventricular function in normal infants and infants with transposition of the great arteries after Senning operation. Circulation 72: 1008, 1985
95. Okuda H, Nakazawa M, Imai Y et al: Comparison of ventricular function after Senning and Jatene procedures for complete transposition of the great arteries. Am J Cardiol 55:530, 1985
96. Backer CL, Ilbawi MN, Ohtake S et al: Transposition of the great arteries: a comparison of results of the Mustard procedure versus the arterial switch. Ann Thorac Surg 48:10, 1989
97. Wong KY, Venables AW, Kelly MJ, Kalff V: Longitudinal study of ventricular function after the Mustard operation for transposition of the great arteries: a long term follow up. Br Heart J 60:316, 1988
98. Musewe NN, Reisman J, Benson LN et al: Cardiopulmonary adaptation at rest and during exercise 10 years after Mustard atrial repair for transposition of the great arteries. Circulation 77:1055, 1988
99. Arensman FW, Bostock J, Radley-Smith R, Yacoub MH: Cardiac rhythm and conduction before and after anatomic correction of transposition of the great arteries. Am J Cardiol 52:836, 1983
100. Gibbs JL, Qureshi SA, Martin R et al: Neonatal anatomical correction of transposition of the great arteries: noninvasive assessment of haemodynamic function up to four years after operation. Br Heart J 60:66, 1988
101. Gibbs JL, Qureshi SA, Wilson N et al: Doppler echocardiography comparison of haemodynamic results of one and two stage anatomic correction of transposition of the great arteries. Int J Cardiol 18: 85, 1988
102. Arensman FW, Radley-Smith R, Yacoub MH et al: Catheter evaluation of left ventricular shape and function 1 or more years after anatomic correction of transposition of the great arteries. Am J Cardiol 52:1079, 1983
103. Vogel M, Smallhorn JF, Trusler GA, Freedom RM: Echocardiographic analysis of regional left ventricular wall motion in children after the arterial switch operation for complete transposition of the great arteries. J Am Coll Cardiol 15: 1417, 1990
104. Cohen M, Fuster V, Steele PM et al: Coarctation of the aorta. Circulation 80:840, 1989
105. Cobanoglu A, Teply JF, Grunkemeier GL et al: Coarctation of the aorta in patients younger than three months. J Thorac Cardiovasc Surg 89:128, 1985
106. Hehrlein FW, Mulch J, Rautenburg HW et al: Incidence and pathogenesis of late aneurysms after patch graft aortoplasty for coarctation. J Thorac Cardiovasc Surg 92:226, 1986
107. Parikh SR, Hurwitz RA, Hubbard JE et al: Preoperative and postoperative "aneurysm" associated with coarctation of the aorta. J Am Coll Cardiol 17:1367, 1991
108. Van Son JAM, Van Austen WNJC, Van Lier HJJ et al: Detrimental sequelae on the hemodynamics of the upper left limb after subclavian flap angioplasty in infancy. Circulation 81:996, 1990
109. Crawford ES, Crawford JL: Diseases of the Aorta. p. 249. Williams & Wilkins, Baltimore, 1984
110. Lieberthson RR, Pennington DG, Jacobs ML, Daggett WM: Coarctation of aorta: review of 234 patients and clarification of management problems. Am J Cardiol 43:835, 1979
111. Chang AC, Farrell PE, Murdison KA et al: Hypoplastic left heart syndrome: hemodynamic and angiographic assessment after initial reconstructive surgery and relevance to modified Fontan procedure. J Am Coll Cardiol 17:1143, 1991
112. Meliones JN, Snider AR, Bove EL et al: Longitudinal results after first-stage palliation for hypoplastic left heart syndrome. Circulation 82(suppl. IV):IV151, 1990
113. Weber HS, Hellenbrand WE, Kleinman CS et al: Predictors of rhythm disturbances and subsequent morbidity after the Fontan operation. Am J Cardiol 64: 762, 1989
114. Fricker FJ, Trento A, Griffith BP: Pediatric cardiac transplantation. p. 223. In Brest AN (ed): Cardiovascular Clinics. Vol. 20. FA Davis, Philadelphia, 1990

115. Starnes VA, Stinson EB, Oyer PE et al: Cardiac transplantation in children and adolescents. Circulation 76(suppl. V):V-43, 1987
116. Trento A, Griffith BP, Fricker FJ et al: Lessons learned in pediatric heart transplantation. Ann Thorac Surg 48:617, 1989
117. Addonizio LJ, Hsu DT, Smith CR et al: Late complications in pediatric cardiac transplant recipients. Circulation 82(suppl. 4):IV-295, 1990
118. Garson A: The Electrocardiogram in Infants and Children: A Systemic Approach. Lea & Febiger, Philadelphia, 1983
119. Dajani AS, Bisno AL, Chung KJ et al: Prevention of bacterial endocarditis. Circulation 83:1174, 1991
120. Moore RA, McNicholas KW, Warran SP: Atlantoaxial subluxation with symptomatic spinal cord compression in a child with Down's syndrome. Anesth Analg 66:89, 1987

# 3
# Hematology and Oncology

# 3

# Hematology and Oncology

*Paul C. J. Rogers*
*Louis D. Wadsworth*

## HEMATOLOGY

### Physiology and Development of Blood

Very early in embryonic life, soon after the fertilized ovum has implanted, blood islands form within the yolk sac. By 14 days' gestation these islands have become hollow, and primitive vascular endothelium and blood cells have developed. These primitive blood cells colonize the liver and spleen, which constitute the main blood-forming organs of intrauterine life, reaching peak activity at 4 to 5 months' gestation. As extramedullary hematopoiesis declines, bone marrow hematopoiesis begins, such that at term, extramedullary hematopoiesis has almost completely disappeared. At the time of birth, red, hematopoietic marrow exists in all the bones of the body, but after birth the red marrow shrinks into the central skeleton and has disappeared from the shafts of the long bones by early adult life. Red marrow is replaced in the limb bones by yellow, fatty marrow. The red marrow eventually exists only in the skull, vertebrae, sternum, ribs, and pelvis. Hematopoietic marrow is normally present in the pelvis at all ages, and for this reason, the posterior iliac crest is the most satisfactory location to perform a bone marrow aspiration and biopsy whatever the patient's age.

Hematopoietic cells develop from stem cells under the influence of various differentiation and growth factors, such as erythropoietin, colony stimulating factor, thrombopoietin, and the interleukins. Differentiation and growth takes place in an optimal stromal microenvironment, which provides suitable conditions for stem cell growth, replication, and maturation. A pluripotent stem cell divides into a series of committed progenitor cells, which in turn mature through a succession of maturation divisions to produce mature red blood cells, granulocytes, monocytes, and platelets.

Developing lymphocytes are not seen in the yolk sac but appear in the liver from 7 weeks' gestation onward, appearing in the thymus at about the same time and in the spleen and bone marrow at about 10 to 12 weeks' gestation. Lymphocytes appear in the blood from 7 weeks' gestation onward, increasingly slowly during the later months of gestation. T lymphocytes, as a rule, are found earlier than B lymphocytes.

## Red Cell Proliferation, Maturation, and Destruction

Of those cells destined to become mature erythrocytes, there are at least three separate stages after differentiation from a pluripotential stem cell before the appearance of a primitive cell form morphologically recognizable as an erythroblast. Subsequently, there are three mitotic divisions during the differentiation of the proerythroblast to the late erythroblast. Each of these maturation steps takes approximately 16 hours. Hemoglobinization occurs during this period and takes 2 to 4 days. Hemoglobinization continues after the late erythroblast has lost its nucleus and becomes a reticulocyte. Reticulocytes mature for 1 to 2 days in the bone marrow, and continue maturing for a further 24 hours in the peripheral blood before becoming mature erythrocytes. Enumeration of reticulocytes gives reasonable measurement of erythropoietic activity, and a reticulocyte count, when corrected for the degree of anemia, can be used to determine whether the marrow erythropoietic response is appropriate for a particular degree of anemia.

Following their development from reticulocytes, mature erythroblasts survive approximately 120 days. Toward the end of this life span, the red cells progressively lose water, increasing their mean cell hemoglobin concentration, and immunoglobulin accumulates on the red cell membrane, until eventually the affected red cells are recognized by the reticuloendothelial system and phagocytosed. This process of normal red blood cell destruction occurs throughout the body, but because the bulk of reticuloendothelial tissue is in the spleen, a significant proportion of normal red cell phagocytosis occurs there. Following phagocytosis of red cells by reticuloendothelial cells, hemoglobin is released, and from this, iron is recycled to the plasma iron pool bound to transferrin. The residual porphyrin ring is degraded to bilirubin, which is carried to the liver for conjugation and excreted into the gastrointestinal tract, where it is converted to urobilinogen.

In response to renal hypoxia, erythropoietin is produced. This agent is the major hormonal stimulus to erythropoiesis. When the normal balance of the rate of red blood cell production and destruction is disturbed in response to hemorrhage or hemolysis, there is an increased production of erythropoietin. In response, increased numbers of marrow stem cells are diverted to the erythroid line and maturation times within the erythroid line are shortened, resulting in the premature release of cells into the circulation that still contain nuclear and ribosomal remnants. These cells are often larger than erythrocytes that have undergone maturation during steady-state erythropoiesis, hence the mild macrocytosis that may be noted in chronic hemolysis.

## Myeloid Proliferation and Maturation

There are at least two divisions after the pluripotent stem cell stage before the appearance of the earliest identifiable precursor of the granulocyte series, which is the myeloblast. Myeloblasts can be seen in normal bone marrow in small numbers, typically less than 5 percent. A series of differentiation steps follows, in which the myeloblasts gradually lose the basophilia of their cytoplasm and become smaller; then specific granules identifying neutrophils, eosinophils, and basophils develop. This process of maturation and differentiation is controlled by a colony stimulating factor known as granulocyte (G)-CSF. It takes approximately 3 days for myeloid precursors to develop from the myeloblast to the myelocyte stage. After this time, the cells enter a postmitotic maturation phase and a marrow storage "pool" before entering the peripheral blood as mature neutrophils. These latter processes take approximately 10 days. The circulating granulocyte pool has two compartments, a circulating and a marginated pool. The marginated pool is comprised of cells that adhere to the walls of small vessels, rather than forming part of the axial stream of blood. Granulocytes are lost from the marginal pool into the tissues, where they die either in inflammatory foci, normal senescence, or by loss into body secretions. The half-life of a neutrophil in the blood is very short, being only a matter of 6 to 8 hours.

### Platelet Production and Maturation

Unlike the other peripheral blood elements, platelets mature as a result of fragmentation of the cytoplasm of a large multinucleated precursor cell, the megakaryocyte. After differentiation of the pluripotent stem cell, the earliest recognizable platelet precursor, the megakaryoblast, can be seen in the marrow. The megakaryoblast matures by endomitosis, and the cell increases dramatically in volume and in nuclear numbers. When an eight-nucleus stage is reached, the cytoplasm becomes granular and platelets begin to be liberated from the cytoplasmic margin. The time interval from the differentiation from the stem cell to the production to mature platelets is approximately 10 days. The lifespan of platelets in the peripheral blood is approximately 7 to 10 days. Approximately 30 percent of normal platelets reside in the spleen. In addition to their function in hemostasis, platelets also have a phagocytic capacity for microorganisms and immune complexes.

## The Blood Count

Automated multiparameter blood counting instruments produce vast amounts of information regarding the peripheral blood elements. This information can be gained from the analysis of a small sample, typically 100 μL of blood. The red cell indices that are usually reported include hemoglobin, hematocrit, mean cell volume (MCV), mean cell hemoglobin (MCH), mean cell hemoglobin concentration (MCHC), and red blood cell distribution width (RDW). The RDW is a numerical measure of variation in red cell size (i.e., anisocytosis). Most modern-day blood counts also include a platelet count and a mean platelet volume (MPV). In addition to a total leukocyte count, most automated blood count analyzers give an automated multipart leukocyte differential. The more up to date machines give a full five-part differential, including eosinophil and basophil counts. The simpler machines separate the leukocytes into granulocytes, lymphocytes, and an intermediate-cell group that consists largely of monocytes. Although many physicians still request manual differentials, in fact, automated leukocyte differentials are probably more accurate and precise, particularly for total granulocyte and lymphocyte numbers.

### Normal Values

Normal blood count values change dramatically and repeatedly during normal childhood growth and development; a full range of normal values for hemoglobin and red blood cell indices is shown in Table 3-1. Hemoglobin, which is at its maximum level within the first 24 hours of life, declines steadily to reach a nadir at 6 months of age. Thereafter, the values slowly increase to reach adult levels by 18 years of age. The MCV is very high at birth and declines to a nadir at approximately 1 year of age, reaching adult levels by 18 years. There are only slight differences between the platelet counts of newborn infants and adults. The normal white blood cell count is high at birth and gradually declines to adult levels by 6 to

**Table 3-1.** Hematology Expected Normal Values

| *Age* | *Red Blood Cell Count (× $10^{12}$/L)* | *Hemoglobin (g/L)* | *Hematocrit* | *Mean Cell Volume (fl)* | *Mean Cell Hemoglobin (pg)* | *Mean Cell Hemoglobin Concentration (g/L)* |
|---|---|---|---|---|---|---|
| Cord[a] | 3.90–5.50 | 140–190 | | 98.0–118 | | |
| 1–7 d[a] | 4.00–6.60 | 150–250 | .410–.730 | 95.0–121 | | |
| 8–28 d[a] | 3.90–6.30 | 149–229 | .420–.600 | 88.0–126 | 31.0–37.0 | 300–366 |
| 29–56 d[a] | 3.30–5.30 | 102–182 | .390–.630 | 86.0–124 | 29.0–36.0 | 280–360 |
| 2–5 mo[a] | 2.70–4.90 | 91–131 | .280–.420 | 77.0–105 | 26.0–34.0 | 290–370 |
| 6–11 mo[a] | 3.10–4.50 | 101–129 | .290–410 | 70.0–86.0 | 25.0–35.0 | 290–360 |
| 1–4 y[a] | 3.70–5.30 | 107–131 | .330–.390 | 70.0–86.0 | 23.0–31.0 | 300–360 |
| 5 y[b] | 3.90–5.30 | 107–147 | .340–.400 | 75.0–87.0 | 24.0–30.0 | 310–370 |
| 6–8 y[b] | 4.05–5.15 | 118–146 | .353–.428 | 77.1–91.5 | 25.8–31.7 | 330–351 |
| 9–11 y[b] | 4.05–5.15 | 118–146 | .353–.428 | 77.1–91.5 | 25.8–31.7 | 330–351 |
| 12–15 y M[b] | 4.43–5.53 | 125–165 | .368–.473 | 77.1–91.5 | 25.8–31.7 | 330–351 |
| 12–15 y F[b] | 4.05–4.98 | 117–149 | .351–.436 | 77.1–91.5 | 25.8–31.7 | 330–351 |
| 16–18 y M[b] | 4.41–5.71 | 131–169 | .380–.489 | 80.0–94.9 | 25.0–33.8 | 330–355 |
| 16–18 y F[b] | 4.00–4.87 | 117–149 | .351–.436 | 80.0–94.8 | 25.0–33.8 | 330–355 |
| Adult M[b] | 4.3–5.5 | 135–170 | .400–.490 | 83.0–97.5 | 27.2–33.4 | 322–362 |
| Adult F[b] | 3.6–5.0 | 114–143 | .330–.440 | 83.0–97.5 | 27.2–33.4 | 322–354 |

[a] (Data from Willoughby (1977), Nathan and Oski (1987), Oski and Naiman (1982), and Williams et al (1983).)
[b] Established by Hematopathology Laboratory, British Columbia's Children's Hospital, Vancouver, British Columbia, Canada.

8 years of age. The increase in leukocytes in the first years of life is largely due to an increase in neutrophils and lymphocytes. Lymphocyte counts reach adult levels by approximately 12 years of age; neutrophil counts reach adult levels by approximately 6 months of age (Table 3-2). Normal ranges for platelet count, MPV, and reticulocyte count are shown in Table 3-3.

## Anemia

Anemia is defined on the basis of the peripheral blood hemoglobin level, in comparison with the reference range for age. It is most convenient to classify anemia further on the basis of the MCV. Consequently, there are three major types of anemia: microcytic, normocytic, and macrocytic, each of which has different etiologies (Table 3-4).

### Classification

**Microcytic Anemia.** Microcytic anemias occur because of an inability to manufacture hemoglobin. There are two major components of hemoglobin: heme, which consists of iron and a porphyrin ring, and globin. Defects can occur in the syntheses of both constituents. Iron deficiency is a major cause of microcytic anemia. Iron deficiency can occur in response to inadequate iron intake. This can result from poor nutrition, particularly in babies fed exclusively on cow's milk; or from malabsorption of iron, which occurs when there are defects of gastric function; or from the presence of various agents such as tetracycline that interfere with iron absorption. Iron deficiency can also result from excessive iron loss, which occurs with chronic hemorrhage or chronic hemosiderinuria, as would occur in chronic intravascular he-

**Table 3-2.** Hematology Expected Leukocyte Normal Values (× $10^9$/L)

| *Age* | *WBC* | *Neutrophils* | *Bands* | *Lymphocytes* | *Monocytes* | *Eosinophils* | *Basophils* |
|---|---|---|---|---|---|---|---|
| Cord[a] | 9.0–30.0 | 3.5–20.0 | 0–1.2 | 2.0–11.0 | 0.5–1.8 | 0.2–0.6 | 0.0–0.6 |
| 1–7 d[a] | 9.0–30.0 | 2.0–20.0 | 0–1.7 | 2.0–10.0 | 0.5–1.8 | 0.2–0.6 | 0.0–0.6 |
| 8–28 d[a] | 5.0–20.0 | 2.0–8.0 | 0.4–1.4 | 2.0–17.0 | 0.5–1.8 | 0.2–0.8 | 0.0–0.2 |
| 29–56 d[a] | 5.0–19.5 | | | | | | |
| 2–5 mo[a] | 5.5–18.0 | | | | | | |
| 6–11 mo[a] | 6.0–18.0 | 2.0–5.5 | 0.2–1.0 | 3.6–12.0 | 0.0–0.9 | 0.0–0.5 | 0.0–0.2 |
| 1–4 y[a] | 6.0–18.0 | | | | | | |
| 5 y[b] | 6.0–16.0 | 2.4–7.5 | 0.2–0.8 | 2.3–8.0 | 0.0–0.8 | 0.0–0.5 | 0.0–0.2 |
| 6–8 y[b] | 3.9–10.2 | 1.7–5.0 | 0.0–0.2 | 1.9–4.3 | 0.1–0.7 | 0.0–0.7 | 0.0–0.1 |
| 9–11 y[b] | 3.9–10.2 | 1.4–5.2 | 0.0–0.2 | 1.5–4.2 | 0.1–0.7 | 0.0–0.7 | 0.0–0.1 |
| 12–15 y M[b] | 3.9–10.2 | 1.5–7.4 | 0.0–0.2 | 1.0–3.6 | 0.1–0.7 | 0.0–0.7 | 0.0–0.1 |
| 12–15 y F[b] | 3.9–10.2 | 1.5–7.4 | 0.0–0.2 | 1.0–3.6 | 0.1–0.7 | 0.0–0.7 | 0.0–0.1 |
| 16–18 y M[b] | 3.9–10.2 | 1.8–6.8 | 0.0–0.2 | 1.0–3.6 | 0.1–0.7 | 0.0–0.5 | 0.0–0.1 |
| 16–18 y F[b] | 3.9–10.2 | 1.8–6.8 | 0.0–0.2 | 1.0–3.6 | 0.1–0.7 | 0.0–0.5 | 0.0–0.1 |
| Adult M[b] | 4.2–10.8 | 2.0–6.0 | 0.0–0.7 | 1.0–4.0 | 0.1–0.8 | 0.0–0.45 | 0.0–0.1 |
| Adult F[b] | 4.2–10.8 | 2.0–6.0 | 0.0–0.7 | 1.0–4.0 | 0.1–0.8 | 0.0–0.45 | 0.0–0.1 |

[a] (Data from Willoughby (1977), Nathan and Oski (1987), Oski and Naiman (1982), and Williams et al (1983).)
[b] Established by Hematopathology Laboratory, British Columbia's Children's Hospital, Vancouver, British Columbia, Canada.

**Table 3-3.** Hematology Expected Normal Values

| Age | *Platelets (× $10^9$/L)* | *Reticulocytes (× $10^9$/L)* | *Mean Platelet Volume (fl)* |
|---|---|---|---|
| Cord[a] | 120–450 | 100–300 | |
| 1–7 d[a] | 120–450 | 100–300 | |
| 8–28 d[a] | 140–350 | 100–300 | |
| 29–56 d[a] | 140–350 | 100–300 | |
| 2–5 mo[a] | 140–350 | 100–300 | |
| 6–11 mo[a] | 180–440 | 40–120 | |
| 1–4 y[a] | 180–440 | 40–120 | |
| 5 y[b] | 180–440 | 40–120 | |
| 6–8 y[b] | 180–440 | 30–180 | 7.4–11.1 |
| 9–11 y[b] | 180–440 | 30–180 | 7.4–1.11 |
| 12–15 y M[b] | 180–440 | 30–180 | 7.4–1.11 |
| 12–15 y F[b] | 180–440 | 30–180 | 7.4–1.11 |
| 16–18 y M[b] | 165–397 | 30–180 | 7.4–1.11 |
| 16–18 y F[b] | 165–397 | 30–180 | 7.4–1.11 |
| Adult M[b] | 160–390 | 40–120 | 8.9–12.6 |
| Adult F[b] | 160–390 | 40–120 | 8.9–12.6 |

[a] (Data from Willoughby (1977), Nathan and Oski (1987), Oski and Naiman (1982), and Williams et al (1983).)
[b] Established by Hematopathology Laboratory, British Columbia's Children's Hospital, Vancouver, British Columbia, Canada.

**Table 3-4.** Causes of Anemia

Microcytic Anemia (usually hypochromic)
- Iron deficiency
- Thalassemia trait (α, β, δβ, others)
- Serious thalassemic syndromes (e.g., hemoglobin H disease)
- Anemia of chronic disease
- Lead poisoning
- Congenital sideroblastic anemia

Normocytic Anemia
- With reticulocytosis
  - Hemorrhage
  - Hemolysis (membrane, enzyme, or hemoglobin disorder)
- Without reticulocytosis
  - Marrow failure syndromes (aplastic anemia)
  - Leukemia[a]
  - Myelodysplastic syndromes[a]
  - Malignant infiltration of marrow (lymphoma, metastatic small blue cell tumors)[a]
  - Storage disorders (e.g., Gaucher's disease)

Macrocytic Anemia
- Chronic hemolytic anemia (membrane, enzyme or hemoglobin disorder)
- Megaloblastic anemia ($B_{12}$ or folate deficiency)
- Liver disease
- Leukemia, lymphoma[a]
- Malignant infiltration of marrow[a]
- Myelodysplastic syndromes[a]
- Aplastic anemia[a]
- Congenital dyserythropoietic anemia

[a] May cause either normocytic or macrocytic anemia.

molysis. Defects in iron metabolism resulting in impaired delivery of iron to the developing erythroblast occur in the anemia of chronic disease found in patients with chronic inflammatory conditions such as arthritis, chronic renal failure, or malignancy. Normal adult hemoglobin (HbA) contains two α- and two β-globin chains. Abnormalities in globin formation occur in the thalassemic syndromes. The thalassemic syndromes are categorized on the basis of the deficient globin chain. In α-thalassemia, there is a decrease in the synthesis of α-globin. In α-thalassemia trait, patients may not be anemic, but typically have a reduced MCV and a mildly increased red blood cell count. In α-thalassemia intermedia, which is hemoglobin H disease, three of the four normal α-globin genes are defective, and large amounts of hemoglobin H are produced. Hemoglobin H is a tetramer of β-globin (β4). This condition occurs typically in patients of southeast Asian origin and results in life-long anemia with hemoglobins in the 70 to 100 g/L (7 to 10 g/dl) range. These patients often have splenomegaly. In α-thalassemia major, (Bart's hemoglobin hydrops fetalis), no α-chain is produced and the condition is incompatible with life. Normal persons have two genes governing β-globin production In the β-thalassemia syndromes, β-globin synthesis is abnormal. The absence or reduced activity of one β-globin gene results in β-thalassemia trait, which is clinically similar to α-thalassemia trait. When there is an absence of both β-globin genes, β-thalassemia major results, producing profound life-long, tranfusion-dependent anemia associated with massive hepatosplenomegaly. Typically, patients become iron overloaded, which gradually results in diminished cardiac, hepatic, and pancreatic function. Various types of β-thalassemia intermedia result from interaction of milder types of β-thalassemia gene abnormalities, or the interaction of β-thalassemia trait with structural hemoglobin variants. Hypochromic microcytic anemia may also occur as a result of lead poisoning and has been reported in rare examples of congenital sideroblastic anemia.

**Normocytic Anemia.** There are many causes of normocytic anemia, which can be roughly divided into two categories on the basis of the reticulocyte count. Normocytic anemia with a significant reticulocytosis occurs in response to recent hemorrhage or hemolysis. Normocytic anemia with a normal or reduced reticulocyte count occurs when there are problems with marrow function, typically in marrow failure syndromes such as aplastic anemia, or when there are maturation problems in erythropoiesis, such as takes place in leukemia, preleukemic syndromes, and congenital dyserythropoietic syndromes. In these latter groups, however, macrocytic anemia may also occur.

There are many causes of hemolytic anemia, due to defects in the red blood cell membrane, hemoglobin, or enzyme and energy supply systems. Congenital defects of the membrane include hereditary spherocytosis, elliptocytosis, and pyropoikilocytosis. Acquired defects of the membrane include the autoimmune hemolytic anemias, fragmentation hemolysis, and the hemolysis associated with *Clostridium welchii* sepsis. Congenital defects of hemoglobin include the clinical syndromes associated with hemoglobin S, hemoglobin C, hemoglobin E, and the unstable hemoglobinopathies. One of the complications of sickle cell anemia is recurrent microinfarction of the liver and spleen. By the teenage years, most sickle cell anemia patients are asplenic. Furthermore, their renal function is often impaired, with an inability to concentrate urine. This latter problem has implications for fluid management, particularly during anesthesia. Inherited defects of the red blood cell reducing potential and energy supply system include G6PD and pyruvate kinase deficiency and a number of very rare enzymopathies. Acquired defects of the red blood cell reducing potential occur in patients with inflammatory bowel disease, dermatitis herpetiformis, and leprosy who are treated with large doses of Salazopyrin and dapsone.

**Macrocytic Anemias.** Macrocytic anemia occurs in patients with megaloblastic anemia (folate or $B_{12}$ deficiency), liver disease, marrow infiltration by leukemia, lymphoma, or metastatic malignancy. Macrocytosis may also be seen in preleukemic syndromes and hypothyroidism and is physiologic in the later stages of pregnancy. Hemolytic anemias may also cause macrocytosis, depending on the degree of reticulocytosis, since reticulocytes are larger than mature red cells.

**Neonatal Anemia.** Anemia in the neonate is usually normocytic for age, but occasionally may be microcytic due to $\alpha$-thalassemic syndromes. Neonatal anemia with a normal MCV may be due to hemolysis or hemorrhage. A not infrequent cause of hemolysis in the neonate is alloimmune hemolytic anemia, which is typified by rhesus immune hemolytic disease of the newborn.

The normal decline in neonatal hemoglobin level can be exaggerated in premature newborn, and is often called "the anemia of prematurity." This anemia seems to result from the sudden drop in erythropoietin production that accompanies the switch from intrauterine life and fetal ($\alpha_2\gamma_2$) hemoglobin production to extrauterine life, and adult hemoglobin ($\alpha_2\beta_2$) production. This decrement in hemoglobin is often exacerbated by concurrent rapid growth and iatrogenic blood loss in the hospitalized, sick, premature infant.

## Approach to Investigation

**Microcytic Anemias.** The essential element in the investigation of a microcytic anemia is the exclusion of iron deficiency. Quantitation of serum iron and iron binding capacity may take moderate amounts of serum, but a serum ferritin requires only tiny serum samples, since the measurement involves the use of an immunoassay. In uncomplicated cases, serum ferritin can be a reliable index of marrow iron stores, and a reduced serum ferritin always indicates iron deficiency. In patients with chronic inflammatory disease or malignancy, the serum ferritin can give a false overestimate of body iron stores, because the assay also measures apoferritin, which is an acute-phase reactant and does not contain iron. In such complicated cases, the serum iron and iron binding capacity should also be measured. If iron deficiency can be excluded, a thalassemia syndrome should be considered next. Investigation should include a hemoglobin electrophoresis and allied studies, such as hemoglobin A2 quantitation, hemoglobin H preparation, and hemoglobin F quantitation.

**Normocytic Anemias.** Normocytic anemias should be primarily evaluated on the basis of the reticulocyte count and the blood smear appearance. Patients with reticulocytosis probably have hemolysis or hemorrhage. If hemolysis is suspected, a direct antiglobulin test should be performed. In the neonate with a positive direct antiglobulin test, further investigation of cord and maternal serum should be directed to the identification of the responsible antibody for the provision of compatible blood for exchange transfusion. If the direct antiglobulin test is negative, subsequent investigation should be directed by a hematologist and the initial direction of this investigation would be determined by peripheral red blood cell morphology. Patients with a normocytic anemia and a reduced reticulocyte count would usually have a primary marrow abnormality, and further investigation would include a bone marrow aspiration and biopsy.

**Macrocytic Anemias.** Investigation of macrocytic anemias revolves around exclusion of a megaloblastic anemia. In megaloblastic anemia, the blood smear will show oval macrocytes and hypersegmented neutrophils. The diagnosis is confirmed by a serum and/or red blood cell folate assay, and a serum $B_{12}$ assay. Once deficiency has been established, it is important to determine the cause for reduced folate or $B_{12}$. Liver disease often causes macrocytic red blood cell morphology, but only rarely causes anemia; the macrocytosis of liver disease is usually accompanied by target cell morphology, and liver disease can be confirmed by chemical and coagulation tests of liver function. If marrow infiltration or myelodysplasia is suspected as a cause of macrocytic anemia, then marrow should be aspirated and biopsied for morphologic examination and ancillary tests including cytogenetics and cell surface marker studies.

## Treatment

**Microcytic Anemias.** Iron deficiency should be managed using oral iron therapy with 3 mg of elemental iron kg/d. In infants, this can be given as a single dose, but in older children and adolescents, the dose should be divided and given two or three times during the course of the day. For patients who are intolerant of oral iron, consideration should be given to the use of parenteral iron therapy given by intramuscular or intravenous injection. Both of these routes of administration have their complications. The intramuscular injection is painful, and skin discoloration can occur unless special precautions are taken. Intravenous iron therapy has been reported to result in severe anaphylactic reactions, but if the appropriate test dose and a graded infusion protocol is followed, complications are usually minimal. Parenteral iron therapy must be reserved for those patients who have proven iron deficiency and proven intolerance or nonresponsiveness to oral iron therapy. The chronic hypochromic microcytic anemia of thalassemia trait does not normally need correction. If a patient with thalassemia trait develops severe anemia, another disease process should be sought, and the degree of anemia is never severe enough to warrant transfusion. The thalassemia intermedia syndromes may require transfusion from time to time, particularly during infection or during pregnancy. Patients with thalassemia major require frequent red blood cell infusion, which should be given in such a way that iron overload is minimized. This can be achieved by infusing iron chelating agents at the same time as the red blood cell infusion and by giving infusions of younger red blood cells (neocytes).

**Normocytic Anemias.** The anemia of blood loss may require blood transfusion. If the patient becomes symptomatic, treatment is usually directed toward the detection and correction of the source of blood loss. Patients with congenital hemolytic anemia may require transfusion support during hemolytic crises, but usually do not require specific treatment other than folate supplementation. Patients with acquired immune hemolytic anemia are usually treated with corticosteroids, other immunosuppressants, or intravenous gammaglobulin, or by splenectomy. Potentially, splenectomy is a dangerous procedure, because of the risk of subsequent septic shock due to encapsulated organisms (i.e., pneumococcus and meningococcus). Splenectomy should not be performed until the patient is over 6 years of age. Patients with hemolytic anemias due to oxidative damage of medications rarely require any form of therapy, other than discontinuation of the offending agent. The management of patients with aplastic anemia, leukemia, lymphoma, and metastatic marrow disease should be conducted by a pediatric hematologist/oncologist.

**Macrocytic Anemia.** Vitamin $B_{12}$ deficiency, should be managed with daily doses of 25 to 100 μg by injection immediately after diagnosis. Once normal counts have been achieved, maintenance with monthly injections of 1,000 μg will usually suffice, but some patients need larger doses to maintain normal blood counts. Patients with folic acid deficiency usually respond rapidly to oral doses of 5 mg/d, although larger doses are often given. It is particularly important to prevent the onset of folate deficiency in patients with increased folate needs, such as those with hemolytic anemia or malignant disease.

## Panic Values for the Anesthetist

In adult anesthesia, it has traditionally been considered that a hemoglobin of less than 100 g/L (10 g/dl) renders a patient unsuitable for anesthesia. There is no evidence to support this figure, and most adolescent and adult patients can easily tolerate anesthesia with hemoglobins of 80 g/L (8.0 g/dl) or more. The individual case must, however, be assessed carefully on its own merits, and the patient with unexplained anemia must be investigated, whenever possible, before anesthesia proceeds. The presence of coexisting cardiac or pulmonary disease may interfere with oxygenation and oxygen delivery by relatively normal amounts of circulating hemoglobin. It is generally advised that rules of thumb regarding hemoglobin levels are best avoided, and that individual consideration of each patient be made before transfusing an anemic patient prior to anesthesia. For patients with sickle cell syndromes, special precautions must be taken. Patients with sickle cell trait typically have 40 to 50 percent of hemoglobin S. No specific preoperative preparation is required, but the patients must remain well hydrated and oxygenated throughout the period of anesthesia. Patients with sickle cell anemia typically have more than 90 percent hemoglobin S, and anesthesia for these patients is potentially very dangerous. It is recommended that the patient be kept warm in the perioperative period and ventilated with 100 percent oxygen before and after intubation and extubation. In the postanesthesia recovery room, the patient should be kept warm and special care should be taken to maintain peripheral circulation. It may be preferable to reduce the percentage of hemoglobin S by simple transfusion to ensure that the hematocrit is above 0.36. For major surgery, it may also be necessary to reduce the concentration of hemoglobin S rapidly, and this can be achieved by exchange transfusion. When this is done, an attempt should be made to keep the hemoglobin S at less than 30 percent of total hemoglobin.

## Bleeding Disorders

### Physiology

An insult to a blood vessel endothelium results in vasoconstriction followed by platelet plug formation and fibrin thrombus formation. The primary hemostatic platelet plug formation is initiated by exposure to collagen. This results in platelet adhesion and a first wave of platelet aggregation, which may be followed by disaggregation. A second irreversible wave of aggregation is induced by the release from platelet granules of substances such as adenosine diphosphate (ADP) and thromboxane $A_2$, which mediate irreversible aggregation. This component of primary hemostasis may be tested in vivo by the bleeding time. The platelet plug must be stabilized by the secondary hemostatic mechanism consisting of the formation of thrombin from prothrombin with the subsequent conversion of fibrinogen to fibrin, which in the presence of factor XIII stabilizes to form a clot. The conversion of prothrombin to thrombin is initiated by either the intrinsic pathway or the extrinsic pathway of the coagulation cascade.

The mechanisms promoting clot formation are opposed by natural inhibitors of coagulation. These include antithrombin III, α-2 macroglobulin, α-1 antitripsin, and the vitamin K-dependent factors protein C and its cofactor protein S. Clot lysis (fibrinolysis) results from the action of plasmin on fibrin. Tissue activators, which are necessary for the conversion of plasminogen into plasmin, initiate fibrinolysis. Plasmin activity is opposed by antiplasmins including α-2 antiplasmin.

Abnormalities in either the initial primary hemostatic mechanism of platelet plug formation or in the secondary hemostatic mechanism can result in an increased bleeding tendency. Abnormalities resulting in decreased activity of the anticoagulant protein or the fibrinolytic system can result in an increased tendency to thrombosis, especially venous thrombosis. Abnormalities such as α-2 antiplasmin deficiency result in increased fibrinolysis activity and consequent hemorrhagic tendency.

### Platelet Disorders

Disorders causing a bleeding tendency may be due to a decrease in platelet numbers or platelet function.

**Decreased Platelet Numbers—Thrombocytopenia.** Thrombocytopenia may result from increased destruction or decreased production of platelets.

*Increased Destruction—Immune Thrombocytopenic Purpura.* Autoimmune thrombocytopenic purpura (ITP) in children is a phenomenon that usually follows viral infection with the production of virus-induced antibodies that recognize glycoproteins on the surface of the platelet. These cause rapid removal of the platelets from the circulation. The majority of children recover spontaneously, but thrombocytopenia may persist for several weeks or months, becoming chronic in about 10 percent of patients. The major clinical concern with this disorder is the small but definite risk of intracranial bleeding. Although the circulating platelets are usually functionally effective, due to their decreased number bleeding remains a risk, particularly at the time of surgery. An immune thrombocytopenia may also follow drug sensitization (e.g., from quinine or thiazide). Autoimmune hemolytic disorders such as those associated with systemic lupus erythematosus may result in antibodies against platelet antigens. The combination of autoimmune hemolytic anemia and autoimmune thrombocytopenia is called Evans syndrome.

Treatment of postviral ITP of childhood is generally undertaken when the platelet count is less than $30 \times 10^9$/L (< 30,000/μl), or when there is mucosal bleeding. The most commonly used treatment consists of corticosteroids at a dosage of 2 mg/kg/d, but more recently, higher doses have been utilized for a shorter period of time. An alternative therapy that is equally efficacious is intravenous gammaglobulin for 1 to 5 days. The standard dosage has generally been 500 mg/kg/d for 5 days, but shorter courses appear to be equally effective. Platelet transfusions are of little use in the bleeding ITP patient and should not be used, except in life-threatening situations in which there is a suspected or proven intracranial bleed. If an intracranial bleed does occur, an emergency splenectomy may also be required.

*Alloimmune Neonatal Thrombocytopenia.* Alloimmunization to fetal platelet antigens is due to the generation of maternal antibodies that cross the placenta and cause severe fetal and neonatal thrombocytopenia, the mechanism being similar to that seen in Rh hemolytic disease. The most common scenario occurs when the mother is PLA-1 negative and the infant is PLA-1 positive. Neonatal immune thrombocytopenia may also occur when the mother has previously had ITP and there is passive transfer of IgG platelet autoantibodies into the infant.

The treatment of choice is to utilize platelets derived from the mother that are negative for the offending platelet antigen. Maternal platelets should be processed to remove the offending antibody present in the maternal plasma. Infants born with severe thrombocytopenia are at risk for an intracranial hemorrhage.

*Nonimmune Thrombocytopenia.* Nonimmune increased destruction of platelets may take place in association with disorders such as hemolytic uremic syndrome, thrombotic thrombocytopenic purpura, giant cavernous hemangiomas, disseminated intravascular coagulation, hypersplenism, sepsis, and cyanotic congenital heart disease. In these situations if the child is bleeding, platelet transfusions produce some clinical benefit.

**Decreased Production of Platelets.** Numerous congenital and acquired disorders can result in the decreased production of platelets, due to decreased or absent megakaryocytes in the marrow, bone marrow depression, or bone marrow infiltration. Management of any bleeding is dependent on raising the platelet count by appropriate platelet transfusion. A rule of thumb is that 1 unit of platelets/m$^2$ of body surface area will produce a platelet count increment of approximately 10 to $12 \times 10^9$/L (10,000 to 12,000/μl). This formula, however, is not effective in the septic patient or in one who is already sensitized to platelet transfusions, when more rapid destruction and removal of platelets from the circulation occurs.

**Functional Platelet Disorders.** Table 3-5 lists the congenital and acquired defects of platelet function. The assessment of suspected disorders of platelet function includes examining the platelet size and

**Table 3-5.** Functional Platelet Disorders

- Congenital
  - Vascular or connective tissue defects, e.g.:
    - Ehlers-Danlos syndrome
    - Hereditary hemorrhagic telangiectasis (Rendu-Osler-Weber syndrome)
  - Adhesion defects, e.g.:
    - Bernard-Soulier syndrome
    - von Willebrand's disease
  - Platelet aggregation defects, e.g.:
    - Glanzmann's disease (thrombasthenia)
    - Afibrinogenemia
  - Defects in release reaction of granules
- Acquired Defects
  - Vascular, e.g.:
    - Scurvy/amyloidosis
  - Uremia
  - Drugs
    - Dipyridamole
    - Aspirin/nonsteroidal anti-inflammatory drugs
    - Heparin
    - Sympathetic blockers
    - Clofibrate
    - Phenothiazine/furosemide
    - Penicillin
    - Reserpine
    - Tricyclic antidepressant
  - Viral infiltrate
  - Hypothyroidism
  - Cardiopulmonary bypass
  - Hepatic disease

morphology on the peripheral smear and performing a bleeding time, which is the standard screening for in vivo platelet function. If the bleeding time is prolonged, platelet aggregation studies may be warranted; such studies examine in vitro platelet aggregation in response to a variety of agents. Tests for von Willebrand's disease are also appropriate. At the time of anesthesia, the potential interactions of drugs that may affect platelet function must be considered. Acquired platelet dysfunction may also be of clinical significance in patients who have uremia, significant hepatic dysfunction, and who are recovering from bypass surgery.

The management of defects of platelet function consists in removing the cause of platelet dysfunction such as the offending medication or treating the underlying acquired disorder. A severe hemorrhagic episode at the time of surgery may necessitate platelet transfusion. DDAVP (a synthetic vasopressin derivative) has been found to shorten the bleeding time in patients with uremia, some of the inherited platelet dysfunction disorders, and von Willebrand's disease. It is usually given approximately 1 hour presurgery at a dose of 0.3 μg/kg in 50 ml N/S (normal saline) over 30 minutes. Antifibrinolytic agents such as epsilonaminocaproic acid and tranexamic acid may also be useful in minimizing mucosal bleeding.

## Secondary Hemostasis

Evaluation of a humoral hemostatic defect is most appropriately undertaken by eliciting a detailed history from the patient and family. If the past history is completely negative and there are no acquired disorders that are associated with any bleeding tendencies, then further screening tests prior to surgery are generally unnecessary. However, if following the history there is any suspicion of a bleeding disorder, the screening tests that are considered appropriate are a complete blood count with platelet count, prothrombin time (PT), activated partial thromboplastin time, (aPTT), fibrinogen, and possibly bleeding time. Based on the results of these tests, further investigations may be required but should be ordered in consultation with a hematologist.

## Inherited Coagulation Disorders

**Hemophilia A and B.** Hemophilia A and B (Christmas disease) are X-linked recessive bleeding disorders attributed to decreased levels of functional procoagulant factor VIII (VIII C) (i.e., hemophilia A), or functional procoagulant factor IX (i.e., hemophilia B). These disorders are variable in their clinical severity. Normal individuals typically have 50 to 150 percent clotting factor activity. A severe hemophiliac is one with less than 1 percent of circulating factor activity. This individual may develop severe spontaneous bleeding, typically hemarthrosis and deep tissue hemorrhage. A moderate hemophiliac has 1 to 5 percent of circulating factor activity and is prone to significant bleeding with mild to moderate trauma. Spontaneous hemarthroses are less common. A mild hemophiliac has between 5 and 25 percent of circulating factor activity and will only have significant bleeds following moderate to severe trauma or surgery.

Hematostasis can be achieved by substituting the appropriate coagulation factor, as indicated in Table 3-6. It must be recognized that 5 to 10 percent of patients with hemophilia may develop inhibitors specific for procoagulant factor VIII C. These patients can be extremely difficult to manage, and patients who continue to bleed despite appropriate substitution therapy must be tested for the presence of acquired inhibitors. An inhibitor screen must always form part of the preoperative workup of the hemophiliac undergoing elective surgery.

**von Willebrand's Disease.** von Willebrand's disease, an autosomal-dominant inherited disorder, caused by a decreased amount of Willebrand factor, which is the large multimeric molecule that binds to and protects the factor VIII C procoagulant factor. This disorder is suspected clinically when a patient with a mild bleeding history has a prolonged bleeding time and a slightly prolonged activated partial thromboplastin time. It is confirmed by assays for functional Willebrand factor activity (ristocetin cofactor) and immunologic Willebrand factor activity. It is a complex entity with several specific variants categorized on the basis of the multimeric structure of the Willebrand factor.

In type I von Willebrand's disease, the most common variant, there is a decrease in the overall amount of Willebrand factor with a normal multimeric structure. These patients usually respond to DDAVP treatment. However, for severe bleeds, cryoprecipitate may be necessary.

In type II, there may be an absence of the large and/or intermediate multimers. Patients with the type II variant with ab-

**Table 3-6.** Treatment of Coagulation Defects Replacement Therapy

| *Factor Deficiency* | *Half-life (h)* | *Level Required for Hemostasis* | *Level Required for Minor Trauma* | *Level Required for Surgery and Major Trauma* |
|---|---|---|---|---|
| I | 56–82 | 100 mg/dl | 150 mg/dl | 200 mg/dl |
| II | 48–60 | 10–20 U/ml | 30 U/ml | 50 U/ml |
| V | 36 | 5 U/ml | 10 U/ml | 25 U/ml |
| VII | 5 | 5 U/ml | 10–15 U/ml | 20 U/ml |
| VIII | 8–12 | 20 U/ml | 25–30 U/ml | >50 U/ml |
| Willebrand | 24–48 | 10 U/ml | 20–30 U/ml | 50 U/ml |
| IX | 24 | 10 U/ml | 15 U/ml | >30 U/ml |
| X | 24–60 | 5 U/ml | 10 U/ml | 25 U/ml |
| XIII | 72 | 2–3 U/ml | 15 U/ml | 25 U/ml |

sent large multimers do not respond to DDAVP. In these patients, cryoprecipitate is indicated.

Patients with the type III variant have severe von Willebrand's disease with a total absence of the Willebrand multimers. This variant may be inherited on an autosomal recessive basis. These patients have no response to DDAVP and cryoprecipitate is the treatment of choice.

## Acquired Hemostatic Disorders

Significant acquired bleeding disorders may be associated with vitamin K deficiency, hepatic dysfunction, or disseminated intravascular coagulation (DIC). Vitamin K deficiency may occur in premature infants with low vitamin K stores. The response of these infants to the administration of vitamin K is not always consistent, due to the immaturity of the liver. Maternal ingestion of drugs may also play a role in inhibiting the synthesis of vitamin K clotting-dependent factors. In the older child, decreased absorption of vitamin K, as seen in cystic fibrosis, or after the prolonged use of antibiotics, may result in a severe acquired bleeding disorder.

Hepatic dysfunction may result in the inability of the liver to manufacture coagulation factors. Hepatic disease will normally be indicated by prolongation of both PT and APTT with a normal platelet count. This same profile will be seen in vitamin K deficiency, but usually the history and routine biochemistry will indicate whether or not the patient has a hepatic disorder.

DIC is due to the consumption of platelets and plasma clotting factors and is initiated by an abnormal stimulus resulting from a wide variety of disorders (Table 3-7). It is generally mediated through tissue injury with the accumulation of fibrin in the microcirculation and subsequent injury and fragmentation of the red blood cells. The coagulation cascade is activated and coagulant factors and platelets are consumed. The abnormal stimulus induces excessive fibrinolysis, which further impairs hemostasis. Hypoxia or a septic stress in the newborn period will result in DIC. Sepsis remains the most common cause of DIC. Uncontrollable, severe DIC may result in the clinical manifestation of purpura fulminans with necrosis of skin and peripheral extremities.

**Table 3-7.** Disease States Associated with Disseminated Intravascular Coagulation

| *Causative Factor* | *Clinical Situation* |
|---|---|
| Tissue damage | Trauma<br>Major surgery<br>Heat stroke<br>Burns<br>Venoms<br>Acute promyelocyte leukemia<br>Fat embolism |
| Abnormal or injured endothelial vascular surface | Infection (bacterial, viral, protozoal)<br>Immune complexes<br>Cardiopulmonary bypass<br>Giant hemangiomata<br>Cirrhosis<br>Respiratory distress syndrome |
| Cell destruction | Incompatible blood transfusion<br>Allograft rejection<br>Hemolytic syndromes<br>Drug hypersensitivity |

The primary management of DIC is to remove and treat the underlying triggering event. It is important that acidosis, shock, and electrolyte imbalance be closely monitored and corrected. Initial replacement therapy in the bleeding DIC patient should include platelet concentrate, fresh frozen plasma (10 to 15 ml/kg); when the fibrinogen is low, cryoprecipitate should be administered. Heparinization remains controversial and is not commonly used in pediatrics, except in DIC associated with acute promyelocytic leukemia, snake venom-induced DIC, and heat stroke.

DIC may be triggered during anesthesia or surgery, and may not be suspected until sites at which hemostasis has previously been secured begin to ooze again. In such circumstances, and when there is uncontrolled bleeding in a shocked patient, a diagnosis of DIC must be considered.

### Thrombotic Disorders

A distinction needs to be made between an arterial and a venous thrombosis. Arterial thromboses are associated with abnormalities or injury to the vascular endothelium. This may be acquired, as in vascular injury due to periarteritis nodosa, systemic lupus erythematosus, Kawasaki disease, and cyanotic congenital heart disease. Inherited causes include homocystinuria, Marfan syndrome, and familial hypercholesterolemia. Venous thrombi consist of platelets and fibrin. These may occur as an acquired problem due to activation of the coagulation system associated with decreased blood flow, or an acquired or inherited hypercoagulability, due to the deficiency of specific inhibiting coagulation factors. Some predisposing causes of venous thrombosis are listed in Table 3-8.

Thrombolytic therapy may be appropriate in some situations for both venous and arterial thromboses. The most commonly used agents are urokinase or streptokinase, and more recently, tissue plasminogen activator. Patients who have recently been exposed to thrombolytic therapy may have bleeding complications at the time of surgery. Patients with deep venous thrombosis are treated by heparinization followed by oral anticoagulant therapy to minimize further expansion of the clot and to prevent embolization. The utilization of aspirin or dipyridamole as a prophylactic agent for arterial thrombosis may be considered for patients at risk.

**Table 3-8.** Predisposing Causes of Venous Thrombosis

| |
|---|
| Acquired |
| Intravenous catheters |
| Surgical or accidental trauma |
| Infections |
| Severe dehydration |
| Immobilization |
| L-asparaginase therapy |
| Cyanotic heart disease |
| Nephrotic syndrome |
| Sickle cell disease |
| Liver disease |
| Neonatal asphyxia |
| Infant of a diabetic mother |
| Lupus anticoagulant |
| Congenital/Inherited |
| Antithrombin III deficiency |
| Protein C deficiency |
| Protein S deficiency |
| Plasminogen deficiency |
| Dysfibrinogenemia |

## Leukocytes

### White Blood Cell Disorders

The white blood cell count and the differential count are useful indicators of a variety of different clinical entities in pediatrics. These tests may detect an increase or decrease in the numbers of specific components of the white blood cells, as well as abnormalities in leukocyte morphology.

**Neutropenia.** Neutropenia is a frequent cause of concern, because of the risk of infection in the profoundly neutropenic patient. Postviral neutropenia is the most common cause of mild to moderate cytopenia followed by marrow suppression from drugs, chemotherapy, and soforth. The patient with a neutrophil count of less than $0.5 \times 10^9$/L (500/$\mu$L) with fever should be regarded as septic until proven otherwise.

**Leukocytosis.** Leukocytosis occurs as a result of stress in a variety of disorders, among which an underlying acute infection always needs to be excluded.

**Eosinophilia.** Allergic disorders, drug reactions, skin disorders such as eczema, or parasitic infestation are associated usually with eosinophilia.

Other disorders of neutrophil function may result from abnormalities of chemotaxis, opsonization, phagocytosis, or intracellular bacterial killing capacity. Typical among these is chronic granulomatous disease, which results in life-long abscess and granuloma formation.

# ONCOLOGY

Although pediatric malignancies are relatively rare, they are still the second most common cause of death in children beyond the neonatal period. In approximately 60 percent of all childhood malignancies, a lifetime cure can now be achieved. Table 3-9 gives the most common malignancies in childhood. It should be recognized that the oncological entities of childhood are distinctly different from those seen in the adult population. The therapeutic approaches are not the same, due to the differences in underlying pathology and concerns of short- and long-term toxicity in the growing, developing child.

**Table 3-9.** Relative Frequency of Major Categories of Malignant Neoplasms in U.S. Children under 15 Years of Age

| *Histologic Category* | *% of Total* |
|---|---|
| Leukemia | 30.9 |
| Central nervous system | 18.3 |
| Lymphoma | 13.8 |
| Sympathetic nervous system | 7.8 |
| Soft tissue | 6.2 |
| Kidney | 5.8 |
| Bone | 4.7 |
| Retinoblastoma | 2.5 |
| Gonadal and germ cell | 2.0 |
| Liver | 1.3 |
| Teratoma | 0.4 |
| Miscellaneous | 6.3 |

## Acute Leukemia

Acute lymphoblastic leukemia (ALL) comprises 80 percent of childhood leukemias, acute myeloblastic leukemia (AML) 15 percent, and chronic leukemias 5 percent. The classification of the leukemias is complex and depends on morphologic appearance, immunophenotyping of the leukemic cells with monoclonal antibodies, detection of cytogenetic markers, and gene rearrangement. The presentation may consist of fever and lassitude, symptoms arising from anemia, neutropenia, and thrombocytopenia. In some patients, there may be lymphadenopathy, splenomegaly, and hepatomegaly. Occasionally, there may also be extramedullary invasion, with central nervous system (CNS) or testicular involvement.

Patients with ALL are usually stratified according to prognostic subgroups. The intensity of their chemotherapy depends on whether they are considered to be at a low or high risk. Poor prognostic factors in ALL include a high white blood cell count at diagnosis, age under 1 year, large bulky disease, specific cytogenetic abnormalities, and the speed with which the leukemic cells respond to initial chemotherapy (induction). Induction usually lasts for 28 days and the intention is to eradicate the leukemia from the bone marrow in order to allow normal stem cells to proliferate. Induction therapy is followed by a period of consolidation therapy with treatments to the CNS for prophylaxis against CNS leukemia. This consists of intrathecal medication with or without cranial irradiation. The 5-year disease-free survival rate for childhood ALL is now in excess of 70 percent and is approximately 40 percent for acute nonlymphocytic leukemia (ANL).

## Hodgkin's Lymphoma

Hodgkin's lymphoma in childhood has a similar presentation to that generally seen in adults. Cervical node enlargement is the most common presentation. Mediastinal adenopathy may cause a superior vena cava syndrome. Pulmonary disease, with or without pleural effusion, may occur in advanced stage IV disease. Treatment is based on clinical staging and may utilize radiotherapy alone or chemotherapy alone; in an advanced stage, a combination of both therapies is used. The trend is to try to minimize therapy to avoid long-term side effects. There is a move away from doing staging laparotomies in children, because of the risk of sepsis following splenectomy. Staging laparotomy may, however, alter the clinical stage of Hodgkin's disease in up to one-third of patients. Currently, 80 percent of children will achieve long-term disease-free survival.

## Non-Hodgkin's Lymphoma

There are several morphologic and immunologic classifications of non-Hodgkin's lymphoma, but for therapeutic purposes in children, they are simply divided into lymphoblastic and nonlymphoblastic varieties. The presenting symptoms depend on the location of the tumor, which may involve an isolated node group, regional disease, or disseminated disease. One-quarter of patients, usually with the lymphoblastic variety, present with mediastinal involvement and may have dyspnea and superior vena cava syndrome. One-third of patients have an abdominal presentation. Intussusception over the age of 6 years is frequently caused by a lymphoma. Aggressive chemotherapy is needed to eradicate the tumor often combined with localized irradiation to the site of bulky tumor. An important complication in the initial chemotherapy may be the tumor lysis syndrome with severe electrolyte imbalance and renal failure. Overall prognosis ranges from 40 to 70 percent long-term survival, depending on the underlying histology and disease stage.

## CNS Tumors

The CNS is the second most common site of malignant tumors in childhood. Two-thirds of CNS tumors manifest as infratentorial tumors, with signs of raised intracranial pressure. They may present as a surgical emergency necessitating early shunt procedure. The most common tumors seen are astrocytoma, medulloblastoma, and ependymoma. Spinal tumors present with localized back pain and/or associated muscle weakness, depending on the level of the lesion. Surgery remains the most important modality of therapy, along with radiotherapy for high-grade tumors. Adjuvant chemotherapy is being used more frequently, especially for medulloblastomas that have been incompletely resected.

## Neuroblastoma

Neuroblastoma arises from neural crest tissue. The most common primary is in the abdomen, with the tumor arising from the adrenal medulla. However, tumor may occur anywhere along the sympathetic chain. This tumor commonly presents under the age of 4 years. Occasionally, spontaneous maturation and involution of the tumor does occur, especially under the age of 1 year. Prognosis is related to age and stage of disease. Recently, the presence of biologic markers such as N-*myc* oncogene and its amplification within tumor cells has been recognized as a poor prognostic factor. Treatment is related to prognostic classification: stages I and II tumors require surgery alone, and stage III and IV surgery and chemotherapy with radiotherapy for unresectable residual tumors. Bone marrow transplantation rescue following high-dose chemotherapy, both autologous and allogeneic, is more frequently being used for this tumor. Children under 1 year old presenting with extensive metastasis to the liver, subcutaneous nodules, with or without bone marrow involvement, but no bony involvement are designated stage IV S. These infants may have considerable mechanical ventilation problems due to the excessive size of their liver, but if they can be managed through this complication, they generally have a good prognosis, as the tumor may involute. The neuroblastoma dumbbell tumor in a paraspinal location may present with neurological signs and weakness of the lower extremities. Prognosis is extremely good for the child under the age of 1 year, if there is no N-*myc* amplification, and over 80 percent of patients recover. Patients over 2 years of age generally have stage IV disease and have a very poor prognosis, with less than 20 percent survival.

## Wilms Tumor

Wilms tumor, or nephroblastoma, is a distinct pediatric entity. There is a relationship with other congenital anomalies such as hemihypertrophy, Beckwith-Wiedemann syndrome, genitourinary anomalies, and congenital aniridia. The Wilms tumor gene has been located on chromosome 11. This tumor is one of the treatment success stories, with over 80 percent of patients cured. Treatment consists of surgical resection of the tumor mass followed by adjuvant chemotherapy. Radiotherapy to the tumor bed is utilized in advanced stages.

## Rhabdomyosarcoma

Rhabdomyosarcoma, a soft tumor, arises from cells of mesenchymal origin. The most common primary occurs in the head and neck, followed by genitourinary and intra-abdominal sites. Extremity and trunk lesions have a poorer prognosis, being associated with the alveolar histologic subtype. Wide excision of the primary tumor is the initial treatment of choice. However, mutilating surgery can be avoided since this tumor may respond to initial chemotherapy and radiotherapy; the tumor can be shrunk in this way and excessive surgery such as a pelvic exenteration can be avoided. Prognosis depends on stage, histologic subvariety, and primary tumor site. The 5-year disease-free survival rate is between 40 and 85 percent.

## Malignant Bone Tumors

### Osteosarcoma

Osteosarcoma occurs with greatest frequency in the adolescent and young adult age group. The most common sites are the distal femur, proximal humerus, and proximal tibia. At presentation there is local pain and swelling. The current approach to therapy consists of diagnostic confirmation by surgical biopsy followed by preoperative chemotherapy to assess the in vivo sensitivity of the tumor to the chemotherapy utilized. Definitive surgery is then undertaken and the degree of necrosis is evaluated to assess whether there is chemotherapy sensitivity or not. Surgery may involve amputation, but limb-sparing surgery is advocated when it does not compromise adequate removal of the tumor. Postoperative adjuvant chemotherapy is then continued, either with the agents utilized presurgery if these were effective, or alternate agents, if there is inadequate tumor necrosis. Overall survival is 55 to 70 percent. Patients with metastatic disease have a significantly worse prognosis.

## Ewing's Sarcoma

Ewing's sarcoma is a small, round-cell tumor. Occasionally, there can be difficulty in differentiating it from the other small, round, blue cell tumors of childhood (i.e., lymphoma, rhabdomyosarcoma, and neuroblastoma). A definitive cytogenic marker is present in Ewing's sarcoma with a translocation between chromosomes 11 and 22. Although this tumor arises in the long bones, it is less frequent than osteogenic sarcoma, and any bone in the body can be affected. Pelvic involvement occurs in approximately one-quarter of patients.

If the removal of the affected bone does not result in a functional deficit, surgery is undertaken. However, Ewing's sarcoma is a radiosensitive tumor and local control can be achieved using this therapeutic modality. Adjuvant chemotherapy is essential, with an overall prognosis of 55 to 75 percent. Patients with metastatic disease have a very poor prognosis.

## Hepatic Tumors

Hepatic tumors are rare in childhood and are subdivided into hepatoblastoma, a tumor of young children, and hepatocellular carcinoma, similar to that seen in adults, which occurs generally in older children. Hepatoblastoma may be associated with other congenital anomalies such as hemihypertrophy and polyposis coli. Hepatocellular carcinoma is frequently associated with hepatitis B virus and occasionally with underlying metabolic disorders such as hereditary tyrosinemia. Complete surgical excision is necessary to achieve a cure. Preoperative chemotherapy is utilized in an attempt to shrink tumors that are initially thought to be nonresectable. Cure is dependent on whether complete resection is eventually attained.

## Complications of Disease or Therapy

Complications may occur because of the tumor itself or as a result of the therapy.

### Mediastinal Mass

A mass may cause airway obstruction and/or superior vena cava (SVC) syndrome. This condition is most commonly associated with anterior mediastinal masses such as these that occur with Hodgkin's disease, non-Hodgkin's lymphoma, or teratoma. Neuroblastoma usually presents as a posterior mediastinal mass. Airway compression may cause dyspnea, especially in the supine position. Ventilation may be sufficiently compromised to necessitate intubation or tracheostomy. The mediastinal mass can occasionally result in the collapse of the trachea, which must be regarded as a medical oncology emergency. Tissue diagnosis is desirable prior to starting therapy, but in an extreme emergency, high-dose steroids should be commenced if there is a strong suspicion of non-Hodgkin's lymphoma. Emergency radiotherapy may also be necessary.

Obstruction of the SVC presenting with headache, neck pain, venous distention, dyspnea, and cardiovascular collapse may also occur.

## Spinal Cord Compression

Compression may be seen in patients with primary or metastatic spinal tumors or paraspinal neuroblastoma. These tumors typically present as back pain that is maximal at the point of compression. Weakness and/or sensory changes in legs, or disorders of bladder or bowel functions may also occur. Emergency laminectomy or laminotomy may be necessary to relieve the symptoms. Some patients may have a rapid response to both radiotherapy and/or chemotherapy.

## Acute Tumor Lysis Syndrome

Acute tumor lysis syndrome occurs in children with leukemia or non-Hodgkin's lymphoma following the institution of chemotherapy. Hyperuricemia results from increased cell breakdown, with subsequent hyperkalemia, hyperphosphatemia, hypocalcemia, and renal failure. These abnormalities can result in tetany and cardiac arrythmia.

This disorder can be prevented by adequate hydration and urinary alkalization. Diuresis is important and mannitol and/or furosemide should be given if urine output drops. Allopurinol should be administered prior to the start of chemotherapy. Hypophosphatemia should be treated with oral aluminum hydroxide. In the presence of hyperkalemia, all exogenous potassium should be omitted. Kayexalate may be necessary as a retention enema. If the patient continues to have increasing renal failure, hemodialysis may be indicated. These patients are obviously at high risk for anesthesia. It is therefore desirable to stabilize their metabolic imbalance prior to anesthesia, whenever possible.

## Syndrome of Inappropriate Antidiuretic Hormone Secretion

Syndrome of inappropriate antidiuretic hormone secretion (SIADH) may occur secondary to the malignancy itself or following the administration of certain chemotherapy agents. Brain tumors or metabolic tumors involving the CNS may present with fluid retention. Vincristine has a specific central antidiuretic hormone (ADH) effect, which may be exacerbated if there is concurrent sepsis. Cyclophosphamide produces similar complications, but its action is on the renal tubule, not central. Fluid retention may be of sufficient severity that the patient has seizures and becomes comatose. The initial treatment should be fluid restriction.

## Hepatic Toxicity

It is important to distinguish toxicity caused by chemotherapy agents from toxicity caused by infections such as viral hepatitis, cytomegalovirus (CMV) or Epstein-Barr virus (EBV) infections. Many drugs are metabolized by the liver. Drugs associated with significant hepatotoxicity include L-asparaginase, 6-MP, methotrexate, BCNU, CCNU, anthracyclines, and actinomycin D.

## Pulmonary Toxicity

Ventilation may be compromised by compression of the airways, a mediastinal mass, widespread parenchymal metastatic disease, or a malignant pleural effusion. Chemotherapy agents such as bleomycin, methotrexate, busulfan, and CCNU may cause pulmonary fibrosis. This drug toxicity may be enhanced by additional external radiation. Radiation therapy alone may cause extensive pulmonary damage when used in high doses. Patients who have received bleomycin should be identified prior to anesthesia, as high concentrations of inhaled oxygen are thought to cause increased fibrosis.

## Cardiac Complications

Encasement of the heart by tumor may result in pericardial tamponade. Pericardial involvement with effusion is often seen in non-Hodgkin's lymphoma of the mediastinum.

The anthracycline group of drugs (consisting of doxorubicin, daunorubicin, epirubicin, and idarubicin) can cause both acute and long-term toxic effects on the heart. There is generally a cumulative dose association before the clinical manifestations become apparent. Cardiotoxicity is most frequently seen when dosages greater than 450 $mg/m^2$ are utilized, and especially if there has been any previous chest irradiation that has included the heart. Patients who have had high-dose anthracyclines prior to anesthesia should be assessed preoperatively by echocardiogram. Patients who are septic and have a decreased cardiac reserve due to previous anthracyclines are more prone to go into congestive failure and frequently become refractory to inotropic support.

## Urinary Tract Complications

Tumor lysis syndrome and metabolic abnormalities have been described above. Drugs that are also associated with urinary tract complications are described below.

**Methotrexate.** High-dose methotrexate used in osteogenic sarcomas may result in renal failure if adequate hydration and alkalization are not utilized appropriately. Monitoring of methotrexate levels and utilization of folinic acid as a rescue is essential when high-dose methotrexate is administered.

**Cisplatinum.** Cisplatinum causes both glomerular and tubular dysfunction. Long-term damage occurs, especially if high doses have been given. This drug is administered with increased intravenous hydration and mannitol diuresis. Hypomagnesemia is a frequent complication, and magnesium supplementation is almost always required. Hypocalcemia may also occur.

**Cyclophosphamide.** Hemorrhagic cystitis occurs due to the effect of the metabolic breakdown product of cyclophosphamide on the bladder mucosa. This complication can be prevented with adequate hydration and frequent urination. Mesna is a drug currently used to detoxify acrolein, the incriminating byproduct of cyclophosphamide that is thought to cause hemorrhagic cystitis.

**Ifosphamide.** Ifosphamide causes complications similar to those of cyclophosphamide.

## Infection

Pediatric patients with malignancy are immunocompromised because of the underlying disorder and, more specifically, because of the antineoplastic therapy administered. Fever should be considered infection until it is proved otherwise. Patients with a neutrophil count of less than $1 \times 10^9/L$ (1,000/μl) should be evaluated for possible sepsis and commenced on broad-spectrum antibiotics.

The increased use of central lines has heightened the risk of systemic infections. Patients who do not respond to initial antibiotics and have persistent fever must be considered to be at risk of having opportunistic infections. Patients who have been on prolonged antibiotic use may have an underlying fungal infection, which is frequently difficult to document by standard culture techniques. *Pneumocystis carinii* usually presents with a dry cough and a slowly increasing respiratory rate. Many centers utilize trimethoprim prophylaxis to diminish the frequency of this infection. Interstitial pneumonia may be caused by viral infections, of which CMV is the most frequently documented.

### Other Complications

Due to both the underlying cancer, as well as the debilitating effects of therapy, nutritional deprivation is frequently encountered. Prolonged calorie protein deprivation may necessitate nasogastric feeding or total parenteral nutrition (TPN). TPN may result in its own complications with lipid disturbance and hepatic dysfunction. Vitamin K depletion should be considered if there has been prolonged malnutrition and concurrent antibiotic usage.

Coagulation abnormalities may be encountered through complications of the disease or of the therapy. Promyelocytic leukemia patients may develop DIC at the commencement of therapy. Impairment of procoagulants and anticoagulants by L-asparaginase may result in both a bleeding tendency and hypercoagulability. Thrombocytopenia is frequently encountered due to marrow suppression from chemotherapy agents.

Nausea and vomiting are common, with severity dependent on the nature of the underlying agent. Highly emetic agents include cisplatinum, cyclophosphamide, cytosine arabinoside, and methotrexate.

Mucositis and esophagitis occur with Adriamycin, actinomycin D, melphalan and high-dose methotrexate. Damage to the mucosal barriers can result in an increased frequency of infection. Patients with poor dental hygiene are more prone to mucosal damage, and neutropenia may exacerbate mouth ulcers. Patients are encouraged to maintain strict mouth hygiene. Local oral symptoms may be treated with sodium bicarbonate or 0.1 percent chlorhexidine. Mucous membrane damage may be exacerbated at the time of intubation, and this may cause local and systemic infections.

## Bone Marrow Transplantation

Bone marrow transplantation is utilized to restore a normal bone marrow population. It is undertaken in congenital or acquired causes of bone marrow aplasia or following high-dose chemotherapy for obliteration of an underlying malignancy. More recent indications include hereditary disorders such as thalassemia or metabolic disorders. In the latter instance, replacement of abnormal stem cells with normal stem cells results in the production of a missing metabolic enzyme. Syngeneic transplantation is a bone marrow transplantation from an identical twin; an allogeneic transplantation is that from a matched HLA donor; an autologous transplant is reinfusion of the patient's own previously harvested marrow.

The procedure of bone marrow transplantation consists of a preparative regime of chemotherapy of varying intensity with or without total body irradiation. The purpose of the preparative regimen is to immunosuppress the patient to receive the new marrow and to eradicate existing bone marrow that may contain a malignant clone of cells or abnormally functioning cells. This is followed by the intravenous infusion of the donated marrow.

### Complications

Complications of bone marrow transplantation may be severe and are as follows:

**Specific Complications.** Specific complications of preparative chemotherapy and/or radiation include renal failure following cisplatinum, severe mucositis, veno-occlusive disease, and cardiac failure.

**Graft Rejection.** Rejection usually occurs because the patient may not have received sufficient immunosuppression to accept the graft, or an inadequate number of stem cells have been administered.

**Infection.** In the early post-bone marrow transplant period, bacterial infection is the major concern. As the bone marrow recovers, viral infection becomes significant and of particular concern is primary or reactivated CMV infection. Patients on long-term immunosuppressive therapy and/or antibiotics are also at risk of severe systemic fungal and other opportunistic infections.

**Bleeding.** Until the bone marrow recovers, the patient is thrombocytopenic. There may be GI bleeding associated with thrombocytopenia. Platelet support is essential during early recovery. Hepatic dysfunction may cause coagulation abnormalities.

**Graft Versus Host Disease.** Acute graft versus host disease (GVHD) accounts for most of the morbidity and mortality associated with allogeneic bone marrow transplant. T cells from the donor attack the recipient cells; symptoms are skin rash, liver abnormalities of rising bilirubin and liver enzymes, and gastrointestinal (GI) symptoms, typically with a profuse mucousy diarrhea. GVHD is graded by severity according to the degree of skin, hepatic, and intestinal tract involvement. It generally occurs only in allogeneic transplantation, but it has occasionally been reported in other immunocompromised patients due to incompatible lymphocytes transfused with blood products. Chronic GVHD occurs after the patient is 100 days post-bone marrow transplant as a multisystem syndrome. Manifestations include esophagitis, skin changes, hepatitis, joint stiffness, chronic intestinal disorders, sicca syndrome, and other symptoms and signs similar to chronic collagen vascular disorders. After allogeneic transplantation, patients receive prophylaxis against GVHD utilizing methotrexate and/or cyclosporine as immunosuppressant agents. In an attempt to prevent GVHD, some centers remove the T cells by monoclonal antibody purging from the donor marrow prior to bone marrow transplantation. All cellular blood products must be irradiated before administration to a bone marrow transplant patient to ensure that lymphocytes present in the product are inactivated.

## TRANSFUSION MEDICINE

### Blood Product Collection, Preparation, and Testing

Blood donations are usually collected by a regional transfusion center, although in larger hospitals, in-house donor collections may be performed. Blood donors should be healthy adults. For first-time donors, the age limits are 16 to 61 years; for established donors the age limits are 17 to 71 years. Donors are required to complete a questionnaire regarding their physical well-being, and, in most centers, are also required to complete a confidential exclusion or self-designation form. This form allows those donors who may in the past have engaged in high-risk sexual activities to exclude themselves from the donor pool and ensures that their blood is used for research purposes only. Using strict asepsis, the donations are collected from an antecubital vein into sealed plastic packs. The donors are required to rest after the collection of the 450 to 500 ml donation, and fluid replacement in the form of liquid refreshment is given. The donations are handled very carefully, because of the danger of damage to plastic bags and are usually stored at 4°C until further processing can be performed. All blood donations are ABO and Rh grouped, and the donor's serum is screened for the presence of atypical red cell antibodies. Infectious disease marker screening is performed, consisting of serologic testing for syphilis, hepatitis B antigen, and antibodies to human immunodeficiency virus (HIV)-1/2, hepatitis C, and human T-cell lymphotrophic virus (HTLV)-1. In centers providing large volumes of blood for pediatric and neonatal units, a significant number of the donors are also subjected to serological testing for CMV antibodies to provide anti-CMV nonreactive units for infusion to premature neonates. Only those units that have proved negative in the syphilis, hepatitis, and retroviral screening can be released from the center. Since blood is an excellent bacterial culture medium, blood and blood products must be handled with great care and with manipulations performed by trained staff under controlled conditions. Packs of red blood cells that have remained at room temperature for 30 minutes must be returned to a properly controlled blood bank refrigerator, if infusion has not started. Particular care should be taken when leaving red blood cells at room temperature for long periods of time in a warm operating room. Domestic refrigerators, which are often used on nursing stations and in operating rooms for the storage of medications, must *not* be used for the storage of blood and blood products.

## Immunohematologic Testing

The basic test in immunohematology is the agglutination test. Hemagglutination is the process by which immunoglobulin molecules link adjacent erythrocytes when these cells carry antigens corresponding to the serological activity of the antibody. The larger immunoglobulin molecules, IgM, are capable of causing agglutination of red blood cells in a saline medium, and are often called saline antibodies. These antibodies always fix complement. IgM antibodies are the first to form following an antigenic challenge, and many of the cold, red blood cell alloantibodies of dubious clinical significance, such as anti-$P_1$, anti-M, anti-N, and anti-Lewis antibodies belong to this category. Smaller immunoglobulin molecules, IgG, are usually not capable of causing red blood cell agglutination in a saline medium, because they are not capable of spanning the distance between two adjacent red blood cells. IgG antibodies form as a secondary response to an antigenic challenge, and may or may not fix complement. The IgG blood group antibodies always form in response to some clear antigenic challenge, such as an injection or infusion of blood or a blood product, or pregnancy. This class of antibody may cause severe hemolytic transfusion reaction, and may also cause alloimmune hemolytic disease in the newborn. It is critical, therefore, that this type of antibody be detected in a patient's serum, but because some of the antibodies do not act in a saline medium, some type of enhancement is necessary to facilitate antibody detection. Common enhancement techniques include the use of albumin or the use of an antiglobulin bridge to link and agglutinate adjacent IgG-coated cells. This immunoglobulin "bridge" is usually an antihuman immunoglobulin raised in another species. This procedure, which traditionally has been called the Coombs test, should be more correctly named the antiglobulin test.

**Direct Antiglobulin Test.** When an antiglobulin reagent is added directly to red blood cells that have been well washed in saline, and a positive result occurs, the patient is said to have a positive direct antiglobulin (Coombs) test (DAT). Such a positive DAT occurs during hemolytic transfusion reactions, in autoimmune hemolytic anemia, alloimmune hemolytic disease of the newborn, or as an immune complication of drug therapy.

**Indirect Antiglobulin Test.** The indirect antiglobulin test (IAT), or indirect Coombs test, is performed by mixing the patient's serum with screening red cells. These screening cells are chosen because they express, in significant dosage, the major red cell antigen systems. After incubation, the screening cells are washed to remove unbound immunoglobulin and the antiglobulin reagent is added. If hemagglutination occurs, the patient's serum is said to have a positive IAT test. This positive result implies the presence of atypical antibodies in the patient's serum. In this way, the technologist and transfusion medicine physician are alerted to the presence of atypical red cell antibodies, and further investigation to identify the nature of the antibodies is required. The IAT is central to the type and screen and the red cell crossmatch.

### Type and Screen

In order to avoid the needless crossmatch of large volumes of blood for surgical procedures that only rarely require red blood cell transfusion, most hospital blood banks operate a type and screen policy. When a type and screen is ordered, the patient is ABO and rhesus grouped and the serum is subjected to an IAT. If no atypical antibodies are found, then no further action is needed. If unexpected surgical complications occur and excessive bleeding results at the time of surgery, then the infusion of group-specific unmatched red blood cells is considered to be a safe and acceptable practice. If, during a type and screen, an atypical red blood cell antibody is detected, this antibody must be identified and appropriately grouped antigen negative units must be available before surgery can proceed safely.

### Maximal Surgical Blood-Ordering Schedule

Many hospitals, in addition to type and screen, operate a maximal surgical blood-ordering schedule system. Such a system designates a maximum order for a specific surgical procedure (e.g., 3 U of blood may be ordered for correction of a tetralogy of Fallot in a 2-year-old child). This system obviates overordering by residents, interns, and medical students for complicated surgeries and ensures the anesthetist and surgeon sufficient blood for the time of surgery. In order for such a system to work, it is essential that the schedules be agreeable to the surgeon, anesthetist, and transfusion medicine physician.

## Blood Products

### Whole Blood

Whole blood is not generally available since almost all blood donations now have the plasma removed for further processing and fractionation. The indications for whole blood infusion are few, but include exchange transfusion for hemolytic disease of the newborn. For clinical use, whole blood is usually reconstituted from red blood cell concentrate and frozen plasma.

### Red Blood Cells

**Red Blood Cell Concentrate.** Red blood cell concentrate, also called packed red blood cells, is the main form of red blood cell product available from a hospital blood bank. A unit contains approximately 200 ml of red blood cells with a hematocrit of 0.75. Red blood cell concentrate can be used whenever red blood cell infusion is required and has the advantage of reduced risk of circulatory overload, reduced transfusion reactions to donor antibodies or plasma components, and reduced infusion of anticoagulant and electrolyte. The drawback to infusing red blood cell concentrate is its viscosity, which interferes with flow rate. This is often troublesome for anesthetists, and is best corrected by using a Y-recipient set and infusing saline along with red blood cells. Red blood cell concentrate should be filtered through a standard blood infusion filter with a nominal pore size of 170 μm. Red blood cell concentrate should be stored at 4°C and has a shelf life, using CPDA-1, the commonly used anticoagulant in North America, of 35 days.

**Leukocyte-Poor Red Blood Cells.** Leukocyte-poor red blood cells are required when patients have had repeated severe febrile reactions directed against the leukocytes, which are inevitably present in a red blood cell concentrate. Such reactions typically occur in massively transfused patients, such as those with hemoglobinopathy, who require frequent red blood cell infusion. Various methods can be used to remove the leukocytes, including washing, which can either be done manually or using an automated instrument. The drawback to washing is that inevitably there is a loss of red blood cells and it is difficult, even with automated instrumentation, to remove more than 85 percent of the leukocytes. Various filtration techniques can be used, and the most efficient of the filters removes 99.9 percent of leukocytes. Such filters are, however, very expensive and should not be used for all patients, but should be reserved for specially selected patients in whom the use of leukocyte blood is critical. Such patients would include patients with life-long transfusion requirements, and patients in whom the infusion of leukocytes will speed up the appearance of alloantibodies against HLA and platelet antigens. These alloantibodies seriously affect the utilization of and response to random donor platelet products. This latter group of patients includes those with AML, and aplastic anemia, as well as bone marrow transplant candidates and recipients.

**Frozen Red Blood Cells.** Red blood cells can be frozen in a mechanical freezer using glycerol as a cryoprotectant. This process is very expensive and should be reserved for the storage of red blood cell units of very unusual phenotype or for autotransfusion to patients with multiple red blood cell antibodies. Reconstituted frozen blood can also be used as a means of providing deleukocyted blood for patients with high-titer HLA antibodies who are having unpleasant febrile reactions. However, the use of modern-day filters is now preferred for these patients. Frozen red blood cells can be stored for many years at −70°C but require deglycerolization prior to infusion; consequently they are not immediately available for the patient.

## Platelet Infusion

Platelet infusions are required for the prevention and treatment of thrombocytopenic bleeding, particularly in the amegakaryocytic patient. They are used extensively for the support of patients with oncologic and hematologic disorders. Platelets should not be used other than in very rare and special circumstances for patients with destructive thrombocytopenia, such as immune thrombocytopenia, drug-induced immune thrombocytopenia, hemolytic uremic syndrome, and thrombotic thrombocytopenic purpura. Platelet infusion may also be occasionally required to treat hemorrhage complications in patients with disorders of platelet function, although they are not thrombocytopenic. The decision to infuse platelets must be taken in conjunction with a hematologist or transfusion medicine physician, and is contingent on the platelet count, the diagnosis, and the specific clinical situation. The infusion of 1 U of platelets will usually cause a platelet increment of 35 to 50 $\times$ $10^9$/L/10 kg of body weight, and this formula should be used in calculating the dosage required. When platelets are infused, it is very important that the platelet count be checked either immediately or 1 hour after the infusion has been completed to determine the increment in platelet count. By following platelet count increments, the hematologist can usually determine when a patient is becoming refractory to random donor platelets.

Platelets are typically available as a platelet concentrate that contains more than 60 $\times$ $10^9$/L (> 60,000/µl) platelets in a volume of approximately 50 ml of plasma. Platelets should be infused through a standard-infusion filter. The various types of microaggregate filters are best avoided for platelet infusion, because these may retain platelets and diminish clinical efficacy. However, special deleukocyting filters are available for platelet concentrate. These decrease the rate of sensitization to random donor platelets, but are very expensive and should be reserved for specific clinical indications.

**Random Donor Platelets.** Random donor platelets are collected from 1 random donor unit of whole blood. The unit is centrifuged, and a platelet-rich plasma is transferred to a satellite pack. This platelet-rich plasma is centrifuged, and the supernatant plasma is transferred to a third pack for further processing, leaving the platelet concentrate behind. Random donor platelet concentrate should be stored at room temperature, ideally at 22°C, and subjected to constant agitation to prevent damage to the platelets, which impairs platelet function. Random donor platelet concentrate has a shelf-life of 3 or 5 days, depending on the type of donor pack that is used.

**Single Donor Platelet Concentrate.** Single donor platelet concentrate is collected by thrombocytapheresis from a single donor. This product is reserved for those patients who become refractory to random donor platelets and is used almost exclusively for patients with oncologic and hematologic disease. These products are only available following a consultation with a hematologist or transfusion medicine physician.

## Plasma

Various types of plasma products were traditionally available: stored, frozen, and fresh frozen; because of concerns regarding the accumulation of plasticizer derived from the plastic pack used for storing the liquid plasma, only fresh frozen and frozen plasma are currently available. Plasma can be used for plasma volume expansion when other products are not available or for infusion of multiple clotting factors, typically in a patient with DIC. Such use is suboptimal, however. Concentrated coagulation factor preparations are available for the treatment of coagulation factor deficiencies. Plasma can also be used for replacement during plasmapheresis, as well as to reconstitute whole blood from red cell concentrate for exchange transfusion.

Plasma is stored frozen at −30°C for up to 12 months, and should be thawed at 37°C immediately before use. Liquid plasma that has not been used within 24 hours should be returned to the transfusion center. Plasma inevitably contains red blood cell fragments that can sensitize the recipient to red blood cell antigens. Rh-negative girls and women of child-bearing age must therefore always receive plasma that has been collected from Rh-negative individuals. If plasma from Rh-negative donors is not available and a patient within this group requires plasma, plasma from donors of any Rh type may be given, provided that Rh immunoglobulin (anti-D) prophylaxis is given at the same time.

## Cryoprecipitate

Cryoprecipitate is prepared from frozen plasma that has been thawed. Plasma thaws under standardized conditions, and fibrinogen and factor VIII remains as a cold insoluble precipitate that can be separated from the rest of the plasma by centrifugation. This cryoprecipitate has a small volume, 5 to 10 ml, and contains significant amounts of factor VIII and fibrinogen from a single-donor unit. Cryoprecipitate is stored at −30°C for up to 12 months and is used for treating mild cases of hemophilia or von Willebrand's disease, or for replacement of fibrinogen and factor VIII in patients with DIC and as a means of replacing fibrinogen in patients with acquired or congenital fibrinogen deficiency. The dose of cryoprecipitate varies with the patient's clinical condition and weight, and dosage should be calculated in conjunction with a hematologist or transfusion medicine physician.

## Anti-CMV Nonreactive Products

Cellular products that have been shown to be nonreactive for anti-CMV should be used only in special clinical circumstances. Since approximately 50 percent of donor blood is CMV seropositive, these products are in short supply and must be reserved only for specific patient groups. Appropriate indications include bone marrow transplant recipients, anti-CMV nonreactive neonates of less than 1,500 g body weight, and anti-CMV nonreactive pregnant women in the second trimester of pregnancy. A case can also be made for the infusion of anti-CMV nonreactive cellular products to CMV-seronegative patients with various oncologic disorders, such as AML, high-risk ALL, and those who have a significant risk of progressing to allogeneic bone marrow transplantation.

## Fractionated Products

By collecting large volumes of plasma that are then subjected to Cohn (cold ethanol) fractionation, various concentrated blood protein fractions can be achieved. The disadvantage of fractionated products is that one contaminated donor may infect an entire pool with an infectious agent. Not all fractionated products, however, can transmit infectious agents. Albumin is pasteurized and does not transmit hepatitis or HIV infection. Gammaglobulin, similarly, has not been shown to transmit viral infection. Viral transmission is a particular risk with clotting factor concentrates, and large numbers of hemophiliacs have been infected with HIV derived from factor VIII concentrate. Factor concentrates are now subjected to a wet-heat treatment that inactivates the retrovirus.

**Albumin.** Albumin is available in 5 percent and 25 percent preparations; they have a physiologic pH and a sodium concentration of approximately 145 mmol/L. Albumin is used for blood volume expansion, particularly in an emergency situation before crossmatched blood is available, for protein and fluid replacement for patients with burns, and for replacement during plasmapheresis. The 25 percent product draws extravascular fluid into the intravascular space and can promote diuresis in patients with hypoproteinemia. Albumin can be stored for long periods of time at room or refrigerator temperature and should be filtered through a standard-infusion filter.

**Intravenous Gammaglobulin.** An expensive blood product with specific clinical indications, intravenous gammaglobulin may be used for patients with inherited immune deficiency, during the management of acute ITP or Kawasaki's disease, and for CMV prophylaxis at the time of bone marrow transplantation. This product is used experimentally in a large variety of conditions, but because of the expense involved, it should only be used following consultation with an immunologist, hematologist, or transfusion medicine physician.

**Specific Immunoglobulins.** Rh immunoglobulin (anti-D) is collected from Rh-negative females who have been immunized to the Rh (D) antigen. It is used in the prophylaxis of Rh sensitization during and after pregnancy and to prevent sensitization to the Rh antigen during inadvertent or unavoidable infusion of Rh-positive cellular products or plasma to Rh-negative patients. This type of prophylaxis is particularly important in female children and women of childbearing age. The product comes in 120- and 300-μg doses. The 300-μg dose is sufficient to prevent sensitization by 30 ml of Rh-positive cells.

**Other Immunoglobulin Products.** Other specific immunoglobulins are available for the prophylaxis of hepatitis B (HBIg), for varicella zoster (VZIG), and CMV hyperimmune globulin. No doubt in the future other specific immunoglobulin products will also become available.

**Clotting Factor Concentrates.** Factor VIII and factor IX concentrates are both available. Both are high-potency products that in the past have been responsible for transmitting hepatitis and retroviruses to recipients. These products should be reserved for the management of severe bleeding or surgical episodes in patients with hemophilia A or B and must be used in consultation with a hematologist or transfusion medicine physician. They are lyophilized and can be stored at refrigerator temperature for long periods of time. Complications include viral transmission, which has now been significantly minimized by heat treatment and immune hemolysis, since this fraction also contains high-titer anti-A and anti-B isoagglutinins.

## Nonhuman Products

### Products Produced by Recombinant DNA Technology

Recombinant DNA technology has been used to produce factor VIII concentrate and albumin. Factor VIII concentrate is currently undergoing clinical trials, and no other recombinant product is currently available. These products have the advantage of considerable purity and zero risk for transmission of viral disease. They will doubtless be initially very expensive, because the development costs have been considerable.

**Porcine Factor VIII.** In hemophiliacs with antibodies to human factor VIII, the use of nonhuman factor VIII may be clinically beneficial and produce sufficient hemostatic activity to allow surgery and recuperation.

**Growth Factors.** As discussed above, hematopoiesis is controlled by a variety of growth factors. Several of these growth factors can now be produced by recombinant DNA technology and used to manage cytopenias in particular situations. Recombinant human erythropoietin is used to manage the chronic anemia of renal failure and may also have benefits in the management of anemia following chemotherapy and bone marrow transplantation. Trials are under way to examine the usefulness of erythropoietin in the management of the anemia of prematurity. If successful, this strategy will minimize the need for neonatal red blood cell transfusion. Granulocyte-macrophage (GM)-CSF produced by recombinant DNA technology is also being used on an experimental basis in the management of severe neutropenic patients following intensive chemotherapy or bone marrow transplantation. It is likely that in the future this type of therapeutic strategy will become more prevalent and will minimize the need for patients' exposure to blood products.

### Nonhuman Plasma Expanders

Several types of nonhuman plasma expanders have been used clinically, including the following: starch derivatives, particularly hydroxyethyl starch and pentastarch; gelatin derivatives, particularly modified fluid gelatin; and dextran products of varying molecular weight. The advantages of these products are zero risk for transmission of infectious disease, easy availability (particularly in times of natural or other disaster), and a relatively low cost of manufacture. They have been used extensively in Europe with considerable success. Literature describing their use in the pediatric age group is almost nonexistent, and research in this area is required. Complications with these factors include allergic reactions and coagulopathies due to dilution and alteration of clotting factors and platelet function.

### Blood Substitutes

Considerable research is ongoing into the development of satisfactory oxygen-carrying blood substitutes. Various types of fluorocarbon molecules have been tried; however, in general, the oxygen-carrying capacity of these products is not significantly greater than that of plasma.

## Autologous Blood Transfusion

Wherever possible, reinfusion of a patient's own blood is much preferred to infusion of homologous product from a random donor. There are several different approaches to autologous transfusion: predeposit, intraoperative salvage, and preoperative hemodilution and venesection. In some centers, autologous blood transfusion programs for children exist. Predeposit autologous donation can be used very successfully for teenaged patients, but can also be used for children as young as 4 years. The principal use of this type of program is for patients undergoing reconstructive spinal surgery. The same approach has also been used for patients undergoing low-risk cardiac surgery or plastic surgery, typically reduction mammoplasty, and for pediatric bone marrow donors. No untoward effects occur, and the procedure is well accepted by patients and parents. Intraoperative salvage can be used for clean surgeries, typically thoracic surgery. Blood is aspirated by the surgeon and anticoagulated. The salvaged blood can be reinfused, ideally after it has been washed. Various types of commercially available salvage and washing instrumentation exist. Preoperative hemodilution and venesection can also be used for patients undergoing reconstructive spinal surgery. Immediately after induction of anesthesia, the anesthetist infuses a large volume of saline, and simultaneously phlebotomizes the patient from another limb. In this way, 2 to 3 U of blood can be obtained; during surgery as hemorrhage occurs, the units are reinfused in reverse order.

Autologous transfusion programs, although very beneficial, are limited for the most part to elective procedures and to patients who are relatively fit and capable of undergoing a phlebotomy and have no long-term transfusion requirements. As a consequence, autologous transfusion programs are of little benefit for the oncology patient.

## Complications of Transfusion

Many complications of transfusion exist; they can be categorized as immune and nonimmune.

### Immune-Mediated Transfusion Reactions

**Hemolytic Transfusion Reaction.** When red blood cells are infused to a patient whose serum contains an antibody that recognizes a foreign antigen on the infused erythrocytes, a hemolytic transfusion reaction occurs. Lysis of the infused donor cells results. When the hemolysis occurs immediately, as is seen when ABO incompatible blood is infused, there is intravascular hemolysis, which may result in hemoglobinemia and hemoglobinuria. There is also a release of vasoactive products, resulting in shock. Circulating cell debris and immune complexes often trigger the coagulation cascade to produce DIC. The combination of hemoglobinuria, shock, and DIC often produces acute renal failure. In the anesthetized patient, the first sign of an acute hemolytic transfusion reaction may be the DIC, which manifests as oozing from sites at which hemostasis had previously been achieved. Acute hemolytic transfusion reactions typically occur from infusion of ABO incompatible blood. This is a rare event and usually follows a clerical error either in the transfusion laboratory or the clinical setting at the time the blood product is infused.

In patients in whom the infusion of foreign red blood cells stimulates an anamnestic antibody response, the production of IgG antibodies directed against the donor red blood cells results in a less aggressive extravascular destruction of donor red blood cells. This phenomenon, the delayed hemolytic transfusion reaction, classically presents as unexpected anemia and jaundice several days following a transfusion in an otherwise well patient. Very rarely, the delayed hemolytic transfusion reaction can be accompanied by renal failure.

Investigators of a hemolytic transfusion reaction include DAT on the patient and a review of all clerical, laboratory, and nursing data regarding the identity of the crossmatched sample, the blood product, and the patient, together with an antibody investigation to detect and identify any atypical red blood cell antibodies.

Hemolytic transfusion reactions can also occur when the red blood cell product has been subjected to thermal stress, as occurs with a faulty blood warmer, or when the blood has been refrigerated inappropriately or inadvertently frozen. Severe hemolytic reactions associated with shock may also occur when bacterially contaminated blood is infused.

*Febrile Reactions.* When a patient who has antibodies to leukocyte antigens receives a blood product (usually red blood cells) containing leukocytes that carry the offending antigen, a febrile reaction is common. The clinical reaction is mild, but consists of fever, without shock, which may be accompanied by rigors. A limited investigation is usually warranted, as this type of reaction can be avoided by infusion of leukocyte-depleted blood (see above).

*Allergic Reactions.* The most common type of immune-mediated transfusion reaction is allergy; its mildest manifestation is urticaria. In its most severe form, urticaria can be associated with bronchospasm and even anaphylactic shock. Allergic reactions occur in patients who are allergic to an allergen present in the infused product. Very occasionally, this type of reaction occurs because an atopic person has given a blood donation and the passively transfused atopic antibody reacts with the corresponding allergen that is present in the patient. This type of reaction is fortunately rare, as patients with a history of severe allergies are unacceptable as blood donors. The most severe types of allergic reactions occur in patients who are IgA deficient. These persons develop antibodies against foreign immunoglobulin A molecules. IgA-related allergic reaction can be very severe and even life threatening. In patients who are IgA deficient, all blood products should be either plasma free, or when plasma products are required, they should be prepared from donations taken from IgA-deficient donors.

## Other Types of Reaction or Complications of Transfusion

Nonimmune transfusion reactions include the transmission of disease and septic shock due to the infusion of blood contaminated with bacteria. Embolism, particle debris, or air or fluid overload may also occur.

Although the risk of transmission of an infectious agent is small, this risk must always be borne in mind when contemplating a transfusion in any patient. This risk is of great importance to parents of sick children, who will invariably raise the matter with the attending and treating physicians. The possibility of infusing a blood product infected with bacteria is remote, but remains a potential problem when infusing platelet concentrate that is stored at 22°C and is often infused to a severely immunosuppressed oncology patient. Of much greater concern, particularly when giving a straightforward infusion of red blood cell concentrate, is the possibility of transmission of a viral agent. The risk of infusing blood that contains infectious HIV particles but is anti-HIV negative is small (calculated at approximately 1/100,000 U). Of much greater concern has been the risk of transmitting viruses that can cause hepatitis, which in turn can cause chronic hepatitis and even cirrhosis. Prior to routine hepatitis C testing of donor units, the risk of transmitting non-A, non-B hepatitis was calculated to be between 1/140 and 1/500 Units. Since the advent of hepatitis C testing, this figure has undoubtedly dropped, but the total elimination of transfusion-associated viral hepatitis remains unlikely until some type of physical or chemical antiviral treatment of blood products is introduced. When considering the risks of disease transmission by blood products, it should always be remembered that the risk increases markedly when using a pooled, fractionated plasma product. Fortunately, most of these products are treated in some way, usually by heat, to eliminate any possible contaminating infectious agents.

## Massive Transfusion

Massive transfusion is defined as the infusion of transfusion fluids with a volume equal to or exceeding the patient's blood volume within a 24-hour period. Massive transfusion typically occurs in the seriously ill, traumatized patient and is accompanied by a variety of specific complications including coagulopathies, citrate toxicity, microembolization, hypothermia, and other metabolic changes. Citrate toxicity occurs because of the infusion of large amounts of citrate. Citrate is an essential ingredient in the anticoagulant mixture used to preserve the donor blood. Hypocalcemia may occur, but only results when very rapid infusions of blood occur. Liver disease and hypothermia can exacerbate the effects of citrate toxicity. Citrate toxicity can be prevented by the infusion of 10 percent calcium gluconate (10 ml/L blood infused). In practice, infusion of too much calcium may cause more problems than citrate toxicity. Calcium gluconate must never be administered through the same line as a blood product, unless it is preceded and followed by a saline flush. Wherever possible, drugs should never be mixed with blood products, but should be infused separately through a different venous access. The recommended solution to mix with red blood cells is normal saline. Five percent dextrose solution and Ringer's lactate must not be infused at the same time as red cells; the best solution to mix with blood may well be a balanced salt solution without added calcium.

Various coagulopathies can complicate massive transfusion. These include thrombocytopenia and reduced levels of all coagulation factors, particularly the labile clotting factors, due to dilution by large amounts of donor blood-depleted platelets and clotting factors. Various "rules of thumb" exist to infuse platelet concentrate and frozen plasma at specific intervals during a massive transfusion episode. If at all possible, these rules should be avoided, and if the hematology laboratory is capable of providing rapid turnaround for platelet counts and coagulation tests, then platelets and plasma should be used empirically as and when indicated by laboratory parameters.

The infusion of large amounts of stored blood invariably results in infusion of large amounts of accumulated particulate debris. This debris may be filtered out in the pulmonary capillary bed; to avoid debris, the use of microaggregate filters is advised for the massive transfusion episode, particularly for the patient with impaired pulmonary function.

Since blood is stored at 4°C, rapid infusion of large volumes of stored blood can result in central cooling, but the use of properly regulated and controlled blood warming devices can prevent this complication. It should be remembered that poorly maintained or faulty blood warming devices may result in excessive warming and hemolysis of donor red blood cells, which may cause the patient even greater problems than hypothermia.

Various other metabolic complications may occur in the massive transfusion situation, including altered acid-based balance, typically acidosis, and impaired oxygen release. Acidosis is usually a consequence of impaired tissue perfusion, rather than the infusion of large amounts of acidified, stored blood, and usually corrects itself once adequate tissue perfusion has been restored. Depletion of 2,3-DPG (diphosphoglycerate) in donor erythrocytes in stored blood may interfere with oxygen release by hemoglobin. Levels of 2,3-DPG return to normal within 24 hours of transfusion. Nevertheless, whenever possible, the infusion of large volumes of older, stored blood should be avoided, and in the massive transfusion situation, if at all possible, the bulk of infused red cells should be not more than 7 to 10 days old.

In the massive transfusion situation, the risk for clerical mixup is significantly increased, and particular care must be taken at these times to maintain the clerical records of when and which blood products were infused. Particular vigilance must be exerted in relation to compatibility and identity of the infused blood products. Such care is of even greater importance after major disasters, when multiple massive transfusion incidents may be occurring simultaneously within an emergency department or operating room.

## SUGGESTED READINGS


Bell A: Hematopoiesis. p. 1. In Harmening Pittiglio D, Sacher R (eds): Clinical Hematology and Fundamentals of Hemostasis. FA Davis, Philadelphia, 1987

Boral LI, Henry JB: The type and screen: a safe alternative and supplement in selected surgical procedures. Transfusion 17:163, 1977

Falk JL, Rackow EC, Weil MH: Colloid and crystalloid resuscitation. Acute Care 10:59, 1984

Friedman BA: An analysis of surgical blood use in the United States hospitals with application to the maximum surgical blood order schedule. Transfusion 19:3, 1979

Friedman BA, Oberman MA, Chadwick AR, Kingdon KI: The maximal surgical blood order schedule and surgical blood use in the United States. Transfusion 16:380, 1976

Glassman AB: Anemia, diagnosis and implications. In Harmening Pittiglio D, Sacher R (eds): Clinical Hematology and Fundamentals of Hemostasis. FA Davis, Philadelphia, 1987

Golde DW, Swisher SH, Petz LD: Predicting the future in transfusion medicine. p. 765. In Petz LD, Swisher SN (eds): Clinical Practice of Transfusion Medicine. Churchill Livingstone, New York, 1989

Herst R: Clinical Guide to Transfusion: Products and Practices. Canadian Red Cross Society, Blood Services, Ottawa, 1987

Hoffbrand AV, Lewis SM: Post Graduate Hematology. 3rd Ed. Heinemann, London, 1989

Holland PV: Risks of red cell transfusion: overview and perspective in perioperative red cell transfusion. NIH Consensus Development Conference, Bethesda, June, 1988

Holland PV: The diagnosis and management of transfusion reaction and other adverse effects of transfusion. p. 713. In Petz LD, Swisher SN (eds): Clinical Practice of Transfusion Medicine. Churchill Livingstone, New York, 1989

Horowitz ME, Pizzo PA: Solid tumours in childhood. Pediatr Clin North Am 38:2, 1991

Johnson FL, Pochedly C: Bone Marrow Transplantation in Children. Pediatric Hematology/Oncology Series. Raven Press, New York, 1990

Kahn RA, Allen RW, Baldassare J: Alternate sources and substitute for therapeutic blood components. Blood 66:1, 1985

Lanzkowsky P: Manual of Pediatric Hematology and Oncology. Churchill Livingstone, New York, 1989

Nathan DG, Oski FA: Hematology of Infancy and Childhood. WB Saunders, Philadelphia, 1987

Oberman MA, Barnes BA, Friedman BA: The risk of abbreviating the major crossmatch in urgent or massive transfusion. Transfusion 18:137, 1978

Oski FA: Disorders of erythrocyte production. In Nathan DG, Oski FA (eds): Hematology of Infancy and Childhood. 3rd Ed. WB Saunders, Philadelphia, 1987

Oski FA, Naiman JL: Hematologic Problems in the Newborn. p. 32. WB Saunders, Philadelphia, 1982

Petz LD, Swisher SH: Clinical Practice of Transfusion Medicine. 2nd Ed. Churchill Livingstone, New York, 1989

Pisciotto PT: Blood Transfusion Therapy: A Physician's Handbook. 3rd Ed. American Association of Blood Banks, Arlington, 1989

Pizzo PA, Poplack DG: Principals and Practice of Pediatric Oncology. JB Lippincott, Philadelphia, 1989

Platt OS, Nathan DG. In Nathan DG, Oski FA (eds): Hematology of Infancy and Childhood. 3rd Ed. WB Saunders, Philadelphia, 1987

Silvergleid AJ: Autologous, directed, and home transfusion programs. p. 327. In Petz LD, Swisher SN (eds): Clinical Practice of Transfusion Medicine. Churchill Livingstone, New York, 1989

Walker RH: Technical Manual. 10th Ed. American Association of Blood Banks, Arlington, 1990

Williams WJ, Beutler E, Erslev AJ et al: Hematology. 3rd Ed. McGraw-Hill, New York, 1983

Willoughby MLN: Pediatric Haematology. Churchill Livingstone, Edenburgh, 1977

# 4

# Gastrointestinal Diseases

# 4

# Gastrointestinal Diseases

*Terrance A. Yemen*

Anesthesiologists commonly encounter infants and children with congenital or acquired gastrointestinal disorders. Sometimes these disorders represent the primary indication for surgery. Not infrequently, they are coexisting disorders in pediatric patients requiring surgery for other reasons. An understanding of the natural history of these disorders and their pathophysiology is essential in order to provide appropriate anesthetic care. In this chapter gastrointestinal problems common in the pediatric patient are reviewed to aid in providing that anesthetic care.

## ANOMALIES AND DISEASES OF NEONATES AND YOUNG INFANTS

### Neonatal Necrotizing Enterocolitis

Necrotizing enterocolitis (NEC) is the most common serious gastrointestinal disorder encountered in neonatal intensive care units. It is second only to the respiratory distress syndrome as a cause of neonatal death.

NEC can occur in both premature and full-term infants. However, the incidence is highest among smaller, more immature neonates at very low birth weights (<1,500 g).[1,2] The overall incidence of necrotizing enterocolitis in an neonatal intensive care unit varies between 1 and 5 percent of neonates, although it can be as high as 15 percent among very low birth weight infants. Some estimates put the number of infants who develop NEC at approximately 2,000 to 4,000 patients per year in America.

Kliegman[3] has referred to NEC as a disease of survivors; approximately 60 percent of patients with the disease have a prior history of respiratory distress syndrome. He speculates that with the introduction of multiple dose surfactant prevention, and rescue surfactant therapy, one can anticipate an increase in very low birth weight infant survival, and therefore more infants at risk of NEC.

The pathogenesis of NEC is not fully understood, but predisposing variables have been identified, including, intestinal ischemia, infectious agents, and neonatal feeding practices. It is probable that multiple factors are responsible, and although one variable may initiate the process, a second or third may accelerate or maintain it.

Particular interest has been focused on mesenteric blood flow. An association has been documented between patent ductus arteriosus, neonates with symptomatic congenital heart disease, and the development of NEC.[4,5] Doppler-determined reductions of diastolic blood flow in the fetal aorta have also been associated with the subsequent development of NEC.[6] However, neonatal ischemic bowel injuries caused by acute asphyxia, respiratory distress syndrome, or umbilical vessel catheterization have not been consistently associated with NEC.

The local effects of bacterial toxins are implicated as initiators in the early stages of bowel injury leading to NEC.[7] Bacteria and viruses have been recovered from patients with NEC, but no consistent pathogen has been found.[8]

Of affected infants, 90 to 95 percent have been fed a commercial formula.[9,10] Infant formula may serve both as a substrate for bacteria proliferation and, in addition, may induce intestinal mucosal injury as a result of high osmolality. The rates and volumes of formula feeding have been investigated as etiologic factors. Anderson and Kliegman[11] have recently proposed that rapid advancement of enteral feeding and excessive volume may predispose premature infants to development of NEC and should be discouraged.

Feeding as a risk factor has also been studied by examining the vascular responses of infants. Term neonates have been shown to respond to enteral feeding by decreasing blood flow to peripheral regions and increasing mesenteric blood flow. Preterm infants demonstrate no significant change in regional blood flow during feeding. This may suggest that premature infants have poor intestinal autoregulation with no increase of intestinal blood flow during feeding. Imbalances among mucosal blood flow, oxygen extraction, and nutrient absorption could thereby result in a mucosal ischemia.[12] It is interesting to note that bacteria isolated from patients with NEC do not produce hydrogen gas unless infant formula is added to the incubation mixture. In patients with NEC, hydrogen gas found in the bowel wall of affected patients is pathognomonic of the disease (pneumatosis intestinalis).

NEC can vary widely in its severity and rate of progression. It can manifest as a relatively benign gastrointestinal (GI) disturbance or have a rapidly fulminating course with intestinal gangrene, perforation, sepsis, shock, and ultimately death.

Typically, the disorder occurs 6 to 10 days after birth and often after the initiating of feeding; abdominal distention is one of the earliest clinical signs. Prematures may also present with bloody stools, apnea, bradycardia, retained gastric contents, lethargy, shock, or temperature instability. Radiologically these infants show evidence of pneumatosis intestinalis, often with evidence of portal or hepatic venous air. Portal vein ultrasonography is more sensitive than radiographs in detecting the presence of portal vein gas, and can potentially lead to earlier diagnosis and therapy.

To allow consistent evaluation of patients, Bell et al.[13] proposed a system of staging. Stage I includes infants with suspected disease or "rule out NEC." Stage II infants have documented NEC with all the nonspecific signs noted in stage I, plus marked abdominal distention and tenderness. Stage II is also characterized by evidence of pneumatosis intestinalis. Advanced, or stage III, disease is characterized by progression to unstable vital signs, respiratory failure, and peritonitis.

Treatment may be both medical and surgical, depending on the stage of the disease. As soon as the diagnosis is suspected, oral feedings are discontinued and an oral gastric tube is inserted to decompress the gastrointestinal tract. Intravenous fluids, including colloid and blood, are given as necessary to maintain an adequate urinary output and hematocrit. Intubation and ventilation are often required to treat lethargy, sepsis, or massive abdominal distention. Broad-spectrum antibiotic therapy is started to cover both gram-positive and gram-negative organisms. Stage III disease can often lead to disseminated intravascular coagulation. Hematocrits, platelets, and clotting parameters need to be followed and treated appropriately. Frequent examination and monitoring of the acid base status, coagulation profile, electrolytes, and abdominal radiographs are essential in assessing the infant's response to treatment and the need for surgery, if any.

Surgery is commonly required in infants with NEC. Kosloske et al.[14] evaluated the clinical, radiologic, and laboratory criteria for surgery. Surgery was recommended for those patients who had pneumoperitoneum, a positive pericentesis, erythema of the abdominal wall, a fixed abdominal mass, or persistently dilated intestinal loops on serial radiographs. Although some centers disagree as to the indications for surgery, a positive pericentesis or pneumoperitoneum always requires an operation. In most cases, the terminal ileum and proximal ascending colon are involved, but the entire bowel may be included in severe cases. In infants with segmental disease, the gangrenous bowel is resected in multiple segments, to preserve as much intestinal length as possible. Exteriorization of the bowel is usually recommended until the disease process abates.

Survival rates of 50 to 75 percent of infants requiring surgery have been described in the past decade.[15,16] The morbidity of infants who survive NEC is related to the development of intestinal strictures, short-bowel syndrome, or complications of total parental nutrition (TPN). In children requiring extensive resection, the problems associated with short-bowel syndrome become most significant. Preservation of terminal ileum and the ileocecal valve are important for the successful introduction of enteral alimentation, and to avoid many of the problems of short-bowel syndrome. In those patients requiring massive resection, intestinal transplants may offer the only hope for survival.

Previous studies indicated that NEC does not appear to affect the growth and neurodevelopment of surviving infants. However, Walsh et al.[17] have recently shown that if the patients are stratified according to Bell's classification, those infants with stage III NEC have a high rate of subnormal body weight and head circumference.

The oral use of IgA and IgG shows promise in decreasing the risk of NEC in premature infants,[18] but prevention must be aimed primarily at the prevention of prematurity. This will not be easily achieved but would result in a massive reduction of those patients at risk.

## Omphalocele and Gastroschisis

Omphalocele and gastroschisis are congenital abdominal wall defects that result in a portion of the infant's gastrointestinal tract remaining outside the abdominal cavity. An omphalocele is a translucent avascular sac consisting of the peritoneum and the amniotic membrane at the base of the umbilical cord. Omphaloceles vary in size. Some are only few centimeters in diameter, containing a few loops of small intestine. Others may be extensive, containing the entire midgut, stomach, and liver. It is important to note that with an omphalocele the amniotic sac is always present, although it may have been ruptured during birth or thereafter. In gastroschisis, the defect is extraumbilical, and an amniotic sac is never present.

The incidence of omphalocele has varied from 1 to 3,200 to 1 in 10,000 live births but has not changed over the last decade.[19] Gastroschisis occurs with a similar incidence of about 1 in 10,000, but the rate for births to mothers less than 20 years old may reach as high as 7 in 10,000 births.[20]

The development of gastroschisis has been attributed to a defect in differentiation of the somatopleural mesenchyme, whereas an omphalocele has been attributed to the failure of embryonic folding at the level of the lateral folds, or to persistent body stock in the region normally occupied by the somatopleura.[21] Most defects that occur in association with gastroschisis appear to be caused by vascular disruption. Investigators have proposed that the condition may result from intrauterine disruption of the right omphalomesenteric artery. This would explain why in the vast majority of cases the defect occurs to the right of the umbilicus.[22] Nonetheless, some investigators believe that gastroschisis and omphalocele are not two separate disorders, but in fact different expressions of a defect with a similar embryologic origin.[23,24] To date, the embryology of gastroschisis is not completely understood or agreed upon. For the purpose of conformity we will consider them two distinct disorders, comparing and contrasting their characteristics.

Congenital anomalies are more commonly associated with omphalocele (30 to 50 percent), compared with gastroschisis (5 to 25 percent).[25–27] Omphaloceles have also been found with greater frequency than expected in families with children affected by other congenital abnormalities.[28] Omphalocele (but not gastroschisis) is often associated with other known syndromes, particularly trisomies 13 and 18, and Beckwith-Wiedemann syndrome, the latter of which consists of umbilical abnormalities, macroglossia, giantism, microcephaly, hypoglycemia and a tendency to develop Wilms tumor.[29,30] These syndromes consist of one-third of the cases of omphaloceles with multiple congenital abnormalities. Greenwald et al.[28] reviewed 159 infants with omphaloceles treated at Boston Children's Hospital, looking for associated congenital defects. Congenital heart disease was found in 19.5 percent of the infants. The most common were tetralogy of Fallot and atrial septal defect. With a large omphalocele, nonrotation of the intestine is always present. Occasionally a Meckel's diverticulum or persistent omphalomesenteric duct are found; other intestinal malformations are rare.

Gastroschisis is associated with prematurity in 22 percent of patients compared with 11 percent for omphalocele. There is an equally higher incidence of prematurity, up to 43 percent, in both conditions when they are associated with other congenital anomalies. In gastroschisis, Moore and Khalid[31] found a 16 percent incidence of gastrointestinal malformations, including intestinal atresia or stenosis. In addition, intestinal perforations are common, and in some patients the entire intestine may be infarcted.

Aside from the difference in the incidence of congenital defects, omphalocele and gastroschisis pose similar problems for the anesthesiologist; infants suffer significant heat losses, and major fluid shifts occur into the exposed bowel. Because of the absence of a protective membrane (i.e., the amniotic sac), an infant with a gastroschisis may have greater fluid losses and an increased risk of infection, as compared with one with an omphalocele. The viscera should be covered with plastic sterile wrap, and towels or bowel bag. This maneuver will help to prevent further infection and limit radiant heat and fluid loss from exposed viscera. A nasogastric tube should be inserted to prevent gastric distension.

The most important aspect of initial management is the restoration of intravascular volume. Excellent IV access must be established. The choice of fluids, colloids as compared with crystalloids, may be less important than establishing adequate hydration. Fluid losses in both gastroschisis and omphalocele are generally isotonic, with some protein loss, particularly in infants with a gastroschisis. Balanced salt solutions are necessary for successful resuscitation and maintenance of plasma electrolytes. The volume of fluid required is high because evaporative losses occur in addition to the third space intestinal losses.[32] It is not uncommon for these infants to require 10 to 15 ml/kg/h of fluid in the initial phase of resuscitation.

The possibility of Beckwith-Weidemann syndrome should be appreciated in patients with omphalocele, and a blood glucose estimation should be performed. Up to 30 to 50 percent of these infants will develop hypoglycemia secondary to pancreatic hyperplasia, which results in hyperinsulinemia.[33] Hypoglycemia may persist beyond the neonatal period. Glucose determinations should be done repeatedly. Titration of glucose infusions should be on the basis of blood glucose levels; bolus doses should not be given.

Cardiac defects are associated with omphalocele, and a preoperative cardiac evaluation should be made. In those children who are unstable and have an associated cardiac defect, an understanding of the cardiac anatomy as detailed by transthoracic echocardiography can be helpful in determining optimal anesthetic management. This may be particularly true in children with cyanotic lesions, or in children with a large septal defect resulting in an unrestricted shunt. The directions of flow in these shunts can shift, depending on the relationship between pulmonary and systemic vascular resistances and the factors that affect both.

Prompt surgery is recommended for both omphalocele and gastroschisis. Both primary and staged repairs have been advocated.[34,35] The decision to perform either will depend on the surgical experience of the institute and the ability to ventilate the child during closure. In cases involving large abdominal wall defects, significant respiratory compromise can occur. There is decreased compliance of the chest as the abdominal wall contents are returned into the abdominal cavity and intrathoracic pressure increases. Herschenson found a 41 percent incidence of prolonged respiratory insufficiency in a study of 22 infants with giant omphaloceles.[36] These infants had narrow chests, with their posterior ribs angulated inferiorly, so they appeared more vertical than normal. Calculated lung volumes in living infants and those found at autopsy showed significant pulmonary hypoplasia. It has been suggested that the failure of the liver to return to the abdominal cavity in utero leaves the lower thoracic inlet of the fetus underdeveloped. Such patients require extensive long-term ventilatory support. Although in gastroschisis the liver is always within the abdomen, the abdominal cavity is often small and underdeveloped. The replacement of bowel into this underdeveloped cavity can also result in respiratory compromise. Staged approaches to closure may be necessary in these patients.

Yaster et al.[37] noted that increases in intragastric pressure greater than 20 mmHg and increases in central venous pressure of more than 4 mmHg during surgical closure of omphaloceles were associated with reductions in venous return and cardiac index. These infants required surgical decompression of the abdomen and a staged closure of the defect. Failure to do so was associated with severe cardiorespiratory compromise and ensuing metabolic acidosis. Decreased hepatic blood flows may lead to delayed metabolism of narcotic analgesics, and impaired kidney perfusion may lead to renal failure. Regardless of surgical technique, the anesthesiologist must be aware of the extensive respiratory and metabolic problems that commonly occur as a result of surgical closure.

The return of bowel function occurs slowly, particularly in gastroschisis patients. Central hyperalimentation is commonly utilized to improve caloric intake while the infant's diet is slowly advanced during the recovery period. Malabsorption and failure to thrive often persist throughout the first year of life in infants with gastroschisis. This may be the result of the associated bowel anomalies common in infants with gastroschisis. In addition, necrotizing enterocolitis can occur in as many as 20 percent of patients following gastroschisis repair and may develop as late as 3 months after surgery. In staged closure, infants often return to the operating room several times over a 1- to 2-week period. The anesthesiologist must be familiar with both the respiratory and nutritional status of the child in order to make an appropriate anesthetic plan. With the improvements in parenteral nutrition and ventilatory support, patients with gastroschisis now have a 95 percent survival rate. There is an 80 percent survival rate in infants with omphaloceles. The poorer success rate in omphalocele is attributed to the presence of associated congenital defects.

## Infantile Pyloric Stenosis

Hirschsprung, a Danish surgeon, first described pyloric stenosis as a distinct diagnostic entity in 1888, although he was unable to offer an effective therapy.[38] It was not until Conrad Ramstedt described his own work in 1912 that an optimal surgical therapy was realized. Since that time improvements in fluid therapy and anesthetic technique have taken his largely unchanged surgical technique from a morbidity of 25 percent or more in 1922 to its current level of 0.1 to 0.01 percent.[39]

No etiology for pyloric stenosis has been described to date, although genetic factors are without doubt important. The incidence in white infants has been cited at 1 in 500 births.[40] Males are two to three times as likely to be affected as females, and whites three to four times as compared with blacks or Asians. Male siblings of females with pyloric stenosis seem to be at particular risk. Pyloric stenosis has been described in identical and nonidentical triplets, raising the possibility that a dominant gene(s) is involved.[41]

Two sphincteric loops of circular muscle fiber encircle the pylorus and converge at the lesser curvature of the stomach. It is the thickening of these circular fibers that obstructs the lumen of the pylorus. Histologic examination shows an increase in number as well as hypertrophy of circular muscle fibers. Electron microscopy has failed to reveal any abnormalities of these cells.[42]

Infants typically become symptomatic at 2 to 3 weeks of age, although the diagnosis is often delayed until 6 to 8 weeks. Initially, parents may notice regurgitation after each meal, which commonly results in a change of formula without the child improving. Eventually regurgitation becomes more pronounced and the vomiting becomes projectile, in rare cases up to 2 or 3 feet. The vomitus contains only stomach contents, milk, and curds. Bilious vomitus suggests duodenal obstruction, and makes the diagnosis of pyloric stenosis suspect. Affected infants are often voracious feeders and will feed again, immediately after vomiting.

Physical examination is often diagnostic, with palpation of an olive-sized mass in the midepigastrium or slightly to the right. The presence of such a mass and a supportive history have been claimed to be diagnostic in 99 percent of cases.[43] Ultrasound has provided noninvasive diagnostic support of the diagnosis when the clinical picture and physical examination are equivocal, and has also provided evidence supporting long-held claims that some infants have a mild form of the disease, without significant symptoms.[44] Barium swallow examinations show elongation and severe narrowing of the pyloric canal. This is commonly known as the "string sign."

Associated abnormalities can occur with pyloric stenosis. Renal abnormalities have been described in a few infants.[45] Additionally elevated levels of unconjugated bilirubin have been noted in one-fifth of patients. Elevated levels of bilirubin have been attributed to a physiologic decrease in glucuronyl transferase activity in the liver. The decrease is believed to be secondary to the vomiting and lack of enteral digestion.[46] However, Gilbert's disease has been raised as an alternative explanation in selected cases.[47] Gilbert's disease is a benign disorder of bilirubin metabolism, periodically resulting in elevated levels of unconjugated bilirubin. The etiology of this disorder is unknown, and liver biopsies of affected individuals are normal. No specific therapy is required. Regardless of the etiology of the hyperbilirubinemia, bilirubin levels usually fall to the normal range after definitive therapy for pyloric stenosis. This is consistent with both Gilbert's disease and nonpathologic hyperbilirubinemia.

Pyloric stenosis is a medical, but not a surgical emergency. Appropriate initial therapy is aimed at correcting metabolic and fluid derangements. The vomitus of babies affected with pyloric stenosis contains varying amounts of chloride, sodium, and potassium, with chloride losses predominating. Chloride concentrations in the vomitus vary from 130 to 160 mEq/L, with the volume of gastric secretions lost as high as 100 ml/d. This has been called a unique situation. Almost all other abdominal surgical conditions result in either isotonic electrolyte losses or sodium depletion.[48] Additionally, with pyloric obstruction, gastric fluid fails to reach the duodenum. Hydrogen cations are then unavailable to buffer the bicarbonate that, under normal circumstances, would be secreted by the pancreas into the duodenum. A increase in plasma bicarbonate occurs that exceeds the absorption threshold of the renal tubule for this anion. As a result, an alkaline urine is produced containing sodium bicarbonate and potassium in exchange for the conservation of hydrogen and chloride anions. Initially the renal system attempts to preserve pH balance. As the vomiting continues, sodium losses in the urine persist and dehydration becomes pronounced. In response, aldosterone levels rise and the kidneys begin to conserve sodium and water, at the expense of pH balance. This results in the excretion of ammonium and acid anions and increased losses of potassium. Serum potassium levels, however, do not decline until intracellular potassium is severely depleted. Without treatment the end result is a metabolic disturbance, with severe dehydration, hypokalemia, hypochloremia, a metabolic alkalosis, and, paradoxically, an acid urine.[49]

The degree of dehydration, starvation, and metabolic derangement depends of the duration and severity of the vomiting. Severe dehydration (15 percent loss of total body water) can result in weight losses exceeding 1 kg. Assessment of the degree of dehydration and duration of disease can be aided by bicarbonate and chloride measurements.[50,51] For infants whose bicarbonate levels exceed 25 mEq/L, or in whom the serum chloride is less than 100 mEq/L, the disease is of greater magnitude, requiring aggressive fluid resuscitation. Initial resuscitation is commonly with normal saline with 5 or 10 percent dextrose. Potassium chloride is added at a rate of 3 to 5 mEq/kg/d, when urine output is restored. The addition of potassium chloride results in a greater replenishment of chloride as well as potassium. In mild cases saline may be given at the rate of 20 ml/kg intravenously as a bolus, followed by 1 to 1.5 times calculated maintenance rates. Within 24 hours most of these children become biochemically normal. In severe cases fluid replacement may take several days. Fluid resuscitation in these cases should be done in a closely monitored environment, as rapid replacement of sodium can result in a CNS disequilibrium syndrome, resulting in seizures and/or death.

Prior to surgery, affected infants should be fully rehydrated and the electrolyte disturbance largely corrected. An increase from the admission weight and normal urinary output should be documented.[52] With adequate electrolyte and fluid replacement urinary chloride levels should be in excess of 20 mEq/L.[53] These infants should be assumed to have a full stomach, regardless of when the last feed occurred. Immediately prior to anesthesia the infant's stomach should be aspirated using an oral gastric tube. Some advise that the stomach should then be lavaged with sodium citrate and emptied again.

Fluid therapy must be continued into the postoperative period until the infant is taking feeds well, usually the next postoperative day. Small feeds should be commenced; aggressive feeding in the immediate postoperative period can result in additional vomiting and resultant fluid losses. Stopping dextrose-containing fluids too early has been associated with severe hypoglycemia.[54] Postoperatively, respiratory depression and apnea have been noted.[55] Although metabolic alkalosis has been repeatedly implicated as a cause of this apnea in pyloric stenosis, there has been little scientific support for such a belief.

## Hirschsprung's Disease

Harald Hirschsprung was the first to describe in detail the clinical entity that bears his name. However, it was not until the late 1940s that Orvar Swenson defined the pathophysiologic mechanism of this disorder and devised effective therapy. Normally the autonomic nervous system of the bowel consists of three distinct plexuses of ganglion cells: Auerbach's, Henle's, and Meissner's. In Hirschsprung's disease, ganglion cells are absent from all three plexuses. In addition, histochemical studies have shown an increase in the number and size of cholinergic and adrenergic fibers in the affected segments of bowel. Affected segments show concentrations of acetylcholine and norepinephrine three to nine times greater than those present in normal bowel.[56,57] The absence of cholinergic ganglion cells prevents coordinated peristalsis. The parasympathetic plexus directly regulates muscle cells in the bowel wall and produces contraction. An imbalance results, involving both the bowel and the internal rectal sphincter. The end result is that the adrenergic system is unable to effect muscle relaxation despite elevated norepinephrine concentrations.

The aganglionosis usually extends proximally into the sigmoid colon. Rarely, the entire colon and a portion of the ileum may be involved. Total intestinal aganglionosis has been reported. At the other extreme, there are reports of ultrashort Hirschsprung's disease. "Skip" lesions have been described; some portions of the bowel are missing ganglion cells and others are not.

The common accepted embryonic explanation for the absence of ganglionic cells in the bowel is the failure of the cranial and caudal migration of the vagal crest neuroblasts between the 5th and 12th weeks of gestation.[58] The cranial and caudal migration of neuroblasts explains both typical Hirschsprung's disease and variants with "skip" lesions.

Hirschsprung's disease occurs in 1 of 5,000 live births.[59] The incidence is four to five times greater in boys than girls and is more likely to occur in siblings of affected individuals, with an incidence as high as 10 percent. For siblings of children with total colon aganglionosis, the incidence is as high as 20 percent. Children with trisomy 21 have a ten times higher incidence of Hirschsprung's disease.[60] Hirschsprung's disease is linked with other anomalies, including small bowel atresia, malrotation, and Waardenburg's syndrome.[61,62] Waardenburg syndrome consists of a characteristic facial deformity, congenital deafness, and extensive areas of white hair.

The clinical picture of Hirschsprung's disease is often evident from birth, but may not be made until later in childhood, or even in early adult life. However, even in older children and adults, review of their medical history will usually show a chronic history of constipation, starting with delayed passage of meconium as a newborn. Infants are typically irritable, have poor feeding, and fail to thrive. Older children present with difficulty in controlling bowel movements, constipation, and partial bowel obstruction. They may have an abnormal history of bowel training. Patients with normal bowel training who are constipated are more likely to have functional constipation.

In newborns, constipation usually results in one of two processes, either severe obstruction or enterocolitis. The incidence of enterocolitis is greatest between 2 and 3 months of age but can occur in the newborn infant. The exact etiology of the enterocolitis is not well understood. Thomas et al.[63] suggested a possible etiology when they isolated *Clostridium difficile* in 10 of 13 children with enterocolitis. Interestingly, infants on breast milk rarely suffer from enterocolitis. Signs and symptoms typically consist of fever, vomiting, progressive abdominal distention, and diarrhea. In previous years, this unrecognized condition had up to an 80 percent mortality. Despite aggressive treatment, morbidity and mortality for acute enterocolitis in the newborn with Hirschsprung's disease still remain significant. Treatment of this condition revolves around adequate fluid and electrolyte resuscitation, broad-spectrum antibiotics, and decompression of the obstructed colon.

The diagnosis of Hirschsprung's disease is based on the triad of clinical presentation, biomedical examination, and rectal biopsy. A barium enema is often used as a diagnostic tool but its interpretation in infants less than 1 month old is difficult. In addition, hypothyroidism and meconium plug syndrome can appear radiologically similar to Hirschsprung's disease. In children over 1 year of age, the diagnosis of Hirschsprung's disease by barium enema can result in a false negative in 5 percent of children examined.

The most reliable diagnostic test is a full-thickness rectal wall biopsy. This procedure requires an anesthetic. In many centers, a frozen section is reviewed immediately at the time of surgery to ensure an adequate specimen. There is normally an absence of ganglion cells 2 cm above the pectinate line. When taking a rectal biopsy the surgeon must be careful to take it above this point. For infants, biopsy of the mucosa and submucosa is easier to perform, and with experience, it offers results comparable to those of a full-thickness biopsy. These biopsies are usually combined with histochemical techniques, adding to the accuracy of the light microscopy.[64,65] In the absence of ganglion cells on the frozen section, the surgeon then proceeds with a colostomy. Intrarectal manonometry to measure internal and external sphincter function has also been described. It is particularly difficult to perform in young infants, as the normal rectal reflex does not occur until 12 days of age. As children get older the test becomes more accurate. However, it is never sufficient alone to make a definitive diagnosis of Hirschsprung's disease; a biopsy is needed as well.

Initially, the bowel can be decompressed by irrigation with normal saline, with care to avoid massive fluid shifts and electrolyte imbalances. Short segments with Hirschsprung's disease have been successfully managed in this manner until a definitive operation can be performed. However, treatment usually requires early surgical decompression of the aganglionic segment by means of a colostomy.

Several types of definitive surgical procedures have been described. Most common are the Swenson, Duhamel, and Soave procedures, which are designed to allow removal of the affected bowel and anastomosis of the normal bowel to the distal rectum, preserving rectal continence. In short segments of Hirschsprung's disease a simple myotomy may be successful; however, failure rates are high.

Sherman et al.[66] reported the largest series of surgical treatments for Hirschsprung's disease using Swenson's procedure. In their study the greatest factors influencing success and mortality were the presence of trisomy 21, the patient's age at the time of operation, and leaks that occurred in the distal colonic anastomosis. At the 5-year followup most of the patients had normal bowel habits. None of these patients had urinary incontinence or impotence. Carcassonne et al.[67] have described 32 infants under 3 months of age with Hirschsprung's disease, including 7 with total colonic aganglionosis. Contrary to the traditional therapy of rectal biopsy and decompression, followed by a definitive procedure at 1 year of age, these infants had a definitive procedure at the time of diagnosis. There was no mortality, and morbidity was not different from that seen with traditional therapy. Therefore, these authors advocated definitive corrective surgery at an early age.

Most of the postoperative complications related to these definitive procedures result from leakage at the anastomotic suture line. It occurs in up to 5 percent of cases and can lead to a pelvic abscess, generalized peritonitis, or sepsis. Enterocolitis is also a significant, although fortunately rare, cause of morbidity and mortality in the postoperative period. Postoperative complications are more common in patients with trisomy 21.

Although Hirschsprung's disease is a serious and life-threatening entity, recent advances in understanding the pathophysiology of the disease (as well as surgical correction) have led to a reduction in the risk such patients face. In addition, definitive therapy has shown that most of these patients live an essentially normal life thereafter.

The anesthesiologist should have an appreciation of the underlying pathophysiology, associated syndromes, surgical objectives, and possible complications. In particular, awareness of the possible septic processes, especially in trisomy 21 patients, is invaluable in planning appropriate anesthetic management.

## Short-Bowel Syndrome

Short-bowel syndrome describes the malabsorptive disorder than results from massive resection of the small intestine.

Although the malabsorption is primarily the result of a decreased mucosal surface area after surgical resection, secondary factors also play a role. In infants, short-bowel syndrome may be the result of either developmental or acquired defects, or a combination of both. Examples include gangrenous mid-gut volvulus, extensive intestinal atresia, necrotizing enterocolitis, and Hirschsprung's disease, particularly when there is total aganglionosis of the colon.

Fifty percent of the newborn small intestine can be resected without need for special postoperative management. This is especially true if the ileocecal valve is retained. In such patients, if diarrhea does develop, it is usually secondary to other complications, including blind loop syndromes, strictures, or a definable disorder of absorption, usually lactose deficiency. For those children suffering more extensive loss of bowel as a result of resection or infection, the amount of remaining bowel that will support survival varies. It is dependent on the quality as well as the quantity of remaining bowel.

Although progress in short-bowel syndrome has been made, the study by Wilmor[68] is commonly quoted when describing the amount of bowel necessary for survival. In this study there were no survivors among infants who had less than 40 cm of small intestine and no ileocecal valve, or in children who had less than 15 cm of small bowel with an intact ileocecal valve. Survival with less than 15 cm of small bowel has been described, but many of these children developed mental and physical handicaps.[69]

The ability of the remaining bowel to adapt and carry on normal function will dependent on the functional reserve left. If the remaining intestine is damaged, as is common in NEC, some of this bowel will recover poorly or not at all.

In understanding the impact of massive resection of small bowel, it is important to appreciate the anatomic and functional differences that exist between the jejunum and ileum. The proximal 40 percent of the small bowel comprises the jejunum, and the rest is ileum. The jejunum has twice the diameter of the ileum and numerous circular folds. Water-soluble substances, sugars, vitamins, and electrolytes are usually absorbed in the jejunum.

Fats, proteins, and fat-soluble vitamins are digested first, and then absorbed in the ileum. The ileum is important for the recirculation of bile salts, with reabsorption occurring in the distal ileum. This recirculation of bile salts plays a critical role in the digestion and absorption of fats. Additionally, the ileum appears to have a greater functional reserve than the jejunum, and is capable of compensating for extensive loss of proximal bowel. At the time of resection, the surgeon attempts to save the ileum rather the jejunum, whenever possible.

The presence of the ileocecal valve is a significant determinant of survival after small-bowel resection. The ileocecal valve is important in preventing bacterial contamination of the small intestine, which further damages the mucosa. In addition, a build-up of bacteria in the terminal ileum will prevent the absorption of bile acids. Bile acids not absorbed produce a cathartic effect. The loss of bile salts is also associated with cholelithiasis.[70]

Gastric hypersecretion has been described in small-bowel syndrome.[71,72] The hypersecretion of gastric acid can cause a number of problems, including further mucosal injury, the prevention of mucosal hypertrophy, and the inactivation of enzymes such as lipase. Interference with fat and protein digestion can produce an osmolar diarrhea with the intestine secreting water and electrolytes rather than reabsorbing them.

Children with short-bowel syndrome may suffer an intolerance to lactose and sucrose, as these disaccharides are normally absorbed in the proximal bowel. The enzymes responsible for the absorption of disaccharides can be disrupted due to bacterial overgrowth or hyperacidity.[73]

In short-bowel syndrome, the ability of the remaining bowel to adapt is important for survival. Experiments have clearly shown that the bowel is capable of increasing its length and caliber.[74] Absorption is enhanced by the growth of villi, which results in a fourfold increase in the absorptive surface.[75] As previously mentioned, the ileum is more able than the jejunum to compensate for a loss of bowel. Specifically, the ileum can increase its absorption of substances that require no special transport mechanisms and still retain its ability to absorb bile acids and vitamin $B_{12}$, which do require special transport systems.[76,77]

The therapy for short-bowel syndrome may consist of three measures. Most important is diet, followed by drug therapy and then surgery. Vanderhoof[78] has described diet therapy in three phases. The first phase of dietary management is to stabilize the patient on TPN. This therapy is a cornerstone for infants with short-bowel syndrome. Many of the advances in the management of these patients over the past 15 to 20 years are directly attributable to improvement in TPN. Since TPN is a long-term therapy, the children must have a permanent indwelling central venous catheter placed early in the treatment.

Following the infant's stabilization on TPN, the patient moves to phase two, continued use of TPN and introduction of enteral nutrition, an important element. Although hyperalimentation is hailed as life-saving in many patients with this syndrome, TPN slows the migration of epithelial cells and leaves a significant reduction in mucosal thickness in laboratory animals.[79] The same is felt to be true in humans. Oral feeding appears to be more effective than TPN in maintaining mucosal protein and disaccharide activity in the bowel mucosa. Enteral feedings are commonly given via a silicone rubber nasogastric feeding tube or through a feeding gastrostomy. Depending on the amount of functional bowel, the second phase may last from several weeks to years. During this phase, parenteral nutrition can usually be given at home, which helps to reduce costs and decrease the risk of infection. Care at home improves the psychosocial development of the child by affording relief from the hospital environment. Evening-only administration of TPN allows the child to live a more normal life during the daytime.

The third phase of dietary therapy is the introduction of solid feeds and the management of long-term micronutrient deficiencies. Poor absorption of vitamin D and calcium can result in rickets or tetany. This is especially true in former preterm infants. Supplementation of water-soluble vitamins, as well as replacement of zinc, is important. The addition of magnesium and iron may be necessary. During this phase, chronic bacterial overgrowth is a frequent problem, especially in the absence of a functioning ileocecal valve. Such patients require long-term treatment with broad-spectrum antimicrobial therapy. Occasionally patients will develop metabolic acidosis due to the production of excess D-lactate by intestinal bacteria. This problem is usually corrected by the elimination of bacterial overgrowth. It should be suspected in patients demonstrating repeated problems with dyspnea and drowsiness.[78]

Drug therapy is usually aimed at solving two problems, the first of which is gastric hypersecretion. As previously mentioned, increased serum gastrin levels often occur following massive small-bowel resection; such hypersecretion can exacerbate the malabsorption problem. $H_2$-blocking agents have been utilized to manage this problem, which is often transient but can persist for several months. Cholestyramine, which is a bile acid binding resin, can reduce the catharteric diarrhea in some patients following ileal resection. It is usually used in conjunction with medium-chain triglycerides or low-fat formulas. Unfortunately, cholestyramine may exacerbate fat malabsorption by reducing the bile acid reabsorption. As such, if bile salt deficiency is a problem, the addition of cholestyramine may in fact exacerbate the malnutrition suffered by these patients. Loperamide, in doses of 0.5 mg/kg/d, has been used as an effective drug to control intestinal motility. This can be useful when rapid transit time is interfering with the absorption of nutrients.

A variety of surgical procedures has been described to improve tolerance of enteral feedings in short-bowel syndrome patients. These include vagotomy and pyloroplasty, recirculating loops, colonic interposition, and the production of various valves, sphincters, and baffles. These have been designed to delay transit and prolong the contact of nutrient elements on the mucosal surface.[80–82] Although these surgical procedures have met with some success in improving outcome, they do not alter the fact that inherent in the survival of short-bowel syndrome, is the need for sufficient length of normal small bowel to provide an absorptive surface for enteral nutrition.

As pointed out by Cooper et al,[83] the prognosis for infants with short-bowel syndrome is improving. Additionally, there are occasional reports of children having survived with less than 15 cm of small bowel.[69] Despite these reports, Hancock and Wiseman[85] have recently pointed out that there may be a definitive limit to how aggressively we treat children with short-bowel syndrome. They call this disorder "lethal short-bowel syndrome," and they reviewed the charts of seven infants with severe short-bowel syndrome. The survival time of the children ranged from 5 days to 18 months. All patients received TPN for 10 days to 6 months. There were no survivors, and a review of the charts suggested that infants with less than 6 cm of small bowel beyond the ligament of Trites will inevitably die, regardless of the etiology or treatment. They suggest that until bowel transplant becomes a viable alternative, operative intervention and nutritional support may prolong life but would not change the final outcome of infants with severe short-bowel syndrome. It was their opinion that aggressive therapy in these children may only contribute to additional morbidity and to needless suffering by patients and parents alike. They concluded that therapy should be withheld once the diagnosis of lethal short-bowel syndrome, as defined in their paper, is made. As small-bowel transplantation becomes an "alternative," the prognosis may improve.[86]

For the anesthesiologist involved in the care of these children, an awareness of multiple problems is called for, most significantly the complications of TPN therapy and catheter-induced infections, which remain the number one cause of death.[86,87] In addition, the anesthetist must be aware of the nutritional deficiencies that exist in these children, must look for evidence of fluid and electrolyte imbalance, and must be prepared for difficulties in acquiring adequate IV access.

## ANOMALIES AND DISEASES OF OLDER INFANTS AND CHILDREN

### Gastroesophageal Reflux

In newborn infants, swallowing-induced peristaltic waves cause a relaxation of the distal esophagus, allowing food to pass into the stomach. This distal or intra-abdominal portion of the esophagus is most critical in preventing the regurgitation of gastric contents into the thoracic esophagus. As the child grows, a high-pressure zone in the abdominal esophagus is created, contributing to the valve-like mechanism in this area. In young children, the abdominal esophagus is about 1.5 cm long.[88] A pressure between 5 and 7 mmHg in this segment is necessary to prevent significant reflux. Maturation of this sphincter mechanism usually occurs around 7 weeks of age. The angle of the gastroesophageal junction is also important, as are mucosal folds that act as a choke valve, further preventing reflux. Should the intra-abdominal esophagus and stomach lie above the diaphragm, as is the situation in hiatal hernia, none of these important mechanisms operate and therefore reflux occurs.[89]

In the past decade, important associations between gastroesophageal reflux and respiratory disease have been identified.[90–94] These associations can be divided into one of three categories. The first is respiratory disease as a result of gastroesophageal reflux. The second is respiratory disease that causes gastroesophageal reflux, and the third is respiratory disease and gastroesophageal reflux in the neurologically impaired child.

Pulmonary aspiration of gastric contents during reflux is clearly the cause of some pneumonias and has been suspected to be a cause of bronchospastic pulmonary symptoms. Reflux with aspiration has been implicated in cases of pneumonia, lung abscess, and "near-miss sudden infant death syndrome."[95–97] Gastroesophageal reflux has been shown to occur in 25 to 80 percent of children with asthma.[98] Studies have also recorded an improvement in bronchospastic symptoms after medical or surgical therapy for reflux.[99]

It has been demonstrated that bronchoconstriction in these asthmatic patients may occur following gastroesophageal reflux without aspiration of acid into the lungs. It appears that intraesophageal acid potentiates the bronchoconstrictor response to other stimuli that may cause bronchospasm.[100] Reflux-mediated laryngospasm by a similar mechanism without actual aspiration of gastric contents into the lungs has been postulated.[101] Although the exact pathways involved in reflex bronchospasm or laryngospasm are not known, they are more common in young children.

Chronic respiratory disease after repair of esophageal atresia has been attributed to aspiration. This aspiration may be a result of either the anastomotic stricture at the site of repair or abnormal distal esophageal peristalsis, which is unrelated to the surgical procedure.

Gastroesophageal reflux can cause a multitude of respiratory symptoms, but also respiratory disorders can provoke reflux. Respiratory activities may increase intra-abdominal pressure, and decrease intrathoracic pressure. Drugs used to treat respiratory diseases decrease the lower esophageal sphincter pressure and increase gastric acid production or counteract the natural gravitational pull of gastric contents caudally, and thus may potentiate gastroesophageal reflux, and its sequelae.

Intra-abdominal pressure is increased by the forced expiration of coughing and wheezing associated with such diseases as cystic fibrosis, bronchopulmonary dysplasia, asthma, or respiratory infection. Negative intrathoracic pressure is accentuated by the forced inspiration occurring in patients with stridor.

Respiratory disorders have not been implicated in relaxing the lower esophageal sphincter tone in humans but the therapy for such disorders may have an effect. Therapy has both a pharmacologic and mechanical effect on the sphincter.

Xanthenes such as theophylline, caffeine, and β-adrenergic agonists such as isoproterenol all reduce lower esophageal tone. Theophylline, in addition to its effect on the lower esophageal sphincter, increases gastric acid secretion.

Nasogastric tubes may cause gastroesophageal reflux. This type of reflux is commonly associated with tube feedings, which are used with increasing frequency (e.g., aggressive nutritional repletion in malnourished patients with cystic fibrosis).

Patients with severe respiratory disease are commonly nursed in the supine position. This is especially true for patients receiving mechanical ventilation. This position slows gastric emptying and increases reflux.[102,103]

The diagnosis of gastroesophageal reflux can be difficult, as it may occur in nonsymptomatic patients. As such, the diagnosis must be based not only on symptomatology, but also on temporal association, and the development of causality. Pathologic gastroesophageal reflux may be diagnosed using endoscopy, histology, pH probes, radiology, or scintigraphy. Reflux that produces endoscopically visible esophagitis is certainly pathologic. However, reflux may be pathologic yet not produce signs of gross or histologic esophagitis. Thus temporal relationships may need to be established. The pH probe identifies several characteristics of gastroesophageal reflux for which norms have been established. It may also define a temporal association between acid reflux episodes and intermittent respiratory symptoms. The disadvantage of the pH probe is that it does not detect the presence of nonacid materials, and therefore it may not pick up gastroesophageal reflux of food particles, as might occur after feeding. In addition, it may not identify a group of patients described as having alkaline gastroesophageal reflux.[104] Scintigraphy and barium esophagraphy may also aid in the diagnosis of gastroesophageal reflux, but neither are particularly sensitive or specific.

Treatment of gastroesophageal reflux in children may be medical or surgical. The initial treatment of reflux usually involves positioning and the use of frequent smaller feedings. Commonly, children are put in a seated position for gastroesophageal reflux. Unfortunately, this position has been shown to increase the incidence of reflux in infants.[105] The optimal position appears to be that in which the child is held upright or placed prone.[106] Pharmacologic therapy consists of using drugs with sphincter-augmenting properties such as metoclopramide, which also augments gastric emptying, and agents to reduce acidity such as cimetidine and ranitidine. The effectiveness of metaclopromide in gastroesophageal reflux has bee somewhat controversial; studies have shown both improvement and worsening of reflux in infants.[107,108] In children with documented esophagitis, the use of $H_2$-blockers such as cimetidine or ranitidine has been effective. Less commonly, bethanechol is used. This drug has the disadvantage that it may exacerbate bronchospasm because of its cholinergic effects.

The majority of children improve in the first year of life, regardless of therapy. The response to medical therapy is usually dramatic. Surgical therapy is usually reserved for neurologically impaired children and those who fail with medical therapy or have life-threatening apnea or severe respiratory problems.

There are two groups of children with reflux-mediated respiratory disease that are likely to require operation. Infants with bronchopulmonary dysplasia form one group.[109] Difficulties in positioning, chronic ventilator dependency, the need for nasogastric feedings, and the disturbance of thoracoabdominal pressure relationships make these patients resistant to the medical management of reflux. The other group resistant to therapy is the neurologically impaired child. Most of these children tend to remain in a supine position, have increased abdominal pressure secondary to spasticity, and have poor oropharyngeal reflexes. They are often susceptible to aspiration while feeding and to reflux-induced respiratory symptoms. Debate still exists over whether or not these patients should have percutaneous gastrostomy alone or in combination with a fundoplication.[110,111]

Anesthesiologists caring for children with gastroesophageal reflux face a number of considerations. The significance of the reflux must be weighed against the risk of pulmonary aspiration and the need for a rapid sequence induction. As mentioned, not all children with a diagnosis of reflux actually aspirate. Antacid prophylaxis should, however, be considered. An understanding of the relationship of reflux to respiratory symptoms is most important in assessing affected children, in order to optimize anesthetic management.

## Intussusception

Intussusception is the result of the invagination of one segment of intestine into another. Most commonly it involves the segment of the bowel just proximal to the ileocecal valve. Typically the ileum, with its mesentery, is drawn into the cecum and the ascending colon. The lead point of this anomaly is termed the intussusceptum. The entrapped bowel becomes compressed and, along with the traction on the mesentery, produces lymphatic and mesentery venous obstruction. If this process persists, the mucosa at the lead point becomes engorged. Increasing edema results in the obstruction of mesenteric arterial flow. The end result of this process is a gangrenous bowel.

The etiology of intussusception is not fully understood. A lead point, such as a Meckel's diverticulum, polyp, intestinal duplication, or lymph node, is sometimes found.[112] More commonly, intussusception in infants appears to be associated with conditions that produce inflammation of the intestinal intramural lymphoid tissue (Peyer's patches). The rotavirus, a major etiologic agent for acute gastroenteritis in children, and adenoviruses have been implicated.[113–115] It is thought that viral gastroenteritis results in increased peristalsis, which predisposes to an intussusception.

Although in most children a lead point relating to a specific disease is not found, a few diseases with specific lead points deserve mention. Meckel's diverticulum is the most common identifiable cause, followed by polyps and duplication of small bowel. In addition, coagulopathies, especially Henoch's purpura, have been implicated. Lymphosarcoma of the intestine is the most common cause of intussusception in children over 6 years of age.[116] In older children, cystic fibrosis has been identified as an etiologic factor.

When no specific lead point is found, the term idiopathic intussusception is used. This occurs most commonly at 5 to 18 months of age, with an incidence of 2 to 4/1,000 live births and a male to female incidence of 3:2, but with no racial predilection at this age. Beyond 5 years of age it occurs as a more chronic and intermittent disease, with a high incidence in black South Africans and Chinese.[117]

Classically, children present with a history of intense abdominal pain associated with an excruciating cry. These periods of pain are usually spasmodic or cyclic in nature and associated with vomiting. With these episodes the baby usually raises his or her knees up toward the abdomen, becomes anxious, and screams. The abdomen may appear distended, with hyperperistalsis audible over the abdomen. Occasionally, a tumorlike mass may be found in the right upper quadrant beneath the liver. In between bouts of spasm and pain, the children are usually listless and pale. Children may appear so listless that they are diagnosed as having meningitis or other central nervous system disorders. The passage of blood and mucus with the stool completes the classic presentation.

When children do not have typical signs and symptoms the disease is called "atypical intussusception." More appropriately, it may be named "nonischemic intussception." This presentation may be more difficult to diagnose, but it is associated with less morbidity, no doubt related to the absence of ischemia in the intussuscepted bowel.

Therapy for affected children is divided into three stages. The first is resuscitation of the child. These children need an intravenous infusion. Fluid resuscitation and the types of fluid given will depend on the state of the child. Obviously, in children who appear septic, or when there is considerable loss of blood per rectum, more aggressive therapy is necessary than for those children identified early in the disease process. Sepsis in children with an intussusception is a late finding and must be treated aggressively with broad-spectrum antimicrobial drugs and intravenous fluids. The children are best managed in an acute care setting prior to radiology or surgery.

After stabilization, a controlled barium enema provides a reliable diagnostic technique and is the definitive treatment in more than 75 percent of cases. In children who are adequately resuscitated and in stable medical condition, a small amount of sedation is appropriate to facilitate reduction of the intussusception. This must be done cautiously in an appropriate setting with adequate resuscitative equipment and appropriate personnel nearby. Barium enema reductions are considered successful when the contrast medium freely flows or refluxes into the terminal ileum. If the reduction is successful most children are able to take a diet the same day. Discharge is within 24 hours. In those children who are not cured by a controlled enema, a second attempt under general anesthesia may be successful.[118] Pneumatic reduction of intussusception is also practiced in some centers with considerable success.

Surgical management is generally reserved for those who have prolonged symptoms, are septic, or have obvious evidence of compromised bowel. In some late or severe cases, a barium enema is not necessary to make the diagnosis, and time is wasted in doing so. In these cases, it is better to prepare the child for surgery. Surgery is occasionally necessary when the barium enema does not reduce the intussusception, or when two or three previous nonsurgical reductions have not been successful. In children over 6 years of age, the high incidence of lymphosarcoma of the bowel will convince many surgeons to proceed directly with surgery. The recurrence rate for nonoperatively reduced intussusception is approximately 4 percent. For operatively reduced intussusception the rate is approximately 2 percent.

## Meckel's Diverticulum

Meckel's diverticulum is the most common congenital anomaly of the intestine. It is present in approximately 2 percent of the population, but only 50 percent are symptomatic.

The omphalomesenteric duct extends from the embryo into the yolk sac and under normal circumstances undergoes complete obliteration. Meckel's diverticulum is the most common persisting remnant should obliteration be incomplete. It is usually found 2 feet from the ileocecal valve, is usually no more than 2 inches in length, and may contain two heterotopic tissue types; hence the rule of twos. Most commonly, it contains pancreatic or gastric mucosal tissues, but colonic, jujunal, or duodenal mucosa have also been identified. The incidence of heterotopic tissue in Meckel's diverticulum is 6 percent.[119]

Usually the diverticulum produces symptoms as a result of associated complications, including intestinal obstruction, perforation, inflammation simulating that of appendicitis, or, more dramatically, hemorrhage. Typically, symptoms occur in children under 2 years of age. Boys are affected more often than girls. Usually the child has a large bloody stool, followed by spontaneous cessation of bleeding. It is unusual for affected children to have perfuse bleeding on the first symptomatic episode. Occasionally affected children can present in a shocklike state, with extensive blood loss or signs of abdominal perforation, sepsis, or obstruction. Bleeding is usually secondary to a peptic ulcer resulting from the heterotopic gastric tissue. Meckel's diverticulum can also commonly present as a lead point in an intussusception, causing intestinal obstruction.

The diagnosis is usually proved by the use of a pertechnetate Tc-99m scan. Although the radioisotope may also be taken up by intussusceptions, hemangiomas, and some duplications of the small bowel, refinements in techniques have improved the accuracy of imaging to nearly 100 percent.[119]

Management depends on the type of presentation. Those with massive blood loss or sepsis require aggressive resuscitation. This must be complete prior to transfer to the operating room. The usual precautions for management of the septic patient should be followed. Death as a result of Meckel's diverticulum is rarely related to hemorrhage, but usually to neglected intestinal obstruction with intestinal infarction and sepsis.[120]

## Appendicitis

Acute appendicitis is the most common indication for exploratory laparotomy in children in North America. Although appendicitis may occur in all age groups, it is most common in the pediatric population (between 6 and 10 years of age). Appendicitis has even been encountered in infants and newborns.

Appendicitis in children presents a unique diagnostic problem. In the past, errors in diagnosis and surgical technique have resulted in approximately 100 pediatric deaths from appendicitis annually in the United States.[121] Recently, with increased awareness of this problem in young children, there has been a decrease in mortality and morbidity.[122] In keeping with the difficulty in diagnosing appendicitis in children, 30 to 47 percent have perforated at the time of diagnosis and surgery.

In order to reduce this risk, it must be appreciated that in children the typical signs and symptoms of appendicitis are often missing. This is especially true in those under 2 years of age, in whom the perforation rate at the time of diagnosis may be as high as 80 percent. Appendicitis should be suspected in any child who presents with fever, malaise, loss of appetite, or other nonspecific constitutional symptoms. Recent improvements in diagnostic ultrasonography have made it possible to use this procedure as a diagnostic tool; it is particularly useful in those with an enlarged appendix, especially those with cystic fibrosis.[123,124]

Undiagnosed complicated appendicitis can lead to generalized peritonitis, subphenic and pelvic abscesses, empyema, and intestinal obstruction. In females, these infectious complications may lead to infertility later in life, as occurs with pelvic inflammatory disease.

It is important for the anesthetist to appreciate that many children with appendicitis present late in the disease. Although children have tremendous physiologic reserve, if they are septic, a great portion of that reserve has been spent. Failure then to initiate aggressive and appropriate management will result in a fulminating course with high morbidity. As with any septic process, recognition and understanding of the disease process, fluid resuscitation with balanced salt solutions, and appropriate antimicrobial therapy are the important cornerstones to prevent morbidity and mortality.[125,126]

## Celiac Disease

The hallmark of celiac disease is chronic intolerance to gluten in the diet. Dietary exclusion of gluten leads to full clinical remission with restoration of the small intestinal mucosa to normal.

The incidence of celiac disease varies from country to country and is highest in Ireland, where 1 in 300 are affected,[127] it is most often found in areas of the world where wheat is a staple food, and there are also genetic considerations.

The majority of patients with celiac disease have an HLA-specific haplotype. For celiac disease the common haplotype is HLA-B8. These genetic subtypes are considered markers of the disease but do not confer disease susceptibility by themselves. Celiac disease is rare in black Africans and the Japanese, which is consistent with the low incidence of the HLA-B8 haplotype in these populations. Concordance and nonconcordance has been reported for celiac disease in monozygotic twins.[128]

As stated, gluten intolerance is the hallmark of celiac disease. Gluten is a large complex molecule made up of four heterogeneous types of protein. Most of the intolerance centers around the alpha-fraction of one of these protein classes. Originally, the disease was considered the result of either an enzyme deficiency or an immunologic mechanism. A peptidase deficiency has been described that is not permanent, since there is restoration of peptidase activity when gluten is removed from the diet.

Elevations in serum IgA and depressions of IgM levels have been described. Additional, IgA deficiency has been noted along with hypogammaglobulinemia. T cells have been implicated in the pathogenesis of celiac disease.[129] Increased density of intraepithelial lymphocytes in the small intestinal mucosa of celiac patients is typical. In addition, there is a change in antigen expression of the T-cell receptor. This change in antigenicity is seen even with the histologically normal mucosa of patients previously diagnosed with celiac disease who are now receiving gluten-free diets.

The proximal small-bowel mucosa in celiac disease is flat, with loss of normal villi. Biopsies show the mucosal surface to be featureless or to have a mosaic appearance. Although this flat mucosal appearance makes the biopsy useful for diagnosis, it is not specific. Milk and soya protein intolerance produce a similar histology. An increased density of intraepithelial lymphocytes is more specific for celiac disease than the flat appearance of the mucosa itself.

Children typically present in the first 2 years of life, although in some areas of the world symptoms may develop at a later age possibly because gluten is introduced into the diet later. Diarrhea is the most common symptom, either acute or chronic. Affected children pass large, bulky, and often offensive stools. Occasionally, children with celiac disease present with constipation, although this is rare. Failure to thrive is common and the children are often short in stature. The classic appearance of celiac disease is an unhappy child with a distended abdomen and wasting of the buttocks and shoulders. Delay in achievement of motor milestones may occur. Height and weight are often below the 10th percentile. Usually celiac disease is diagnosed on the basis of a biopsy of small intestinal mucosa and an improved clinical course upon withdrawal of gluten from the diet. Strict adherence to a gluten-free diet is difficult. It is recommended that celiac disease not be diagnosed without a confirmatory small bowel biopsy. Because the histologic picture is not specific, the reintroduction of gluten at a later time after the small intestinal mucosa becomes normal is recommended. Should the child's clinical situation then deteriorate, the diagnosis is definitively established.[130]

It has recently been shown that circulating IgA antigliadin antibodies have a high degree of sensitivity and specificity for this disorder.[131,132] If these antibodies are present at the time of diagnosis in a child with a confirmatory small intestinal biopsy, and if they disappear parallel to exclusion of gluten from the diet, a diagnosis of celiac disease is established.

The exclusion of wheat, rye, barley, and oats from the diet must be maintained for life. There is an increased risk of cancer of the mouth, pharynx, and esophagus and also lymphoma in celiac patients receiving an unrestricted diet. Adherence to a gluten-free diet for 5 years or more decreases the risk for these types of malignancy to normal levels.[133]

## TOTAL PARENTERAL NUTRITION

TPN is commonly used for the treatment of patients with severe gastrointestinal disorders. It can be used as a substitute for enteral feedings in patients unable to take feedings orally, or as a supplement to enhance feedings when oral intake alone is insufficient to meet caloric requirements. The principle gastrointestinal indications for the use of TPN in pediatric patients include short-bowel syndrome, diarrhea secondary to inflammatory bowel diseases, or conditions such as omphalocele and gastroschisis in which bowel function does not return to normal levels for several days to weeks after surgical repair.

The goal of TPN is to maintain body tissues and to provide for appropriate growth and the healing of wounds. TPN must provide adequate fluid, energy, fat, protein, electrolytes, minerals, vitamins, and trace elements to meet each individual patient's requirements. Intravenous nutrition requirements are not precisely defined. Consequently, nutrient needs are based on estimates of oral intake requirement, nitrogen balance studies, and accepted standards. Fluid and energy requirements are calculated for weight and ages.

Energy is usually supplied in the form of glucose, commonly in conjunction with a lipid emulsion. Glucose is usually given in the form of dextrose monophosphate. Premature infants are often unable to metabolize glucose, even at relatively low doses, and require lower concentrations and slower increases in dextrose infusions, compared with their older counterparts. The addition of insulin, in conjunction with glucose infusions, has been advocated in extremely low birth weight infants with hyperglycemia.[134] The goal is to avoid glucosuria.

Lipid emulsions are given as either a 10 percent or 20 percent solution. They consist of a triglyceride stabilizer with eight phospholipids isotonically balanced with glycerol. Lipid emulsions provide a concentrated caloric source with a relatively low osmolality. With these solutions, 25 to 40 percent of the calories provided come from the lipid infusion. Tolerance is assessed by monitoring serum triglyceride levels 48 hours after the completion of the lipid infusions. Lipid emulsions may cause hyperlipidemia, resulting in decreased oxygenation and displacement of unconjugated bilirubin from albumin binding sites.[135]

Protein requirements are estimated from studies of fetal nitrogen accumulation or by analysis of breast-fed infant data. Most amino acid solutions currently available are not made specifically for infants and children. Newer formulas are being developed to yield a plasma amino acid pattern resembling that seen in breast-fed infants. Specific amino acid formulas for patients with renal or hepatic failure are also being introduced.

Electrolyte and mineral requirements must also be considered. Specifically, potassium, magnesium, and phosphorus should be monitored carefully when parenteral nutrition is given, as there is a flux of these minerals intracellularly as the patient become anabolic. Symptoms of hypophosphatemia, hyperkalemia, and hypermagnasemia can be severe and life threatening. Precipitation of calcium phosphate in solutions is a special problem for premature or term infants and for young children. Currently available solutions often do not meet the metabolic requirements of these minerals. The result is that infants on long-term parenteral nutrition have a high prevalence of bone demineralization, rickets, and fractures.

Four trace elements have been associated with documented deficiency states in humans and are routinely provided in parenteral nutrition solutions. They are zinc, copper, chromium, and magnesium.

Complications of TPN therapy may be divided into three main categories: infectious, metabolic, and mechanical. Infections are the most common and serious complications and are usually caused by streptococcus or gram-negative organisms. Neonates who have had stable glucose measurements on TPN and who become intolerant to this infusion should be suspected of having sepsis.

Long-term TPN can lead to hepatobiliary disorders. Cholestatic jaundice is recognized as one of the more serious complications. Microscopic examination of liver biopsies from patients developing cholestatic jaundice in the early stages has shown only minimal hepatocellular damage.[136] Although no specific cause and effect relationship has been found between a specific component of parenteral nutrition solutions and liver disease, amino acids have come under the most suspicion.[137,138] It should be noted that cholestasis has been observed in some neonates prior to receiving parenteral nutrition.[139,140] Cholestasis may be part of a normal phase that persists when normal enteral feeding must be withheld. Mechanical problems relate to the inability to maintain adequate intravenous access. Both peripheral and central access have been used in children. Peripheral access can be used when the total osmolar load does not exceed 900 mOsm. For larger osmolar loads, central venous access is required. Complications relating to the insertion of central catheters include pneumothorax, hemothorax, hydrothorax, arterial puncture, myocardial perforation, air embolization, cardiac arrhythmias, cardiac tamponade, and thrombosis. In children requiring long-term catheter placement, such as those with short-bowel syndrome, thrombosis of veins in the central system becomes a dominant problem. The metabolism of glucose and intralipid results in the production of carbon dioxide. Infants with respiratory dysfunction may be unable to cope with the need for increased ventilation as $PCO_2$ rises. With increased understanding of the metabolic requirements of infants, the advent of "TPN teams" (which allows standardization of protocols), and the use of skilled personnel to insert and care for central venous catheters, many of the complications described can be avoided.

Many additives, and a variety of other medications, can be safely added to parenteral nutrition solutions. However, the compatibility of each drug with the solution must be checked with the pharmacy before use. Antibiotics are commonly infused in piggyback fashion, so that parenteral nutrition infusions do not continue while they are given.

Whenever possible, children who require surgery should have their TPN continued in the operating room. This will allow the child to receive those calorie requirements that may be interrupted by long periods of time in the operating room. Whenever possible, TPN lines should not be used as an access and should be left undisturbed to limit the risk of infection. With severely ill children, or children on long-term TPN, this is often impossible, as IV access becomes a priority. In either situation the anesthesiologist should be familiar with the drugs that are compatible with TPN infusions and those that are not. As a general rule, intralipid solutions should be discontinued if other drugs are going to be inserted into the same line.

The stress of surgery and anesthesia may alter glucose homeostasis; therefore, monitoring glucose levels before and during surgery is strongly recommended. When TPN is continued into the operative period serum glucose levels may rise significantly, placing the patient at risk for the complications of hyperglycemia. If the decision is made to discontinue TPN before operating, the patient will need to be maintained on a 5 to 10 percent glucose infusion. Serum glucose determinations are then made at frequent intervals, in order to avoid hypoglycemia.

## REFERENCES


1. Kliegman RM, Fanaroff AA: Neonatal necrotizing enterocolitis: a nine year experience. Am J Dis Child 135:603, 1981
2. Kanto WM, Wilson R, Breart TL et al: Perinatal events in necrotizing enterocolitis in premature infants. Am J Dis Child 141:167, 1987
3. Kliegman RM: Neonatal necrotizing enterocolitis: bridging the basic science with the clinical disease. J Pediatr 117: 833, 1990
4. Palder SB, Schwartz MZ, Tyson K et al: Association of closure of patent ductus arteriosus and the development of necrotizing enterocolitis. J Pediatr Surg 23: 422, 1988
5. Leung MP, Chau K, Mui P et al: Necrotizing enterocolitis in neonates with symptomatic congenital heart disease. J Pediatr 113:1044, 1988
6. Hackett GA, Campbell S, Gamsu H et al: Doppler studies in the growth retarded fetus and the prediction of neonatal necrotizing enterocolitis, hemorrhage and neonatal morbidity. Br Med J 294:13, 1987
7. Scheifele DW, Bjornoson GL, Dyer RA et al: Delta like toxin produced by coagulase-negative stalphylococci is associated with neonatal necrotizing enterocolitis. Infect Immun 55:2268, 1987
8. Gerber AR, Hopkins RS, Lauer BE et al: Increased risk of illness among nursery staff caring for neonates with necrotizing enterocolitis. Pediatr Infect Dis 4:246, 1985
9. Kliegman RM, Fanaroff AA: Necrotizing enterocolitis. N Engl J Med 310:1093, 1984
10. Kliegman RM, Pittard WB, Fanaroff AA: Necrotizing enterocolitis in neonates fed human milk. J Pediatr 95:450, 1979
11. Anderson DM, Kliegman RM: The relationship of neonatal alimentation practices to the occurrence of endemic necrotizing enterocolitis. Am J Perinatol 8: 62, 1991
12. Neu J: Necrotizing enterocolitis. p. 1021.

In Rudolph AM (ed): Rudolph's Pediatrics. 19th Ed. Appelton & Lange, East Norwalk, CT, 1991

13. Bell MG, Ternberg JL, Feigin RD et al: Neonatal necrotizing enterocolitis: therapeutic decisions based upon clinical staging. Ann Surg 187:1, 1978
14. Kosloske AM, Papile LA, Burnstein J: Indications for operation in acute necrotizing enterocolitis of the neonate. Surgery 87:502, 1980
15. Ricketts RR: Surgical therapy for necrotizing entercolitis. Ann Surg 200:653, 1984
16. Cikrit D, Mastandrea J, West KW et al: Necrotizing enterocolitis: factors affecting mortality in 101 surgical cases. Surgery 96:648, 1984
17. Walsh M, Klievman R, Hack M: Severity of necrotizing enterocolitis: influence on outcome at 2 years of age. Pediatrics 84: 808, 1989
18. Eibl MM, Wolf HM, Furnkranz H et al: Prevention of necrotizing entercolitis in low birth weight infants by IgA and IgG feeding. N Engl J Med 319:1, 1988
19. Torfs C, Curry C, Roepper P: Gastroschisis: a review. J Pediatr 116:1, 1990
20. Bugge M, Hague M: Gastroschisis OG, Omphalocele I Denmark. Ugeskr Laeger 145:1323, 1983
21. Duhamel B: Embryology of exothalmus and allied malformations. Arch Dis Child 38:142, 1963
22. Hoyme HE, Jones MC, Jones KL: Gastroschisis: abdominal wall disruption secondary to early gestational interruption of the omphalomesenteric artery. Semin Perinatol 7:294, 1983
23. Shaw A: The myth of gastroschisis. J Pediatr Surg 10:235, 1975
24. Glick PL, Harrison MR, Adzick MS et al: The missing link in the pathogenesis of gastroschisis. J Pediatr Surg 20:406, 1985
25. Lindham S: Omphalocele and gastroschisis in Sweden 1965–1976. Acta Pediatr Scand 70:55, 1981
26. Roeper PJ, Harris J, Lee G, Neutra R: Secular rates and correlates for gastroschisis in California (1968–1977). Tetrology 35:203, 1987
27. Baird PA, MacDonald EC: An epidemiologic study of congenital malformations of the anterior abdominal wall in more than half a million consecutive life births. Am J Hum Genet 33:470, 1981
28. Greenwald RD, Rosenthal A, Nada AS: Cardiovascular malfunctions associated with omphalocele. J Pediatr Surg 85:181, 1974
29. Irving J: Exothalmus with macroglossia: a study of 11 cases. J Pediatr Surg 2:499, 1967
30. Roe TF, Kershnar AK, Weitzman JJ, Madrigal LS: Beckwith's syndrome with extreme organ hyperplasia. Pediatrics 52:372, 1978
31. Moore T, Khalid N: An international survey of gastroschisis and omphalocele (490 cases). 1. Nature and distribution of additional malformations. 2. Relative incidence, pregnancy and environmental factors. Pediatr Surg Int 1:46, 109, 1986
32. Philippart AI, Cantry TG, Filler RM: Acute fluid volume requirements with anterior abdominal defects. J Pediatr Surg 7:553, 1972
33. Schiff D, Colle E, Wells D et al: Metabolic aspects of the Beckwith-Wiedemann syndrome. J Pediatr 82:258, 1973
34. Canty TG, Collins DL: Primary facial closure in infants with gastroschisis and omphalocele: a superior approach. J Pediatr Surg 8:707, 1983
35. Schwartz MZ, Tyson KRT, Milliorn K et al: Stage reduction using a silastic sac as a treatment of choice for large congenital abdominal wall defects. J Pediatr Surg 18:713, 1983
36. Herschenson M, Brouillette R, Klemka L et al: Respiratory insufficiency in newborns with abdominal wall defects. J Pediatr Surg 20:348, 1985
37. Yaster M, Buck JR, Dudgeon DL et al: Hemodynamic effects of primary closure of omphalocele/gastroschisis in human newborns. Anesthesiology 69:84, 1981
38. Ravitch MD: The story of pyloric stenosis. Surgery 48:1117, 1960
39. Wollstein M: Healing of hypertrophic pyloric stenosis after Fredit-Ramstedt operation. Am J Dis Child 23:511, 1922

40. Laron, Horne: The incidence of infantile pyloric stenosis. Am J Dis Child 94:151, 1957
41. Janik JS, Hirikati NS, Lehocky R: Pyloric stenosis in identical triplets. Pediatrics 70:282, 1982
42. Jona JZ: Electron microscopic observation in infantile hypertrophic pyloric stenosis. J Pediatr Surg 13:17, 1978
43. Stevenson RJ: Non-neonatal intestinal obstruction in children. Surg Clin North Am 65:1224, 1985
44. Stunden RJ, LeQuesne GW, Little KE: The improved ultrasound diagnosis in hypertrophic pyloric stenosis. Pediatr Radiol 16:200, 1986
45. Atwell JD, Levick P: Congenital hypertrophic pyloric stenosis and associated anomalies in the genitourinary tract. J Pediatr Surg 16:1029, 1981
46. Wooly MM, Bertram FF, Asch JM: Jaundice, hypertrophic pyloric stenosis and glucuronyl transferase. J Pediatr Surg 9: 359, 1974
47. Roth B, Statz A, Heinisch H: Jaundice with hypertrophic pyloric stenosis: a possible manifestation of Gilbert Syndrome. J Pediatr 116:1003, 1990
48. In Raffensperger JG (ed): Swenson's Pediatric Surgery. 5th Ed. Appleton & Lange, East Norwalk, CT, 1990
49. Rose BD: Clinical Physiology of Acid-Base and Electrolyte Disorders. 2nd Ed. McGraw-Hill, New York, 1984
50. Breaux CW, Hood JS, Georgeson KE: The significance of alkalosis and hypochloremia in hypertrophic pyloric stenosis. J Pediatr Surg 24:1250, 1989
51. Goh DW, Hall SK, Gornall P: Plasma chloride and alkalemia in pyloric stenosis. Br J Surg 77:922, 1990
52. Dawson K, Graham D: The assessment of dehydration in congenital pyloric stenosis. NZ Med J 104:162, 1991
53. Bissonnette B, Sullivan P: Pyloric stenosis. Can J Anaesthe 38:668, 1991
54. Shumake LB: Postoperative hypoglycemia in congenital hypertrophic pyloric stenosis. South Med J 68:223, 1975
55. Daly S, Conn A: Anaesthesia for pyloromyotomy: a review. Can Anaesth Soc J 16:316, 1969
56. Ikawa H, Yokoyama J, Morikama Y: A qualitative study of cetocholine and Hirschsprung's disease. J Pediatr Surg 15:48, 1980
57. Touloukian RJ, Aghajanian G, Roth RH: Adrenergic hyperactivity of the aganglionic choline. J Pediatr Surg 8:191, 1973
58. Okamoto E, Veda T: Embryogenesis of intramural ganglia of the gut and relation to Hirschsprung's disease. J Pediatr Surg 2:437, 1967
59. In Raffensperger JG (ed): Swenson's Pediatric Surgery. 5th Ed. Appleton & Lange, East Norwalk, CT, 1990
60. Hart MH: Congenital aganglionic megacolon. p. 1039. In Rudolph AM (ed): Rudolph's Pediatrics. 19th Ed. Appleton & Lange, East Norwalk, CT, 1991
61. Gauderer M, Rothstein F, Izant R: Ileoatresia with long segment Hirschsprung's disease in a neonate. J Pediatr Surg 19:15, 1984
62. Curie A, Haddad M, Honeyman M, Buddy S: Associated developmental abnormalities of the anterior end of the neural crest: Hirschsprung's disease-Wardenburg's syndrome. J Pediatr Surg 21:248, 1986
63. Thomas D, Freino D, Bayston R et al: Enterocolitis and Hirschsprung's disease: a controlled study of the etiological role of *Clostridium difficile*. J Pediatr Surg 21:22, 1986
64. Meier-Ruge W, Lutterbeck P, Harsog B et al: Acetylcholinesterase in suction biopsies of the rectum in the diagnosis of Hirschsprung's disease. J Pediatr Surg 7:11, 1972
65. Schofield D, Devine W, Yunis E: Acetylcholinesterase stained suction rectal biopsies in the diagnosis of Hirschsprung's disease. J Pediatr Gastroenterol Nutr 11:221, 1990
66. Sherman JO, Synder ME, Weitzmann JJ et al: A 40-year multinational retrospective study of 880 Swenson's procedures. J Pediatr Surg 24:833, 1989
67. Carcassonne M, Guys JM, Morrison IG et al: Management of Hirschsprung's disease: curative surgery before 3 months of age. J Pediatr Surg 24:10, 1989

68. Wilmore DW: Factors correlating with successful outcome following extensive intestinal resection in newborn infants. J Pediatr 80:88, 1977
69. Kurz R, Saver H: Treatment and metabolic findings in extreme short-bowel syndrome with 11 cm of jejunal remnant. J Pediatr Surg 18:257, 1983
70. Pellerin D, Bertin P, Nihoul-Fekete CL, Ricour CL: Cholelithiasis ileal pathology in childhood. J Pediatr Surg 10:35, 1975
71. Aber GM, Ashton F, Carmalt MH, Whitehead TP: Gastric hypersecretion following massive small bowel resection in man. Am J Dig Dis 12:785, 1967
72. Straus E, Gerson CD, Valow RS: Hypersecretion of gastrin associated with short-bowel syndrome. Gastroenterology 66:175, 1974
73. Howat JM, Aronson I: Sugar intolerance in neonatal surgery. J Pediatr Surg 6:719, 1971
74. Bel MJ, Martin LW, Schubert WK: Massive small-bowel resection in an infant: long-term management and intestinal adaption. J Pediatr Surg 8:197, 1973
75. Flint JM: The effect of extensive resections of the small intestine. Bull Johns Hopkins Hosp 23:127, 1962
76. Dowling RH, Booth CC: Functional compensation after small bowel resection in man. Lancet 2:146, 1966
77. MacKinnon AM: Intestinal adaption of vitamin $B_{12}$ absorption. Clin Sci 42:29, 1972
78. Vanderhoof JA: Short-bowel syndrome. In Rudolph AM (ed): Rudolph's Pediatrics. Appelton & Lange, East Norwalk, CT, 1991
79. Feldman EJ, Dowling RH, McNaughton J: Effects of oral versus intravenous nutrition on intestinal adaption after small bowel resection in the dog. Gastroenterology 70:712, 1976
80. Mitchell A, Watkins RM, Collin J: Surgical treatment of the short bowel syndrome. Br J Surg 71:329, 1984
81. Garcia BF, Templeton JM, Eichelberger MR: Colon interposition for short-bowel syndrome. J Pediatr Surg 16:994, 1981
82. Wang KL, Heller K: Surgical techniques in short-bowel syndrome. Prog Pediatr Surg 25:81, 1990
83. Cooper A, Floyd T, Ros A: Morbidity and mortality of short-bowel syndrome acquired in infancy: an update. J Pediatr Surg 19:711, 1984
84. Postuma R, Moroz S, Friesen F: Extreme short-bowel syndrome in an infant. J Pediatr Surg 18:264, 1983
85. Hancock BJ, Wiseman NE: Lethal short-bowel syndrome. J Pediatr Surg 25:1131, 1990
86. Okada A, Takagi Y: Home parenteral nutrition: an indication for small bowel transplantation. Transplant Proc 22: 2431, 1990
87. Grossfeld JL, Rescoria FJ, West KW: Short-bowel syndrome in infancy and childhood: analysis of survival in sixty patients. Am J Surg 151:41, 1986
88. Botha CS: The gastroesophageal region of infants. Arch Dis Child 33:78, 1958
89. Chrispin AP, Freidland GW: Functional disturbances in hiatal hernia in infants and children. Thorax 22:422, 1967
90. Barish CF, Wu WC, Castell TO: Respiratory complications of gastroesophageal reflux. Arch Intern Med 145:1882, 1985
91. Nelson HS: Gastroesophageal reflux in pulmonary disease. J Allergy Clin Immunol 73:547, 1984
92. Allen CJ, Newhouse MT: Gastroesophageal reflux in chronic respiratory disease. Am Rev Respir Dis 129:645, 1984
93. Christie DL: Respiratory disease associated with gastroesophageal reflex. Pediatrics 53:344, 1979
94. Orenstein SR, Orenstein DM: Gastroesophageal reflex and respiratory disease in children. J Pediatr 112:847, 1988
95. McVeagh P, Howman-Giles R, Kemp A: Pulmonary aspiration studied by radionucleotide milk scanning and barium swallow roetenography. Am J Dis Child 141:917, 1987
96. Walsh JK, Farrell MK, Keenan WJ et al: Gastroesophageal reflux in infants: relation to apnea. J Pediatr 99:196, 1981
97. Veereman-Wauters G, Bochner A, Caillie-Bertrand M: Gastroesophageal reflux in infants with a history of near-miss sudden infant death. J Pediatr Gastroenterol Nutr 12:319, 1991

98. Berquist WE, Rachelefsky GS, Kadden M et al: Gastroesophageal reflux-associated recurrent pneumonia and chronic asthma in children. Pediatrics 68:29, 1981
99. Hoyoux C, Forget P, Lambrechts L, Geubell F: Chronic bronchopulmonary disease and gastroesophageal reflux in children. Pediatr Pulmonol 1:149, 1985
100. Herve P, Denjaen A, Jian R et al: Interesophageal perfusion of acid increases the bronchial motor response to methocholine and to isocapnic hyperventilation in asthmatic patients. Am Rev Respir Dis 134:986, 1986
101. Spitcer AR, Boyle JT, Tuchman DN, Fox WW: Awake apnea associated with gastroesophageal reflux: a specific clinical syndrome. J Pediatr 104:200, 1984
102. Myers WF, Herbst JJ: The effectiveness in positioning therapy for gastroesophageal reflex. Pediatrics 69:768, 1982
103. Yu VTH: Effective body positioning on gastric emptying in the neonate. Arch Dis Child 50:500, 1975
104. Vandenplas Y, Loeb H: Alkaline gastroesophageal reflux in infancy. Pediatr Gastroenterol Nutr 12:448, 1991
105. Orenstein SR, Whitington PF, Orenstein DM: The infant seat as treatment for gastroesophageal reflux. N Engl J Med 309: 760, 1983
106. Orenstein SR, Whitington PF: Positioning for the prevention of infant gastroesophageal reflux. J Pediatr 103:534, 1983
107. Tolia V, Calhoun J, Cuhns L, Kauffman RE: Randomized prospective double-blind trial of metaclopromide and placebo for gastroesophageal reflux in infants. J Pediatr 115:141, 1989
108. Machida HM, Forbes DA, Gall DG, Scott RB: Metaclopromide and gastroesophageal reflux of infancy. J Pediatr 112:483, 1988
109. Giuffre RM, Rubin S, Mitchell I: Antireflux surgery in infants with bronchopulmonary dysplasia. Am J Dis Child 141:648, 1987
110. Stringel M, Delgado AG, Cook JD et al: Gastroscopy: initial fundoplication in neurologically impaired children. J Pediatr Surg 24:1044, 1989
111. Flake AW, Shopene C, Ziegler MM: Antireflux gastrointestinal surgery in a neurologically handicapped child. Pediatr Surg Int 6:92, 1991
112. Gross RE: The Surgery of Infancy and Childhood. p. 381. WB Saunders, Philadelphia, 1953
113. Koono T, Suzuki H, Kutsuzawa T: Human rotavirus and intussception. N Engl J Med 297:945, 1977
114. Gardner PS, Know EG, Court SDM: Virus infection and intussception in childhood. Br Med J 2:697, 1962
115. Clarke Jr EG, Phillips IA, Alexander ER: Adenovirus infection in intussception in children in Taiwan. JAMA 208:1671, 1969
116. Wayne ER, Campbell JB, Kosloske AM, Burrington JD: Intussception in the older child: suspect lymphosarcoma. J Pediatr Surg 11:79, 1976
117. Colombani PM, Dudgeon DL, Beaver BL et al: Jejunoileal anomalies. p. 1032. In Rudolph AM (ed): Rudolph's Pediatrics. 19th Ed. Appleton & Lange, East Norwalk, CT, 1991
118. Collins DL, Pinckney LE, Miller KE et al: Hydrostatic reduction of ileocolic intussusception: a second attempt in the operating room with anesthesia. J Pediatr 115:204, 1989
119. Rutherford RB, Akers DR: Meckel's diverticulum: a review of 148 pediatric patients with special reference to the pattern of bleeding and to the mesodiverticular bands. Surgery 59:618, 1966
120. Ho JE, Konieczny KM: The sodium pertechnetate Tc-99m scan: an aid in the evaluation of gastrointestinal bleeding. Pediatrics 56:34, 1975
121. Raffensperber JG: Meckel's diverticulum. p. 491. In: Swenson's Pediatric Surgery. 5th Ed. Appleton & Lange, East Norwalk, CT, 1990
122. Vital Statistics of the United States. DHEW, Washington, DC, 1950–1973
123. Gamal R, Moore TC: Appendicitis in children aged 13 years and younger. Am J Surg 159:589, 1990
124. Coughlin JP, Michael WL, Gauder ER: The spectrum of appendicele disease in cystic fibrosis. J Pediatr Surg 25:835, 1990

125. Puylaert J, Rutgers P, Lalisang R: Prospective study of ultrasonography in the diagnosis of appendicitis. N Engl J Med 317:666, 1987
126. Neve R, Quenvill N: Appendicitis with perforation in a 12-day-old infant. J Can Med Assoc 94:447, 1966
127. Hardman RP, Bowerman D: Appendicitis in the newborn. Am J Dis Child 105: 99, 1963
128. Mylott N, Eagan-Mitchell B, McCarthy C et al: Incidence of celiac disease in the west of Ireland. Br Med J 1:703, 1973
129. Kamath KR, Dorney SFA: Is discordance for celiac disease in monozygotic twins permanent? Pediatr Res 17:423, 1983
130. Spencer J, Diss TC, Issacson PG et al: Expression of the disulfide linked and nondisulfide linked to forms of the gamma delta T cell receptor in human small intestinal epithelium. Eur J Immunol 19:1335, 1989
131. Neeuwissee G: Diagnostic criteria in celiac disease. Acta Paediatr Scand 59:461, 1970
132. Scott H, Johan E, Havnen J et al: Serum antibodies to dietary antigens: a prospective study of the diagnostic usefulness in celiac disease of children. J Pediatr Gastroenterol Nutr 11:215, 1990
133. Troncone R, Ferguson A: Anti-gliadin antibodies. J Pediatr Gastroenterol Nutr 12:150, 1991
134. Heyman MB: Enteral and parenteral nutrition. p. 257. In Rudolph AM (ed): Rudolph's Pediatrics. 19th Ed. Appelton & Lange, East Norwalk, CT, 1991
135. Binder ND, Raschko PK, Benda GI, Reynolds JW: Insulin infusion with parenteral nutrition in extremely low birth weight infants with hyperglycemia. J Pediatr 114:273, 1989
136. Dahlstrom KA, Goulet OJ, Roberts RL et al: Lipid tolerance in children receiving long-term parenteral nutrition: a biochemical and immunological study. J Pediatr 113:985, 1988
137. Bernstein J, Chang CH, Borough AJ et al: Conjugated hyperbilirubinemia in infancy associated with parenteral alimentation. J Pediatr 98:361, 1977
138. Black D, Suttle E, Whitington P et al: The effect of short term total parenteral nutrition on hepatic function in the human neonate: a randomized study demonstrating alteration of hepatic canicular function. J Pediatr 99:445, 1981
139. Vileisis RA, Inwood RJ, Hunt CE: Prospective controlled study of parenteral nutrition associated with cholestatic jaundice and effective protein uptake. J Pediatr 96:893, 1980
140. Rager R, Finegold MG: Cholestasis in mature newborn infants: is parenteral alimentation responsible? J Pediatr 86: 264, 1975

# 5
# Liver Diseases

# 5

# Liver Diseases

*Charles M. Haberkern*
*John J. Mulroy, Jr.*

The anesthetic management of pediatric patients with liver disease requires an understanding of the disease and its effect on liver function, plus appreciation of the impact of this liver dysfunction on the anesthetic course. Many issues are similar to those in adults with liver disease; however, given the different profile of diseases affecting children, consideration is directed primarily to the pediatric population.

In this chapter, the effects of surgery and anesthesia on liver function, the effects of liver dysfunction on anesthesia, and the means of assessing liver function in children are discussed. Then the individual diseases affecting the liver in neonates, infants, and older children are discussed, highlighting the potential effects of the diseases and their treatment on anesthetic management.

## GENERAL CONSIDERATIONS

### Anesthesia, Surgery, and Liver Function

In adults it has been shown that surgery performed under any kind of anesthesia is followed by detectable changes in liver function tests. These changes are generally transient and unimportant in the otherwise healthy patient, although they may be significant in the patient with underlying liver disease.[1–3] This transient liver dysfunction is thought to be the result of factors related to surgery and anesthesia that contribute to the compromise of oxygen delivery to the liver by either decreasing systemic arterial pressure or increasing splanchnic vascular resistance.[4–10] These factors include the direct effects of anesthetic agents (e.g., halothane lowers cardiac output, regional anesthetics lower perfusion pressure), positive pressure ventilation, hypocarbia or hypercarbia, surgical blood loss, surgical retraction, and stress-induced release of catecholamines and vasopressin. There is some evidence to suggest that isoflurane preserves hepatic blood flow and hepatic functions better than halothane.[11] The alterations in both liver perfusion and biochemical tests of liver function have been shown to be greater after abdominal surgery than after superficial or peripheral procedures.

Anesthesia and surgery affect liver perfusion and function in children as well as adults. Wark and colleagues[12] have demonstrated that 4 to 10 percent of children anesthetized with halothane on multiple occasions within a period of a year have minor alterations of serum liver enzymes. However, they also showed that those with preexisting chronic liver disease are not predisposed to significant deterioration in liver function following surgery under halothane anesthesia.[13] It has been demonstrated that children repeatedly anesthetized with isoflurane for brief periods of time for radiotherapy show no alterations in liver function tests.[14]

In addition to the general effects of surgery and anesthesia on liver function and hemodynamics, specific anesthetic agents may have direct hepatotoxic effects.[3] Chloroform and trichloroethylene have been implicated as direct hepatotoxins; more significantly, halothane, enflurane, and possibly isoflurane are thought to be potentially toxic to the liver, with the ability to produce liver dysfunction and failure.[6,15–17] This volatile agent-induced "hepatitis" is thought to be mediated through reductive metabolites of the agent and/or an immunologic response.[3,18] Halothane hepatitis is rarely reported in children.

## Liver Dysfunction and Anesthesia

Adults with acute or chronic liver disease are known to have an increased risk of complications with surgery and anesthesia.[19,20] Child and Pugh[1,8] devised a classification of this risk for patients with cirrhosis, based on serum bilirubin, albumin, and prothrombin time (PT); plus the presence of ascites and encephalopathy and the general nutritional status. While there is no apparent equivalent risk classification for children with liver disease undergoing surgery, the same factors must be considered.

Liver disease in children poses many potential problems that affect their anesthetic management.[1,8,21,22] These problems will be discussed below in the context of specific disease entities, but some general comments may be made here. Cardiopulmonary function may be compromised by ascites, intrapulmonary shunting, edema, and intravascular repletion (secondary to hyperaldosteronism and hypoalbuminemia) or depletion (secondary to blood loss or diuretic therapy). Abdominal distention from ascites may increase the risk of aspiration of gastric contents. Nutritional status may be compromised, with generalized body wasting, and there may be potassium, magnesium, and zinc depletion. The alteration of both nutritional and mental status in advanced liver disease may affect the response to anesthesia. Renal function may be compromised by heart failure, hypovolemia, infection, or the poorly understood "hepatorenal syndrome." Immune function may also be significantly impaired in chronic liver disease, and the risk of bacterial and other infections is increased. The anesthetic implications of drug therapy used for individual liver diseases is discussed below.

Coagulopathy is a problem associated with liver disease that merits specific attention. The hemostatic profile can be affected in liver disease by altered hepatic synthesis and clearance of coagulation factors and their inhibitors, altered platelet number and function, and disseminated intravascular coagulation.[22,23] All the coagulation proteins except Willebrand factor are synthesized in the liver; in addition, absorption of vitamin K, necessary for the activation of the nonfunctional precursor forms of factors II, VII, IX, and X, depends on biliary function. Similarly, protein inhibitors of blood coagulation, notably antithrombin III, are synthesized by the liver. Platelet survival is compromised by hypersplenism, and platelet-associated antibodies are present in chronic liver disease. Platelet aggregation and adhesion may also be compromised.[24] Disseminated intravascular coagulation may accompany liver disease as a result of acquired dysfibrinogenemia, release of tissue thromboplastin, reduced clearance of activated coagulation factors, reduced synthesis of coagulation inhibitors, and reduced clearance of fibrinolysins.

The alteration of pharmacokinetics and pharmacodynamics of anesthetic drugs is another problem that merits specific attention.[25] The liver plays a central role in the handling of administered drugs from absorption to metabolism and excretion; liver dysfunction alters pharmacokinetics in multiple ways.[26] While most of the information concerning alterations in pharmacokinetics is based on data from adults with cirrhosis and acute hepatitis, some of this information is applicable to children with other liver diseases. Reduction in hepatic blood flow, which accompanies cirrhosis and other chronic liver conditions, leads to a reduction of hepatic clearance of drugs, particularly those that are efficiently extracted by the liver (e.g., morphine, meperidine, lidocaine, and propranolol); reduction in hepatic blood flow also reduces clearance of orally administered drugs that normally undergo substantial first-pass metabolism in the liver.[27] Hepatocellular dysfunction reduces metabolism of drugs by some pathways (e.g., oxidation) while sparing other pathways (e.g., glucuronidation). Hepatocellular dysfunction may also alter protein binding by reduced production of albumin and α-1-acid glycoprotein and by displacement of drugs by endogenous substances produced in the damaged liver. This alteration in protein binding may affect the pharmacodynamics of efficiently extracted drugs and the clearance of poorly extracted drugs. Liver disease may also be accompanied by impaired biliary excretion of unchanged drug and/or drug metabolites and by altered enterohepatic circulation of excreted drugs. All of these changes accompanying liver disease produce a complicated and frequently unpredictable effect on the action and metabolism of particular drugs.

**Table 5-1.** Use of Some Common Anesthetic Agents in Patients in Liver Diseases Based on Pharmacokinetic Changes

| *Agent* | *Use in Liver Disease* |
|---|---|
| Narcotics[a] | |
| Alfentanil | Caution[29] |
| Fentanyl | Okay[30] |
| Meperidine | Caution[25] |
| Methadone | Okay[25] |
| Morphine | Okay[25] |
| Sufentanil | Okay[28] |
| Hypnotics/sedatives[a] | |
| Thiopental | Okay[33] |
| Propofol | Okay[34] |
| Diphenhydramine | Probably okay[32] |
| Diazepam | Caution[25] |
| Lorazepam | Okay[25] |
| Midazolam | Caution[25] |
| Muscle relaxants | |
| Atracurium | Okay[25] |
| Doxacurium | Caution in liver transplantation |
| Metocurine | Okay[31] |
| Mivacurium | Caution in end-stage liver disease |
| Pancuronium | Probably okay[25] |
| Succinylcholine | Caution in end-stage liver disease |
| Tubocurare | Caution[31] |
| Vecuronium | Caution[25] |
| Miscellaneous | |
| Lidocaine | Caution[25] |
| Propanolol | Caution[25] |
| Cimetidine | Caution in end-stage liver disease[25] |
| Metoclopramide | Probably okay[25] |
| Ketorolac | Okay[31] |

[a] Use of agent may need to be reduced in patient with liver disease if neurologic status is compromised.

Table 5-1 summarizes available information concerning the effect of liver disease on drugs commonly used in pediatric anesthesia.[25,28–34] Most of the data upon which this information is based comes from work in adults with alcoholic cirrhosis or acute hepatitis, and very little comes from infants and children. However, this data should be applicable in a general sense to our consideration of the pediatric population.

## ASSESSMENT OF LIVER FUNCTION

### Physical Examination

The presenting signs and symptoms of liver disease in infants and children are described below in the context of specific diseases. In general, children with liver disease often appear generally well on initial presentation but on closer examination are noted to have abdominal distention, hepatomegaly, and/or jaundice. As a disease process progresses, other signs and symptoms become more evident: failure to thrive; weakness, apathy, malaise; bleeding; hyperventilation; and encephalopathy.

### Laboratory Assessment

The liver performs three general functions: synthesis, metabolism, and excretion. These functions can be assessed by both specific and nonspecific laboratory tests as described below. In adults, preoperative multiple laboratory screening has demonstrated an incidence of unsuspected elevation of liver function tests of 1/700,[35,36] largely due to undiagnosed infectious or alcoholic hepatitis. There are no comparable data for children, but presumably the incidence of unsuspected liver dysfunction is lower.

#### Serum Proteins

A useful measure of liver function is the concentration of serum proteins produced by the liver. Serum concentrations of coagulation factors I, II, V, VII, IX, and X are a measure of liver synthetic function. Similarly, PT, which measures the conversion of prothrombin (II) to thrombin, is an index of liver synthetic function. Since factors II, VII, IX, and X are vitamin K dependent, PT itself does not distinguish between hepatocellular dysfunction and vitamin K deficiency, although factor V concentration does provide this distinction. Serum albumin is synthesized by the liver and constitutes the major determinant of plasma colloid oncotic pressure. Serum albumin has a longer half-life than that of the coagulation proteins, so its concentration is less helpful in assessing acute hepatocellular dysfunction. Serum albumin concentration is affected by a patient's nutritional status, and markedly depressed concentrations suggest prolonged or severe malnutrition and/or liver dysfunction. The liver is responsible for the production of other proteins (e.g., globulins and lipoproteins) as well as important nonprotein substances like cholesterol, bile acids, and glucose, the concentration of the latter being affected only in end-stage liver disease.

#### Transaminases

The transaminases, aspartate aminotransferase (AST) and alanine aminotransferase (ALT), are not specific measures of liver function. Both enzymes, especially AST, are present in many different kinds of cells and are released into the circulation during any acute cell injury. The serum concentrations of both transaminases are elevated in almost all liver diseases. However, since the elevation of their concentrations reflects sudden release of cellular contents into the circulation, the degree of elevation is affected by the acuteness of the disease process, not necessarily by the amount of liver dysfunction or the disease prognosis.

### Alpha-fetoprotein

Alpha-fetoprotein (α-FP) is a protein that is similar in size to albumin and whose function is undefined. It is normally produced by the fetus and is found in significant concentrations in the fetus and in pregnant women; it is detectable only in minute concentrations after infancy. However, as noted below, serum concentrations of α-FP are elevated in certain hepatic diseases, especially hepatoblastoma and hepatic carcinoma.

### Ammonia Conversion

Metabolic function of the liver can be assessed by examination of the liver's ability to convert ammonia to urea. Although the rate of urea formation cannot be determined easily, one can measure serum concentrations of ammonia ($NH_3$). This is largely produced from the breakdown of protein and amino acids by colon bacteria. It is then absorbed into the circulation and normally converted to urea in the liver. Ammonia is also metabolized in skeletal muscle to glutamate; in general, arterial concentrations are higher than venous concentrations. There is a strong correlation between elevation of serum ammonia and liver disease, both acute and chronic: hepatocellular dysfunction decreases the ability of the liver to convert ammonia to urea; intestinal blood accompanying varices increases the amount of ammonia to be metabolized; portosystemic shunting associated with chronic liver disease decreases the delivery of ammonia to the liver for metabolism; and muscle wasting accompanying chronic disease decreases the peripheral metabolism of ammonia.

### Cholestasis Indicators

Certain biochemical tests suggest the impairment of liver excretory function that accompanies cholestasis. Alkaline phosphatase is an enzyme that is present in many tissues, including liver, bone, and intestines. The serum concentration of this enzyme reflects all of its isoenzymes, predominantly that derived from bone. Thus the concentration of alkaline phosphatase has a wide range of normal values during the period of rapid bone growth in childhood, and elevations of the enzyme are nonspecific. However, in association with liver disease, an elevation of this enzyme usually reflects cholestasis, presumably because of its altered production or release by canalicular cells. Gamma-glutamyl transpeptidase (GGTP) is another enzyme that is found in many different cells, but especially in those lining the hepatobiliary system. Thus its concentration is also very frequently elevated in disease processes affecting this system. 5′-Nucleotidase (5′-NT) is another enzyme that is rather specific for the hepatobiliary system and is therefore helpful in the diagnosis of cholestasis in childhood.

## Other Diagnostic Studies

A host of other diagnostic studies and procedures are performed in children to investigate liver disease. Some of these will be mentioned below in the context of specific diseases and include duodenal intubation for examination of bilirubin content; endoscopic retrograde cholangiopancreatography (ERCP); percutaneous transhepatic cholangiography (PTC); ultrasound; laparoscopy; excretion of rose bengal sodium iodine-131; hepatobiliary scintigraphy; and liver biopsy.[37]

# HEPATITIS, NEONATAL AND POSTNATAL

## Neonatal Hepatitis

*Neonatal hepatitis* (or the neonatal hepatitis syndrome) is a term used to describe a category of noninfectious disorders characterized by intrahepatic cholestasis in the newborn accompanied by primary pathologic disturbance of the liver parenchymal cells.[37] Neonatal hepatitis is an idiopathic cause of neonatal cholestasis, also referred to as infantile obstructive cholangiopathy and idiopathic or cryptogenic neonatal cholestasis. It is to be distinguished from extrahepatic bile duct atresia (biliary atresia), from conditions characterized by a paucity of intraheptic bile ducts (e.g., Alagille syndrome and Byler syndrome), and from a variety of infectious, metabolic, toxic, and other causes of neonatal cholestasis, some of which are discussed in this chapter.

Neonatal hepatitis is the most common cause of cholestasis in newborns and has a reported incidence of 1/2,500 to 1/9,000 live births.[38] It presents with prolonged, conjugated hyperbilirubinemia in the newborn, frequently affecting males of low birth weight. The course is variable depending upon whether the case is sporadic or familial: cirrhosis and/or death may occur in about 30 percent of the former and 70 percent of the latter. Surgical exploration of the bile ducts may adversely affect the outcome of infants with neonatal hepatitis,[39] but laparotomy without biliary exploration in sporadic cases may not affect outcome.[40] However, as is true for postnatal viral hepatitis, it is generally recommended that all nonemergency surgery be avoided in infants with this disease until it has become quiescent.

## Hepatitis in the Newborn

Infectious causes of neonatal hepatitis account for only a small portion of all the total cases in the newborn. The infecting agents include bacteria (especially *E. coli* and *Listeria monocytogenes*) and viruses [including the hepatitis viruses discussed below, the human immunodeficiency virus (HIV), and the TORCH complex of agents]. Discussion here will be limited to a brief consideration of the latter.

The term TORCH refers to a group of infectious agents that can affect the fetus and newborn: toxoplasmosis, syphilis, rubella, cytomegalovirus (CMV), and herpes simplex.[41] The liver is involved in all these infections, although other organ systems may also have significant involvement (Table 5-2). All the agents may cause intrauterine infection, while CMV and herpes simplex may also infect the newborn at the time of delivery or in the immediate postpartum period. Hepatomegaly, jaundice, and nonspecific impairment of liver function are commonly present. Calcification of the liver may be evident on radiographic examination of patients with toxoplasmosis and CMV infections. Chronic liver changes are uncommon, although cirrhosis and noncirrhotic portal fibrosis have been described in association with CMV infection.

While there are no specific recommendations concerning anesthesia and surgery for infants with TORCH infections, avoidance of nonurgent surgery during the period of acute inflammation of the liver is prudent. In addition, consideration of the implications of possible central nervous system and/or cardiac involvement in some of these infections is necessary.

## Postnatal Viral Hepatitis

Infants and children are susceptible to the same viruses that cause hepatitis in adults: hepatitis A virus (HAV); hepatitis B virus (HBV); non-A, non-B hepatitis viruses (NANB), including two identified blood-borne agents [one of which is the hepatitis C virus, (HCV)] and one enterically transmitted agent; and hepatitis D (HDV), the delta agent that requires con-

**Table 5-2.** Torch Infections: Physical Manifestations and Treatment

| *Agent* | *Clinical Findings* | *Drug Therapy* |
|---|---|---|
| Toxoplasmosis | Hydrocephalus with intracranial calcifications<br>Microcephaly<br>Chorioretinitis | Pyrimethamine isethionate<br>Sulfadiazine |
| Syphilis | Rhinitis<br>Rash<br>Osteitis | Penicillin |
| Rubella | Cataracts, cloudy cornea<br>Deafness<br>Petechiae<br>Cardiac malformations[a] | — |
| Cytomegalovirus | Microcephaly with periventricular calcifications<br>Deafness | — |
| Herpes | Vesicular rash<br>Keratoconjunctivitis<br>Acute central nervous system disease | Acyclovir<br>Vidarabine |

[a] Patent ductus arteriosus, peripheral pulmonic stenosis, atrial and ventricular septal defects.
(Adapted from Alpert and Plotkin,[79] with permission.)

comitant hepatitis B infection.[42] None of the hepatitis viruses are significant causes of neonatal hepatitis, although all except HAV have been shown to be transmitted from mother to newborn. Transmission of HBV from mother to infant is most likely to occur when the mother carries the hepatitis B e antigen ($HB_eAg$), or when she is acutely infected in the third trimester of pregnancy or early postpartum. Table 5-3 shows some important aspects of the different postnatal virus infections.

The clinical presentation of viral hepatitis is variable: it may be symptomatic with or without jaundice (i.e., icteric or anicteric, respectively), or asymptomatic with detectable liver enzyme and serologic changes or with serologic changes only (i.e., subclinical or inapparent, respectively). In general, younger patients are more likely to have asymptomatic HAV and HBV infections. The signs and symptoms of infection are varied and generally nonspecific. The prodromal period may be characterized by fatigue, anorexia, fever, headache, abdominal discomfort, loss of appetite, vomiting, weight loss; sore throat and cough; arthralgias, arthritis, myalgias, rash, urticaria, hematuria, proteinuria; and neuritis and other neurologic changes. The icteric period may be marked by darkening of the urine, lightening of the stool, jaundice, pruritus, enlargement and tenderness of the liver, splenomegaly, and lymphadenopathy. Elevation of serum aminotransferases accompanies the late prodrome, peaks after the onset of jaundice, and may persist for a few months. Jaundice and the rise of serum bilirubin follow the elevation of serum aminotransferases, and they persist for about 6 weeks. Indices of synthetic function (e.g., PT and serum albumin concentration) are normal or only minimally abnormal. Seroconversion generally occurs at the end of incubation or at the onset of symptoms for the various viruses, except for HCV, whose presently available serologic tests may not convert until weeks after clinical symptoms. The listed complications of acute viral hepa-

**Table 5-3.** Postnatal Viral Hepatitis Infections

| *Virus* | *Type* | *Transmission* | *Incubation (weeks)* | *Complication* |
|---|---|---|---|---|
| A | RNA | Enteric | 4 | Cholestatic hepatitis<br>Relapsing hepatitis<br>Fulminant hepatitis |
| B | DNA | Blood, saliva, semen, vaginal fluid, urine, breast milk | 4–26 | Chronic antigen carrier<br>Chronic hepatitis<br>Cirrhosis<br>Hepatocellular carcinoma<br>Fulminant hepatitis |
| Non-A, non-B | | Enteric<br>Blood | 2–9<br>2–26 | Chronic hepatitis<br>Cirrhosis<br>Hepatocellular carcinoma<br>Aplastic anemia |
| Includes: | | | | |
| C | RNA | Blood | | |
| D | RNA | Blood (with HBV) | > 4 | Chronic antigen carrier<br>Chronic hepatitis<br>Cirrhosis |

titis in children are generally rare. However, children under 3 years of age who are infected with HBV are particularly prone to become chronic HBV carriers, with persistence of the HBV surface antigen ($HB_sAg$) and of the antibody to the HBV core antigen (anti-HBc), and to develop chronic hepatitis.

Acute viral hepatitis poses problems for surgery and anesthesia in addition to the general considerations described previously. The risk of transmission of a virus to the health care provider during the acute phase of an infection is naturally magnified.[43] Based on information from adults, the risk of perioperative morbidity and mortality for the patient is generally recognized to be significantly increased by the presence of acute viral hepatitis,[44–47] and all elective surgery should be delayed until at least 1 month after liver function tests have returned to normal.[1,3,6,8] Patients with chronic hepatitis (either chronic persistent hepatitis or chronic active hepatitis) who have been asymptomatic for at least 3 months tolerate anesthesia well.[48,49] Patients on chronic corticosteroid therapy for chronic hepatitis should receive appropriate additional "stress" coverage during the perioperative period. Patients with symptomatic chronic active hepatitis should have all nonemergency surgery deferred until there is clinical improvement.

## Biliary Atresia

Biliary atresia or extrahepatic bile duct atresia is the cause of about one-third of the cases of neonatal cholestasis, with a reported incidence of 1/8,000 to 1/25,000.[37,38] Biliary atresia is slightly more common in girls and has no familial predilection, but may be associated in about 10 percent of cases with other significant anomalies (i.e., cardiovascular defects, polysplenia, intestinal malrotation, and situs inversus). Based on clinical and pathologic characteristics, there appear to be two general types of this disorder: (1) an embryonic or fetal type, characterized by an immediate onset of jaundice after birth, the presence of no identifiable bile duct remnants in the porta hepatis, and the presence of other defects; and (2) a perinatal type, characterized by later onset of neonatal jaundice after a jaundice-free period, the presence of bile duct remnants, and the absence of associated defects. The latter type accounts for about two-thirds of cases.

Newborns with biliary atresia usually have normal birth weight and appear well, but develop jaundice and acholic stools between the first and sixth weeks of life. Hepatosplenomegaly becomes apparent and the disease progresses to biliary cirrhosis and portal hypertension. Without surgery, the average life expectancy of an infant with biliary atresia is about 2 years; even with surgical intervention, cirrhosis and portal hypertension are common as the intrahepatic process progresses.

Early diagnosis is essential in the management of newborns with cholestasis. This will define easily correctable lesions like choledochal cysts, and it will distinguish nonsurgical causes of intrahepatic cholestasis like neonatal hepatitis from biliary atresia. This distinction can sometimes be suggested by the general clinical picture: liver function tests, viral serology, cultures, metabolic screens, and other diagnosis-specific tests. The distinction can be made by investigative tools specific for the hepatobiliary system (e.g., duodenal intubation for fluid analysis, real-time hepatic ultrasound, and hepatobiliary scintigraphy with technetium-labeled iminodiacetic acid analogues). Ultimately, the diagnosis depends upon liver biopsy and intraoperative cholangiography. For infants with distal atresia of the extrahepatic biliary duct and a patent proximal portion, surgical intervention can provide correction of the defect. For infants with the much more common problem of biliary obstruction at or above the porta hepatis, surgical intervention with hepatoportoenterostomy (Kasai procedure and its modifications) offers only palliation. Even if this procedure is performed before 2 months of age, when bile flow can be established in about 80 percent of cases, long-term complications are common. Orthotopic liver transplantation may now offer a better option for these infants.

While there are no predictors of perioperative outcome for infants with liver disease similar to those developed by Child and Pugh[1,37] for adults with cirrhosis, anesthetic care should address the many problems of infants with biliary atresia. These include poor nutritional status, recurrent ascending cholangitis and other infections, coagulopathy secondary to hypersplenism and malabsorption of the fat-soluble vitamins, and esophageal and gastric varices. Pruritus may occur and may be treated with cholestyramine and/or phenobarbital. Ascites when present may be treated with salt restriction and diuretics.

## TUMORS OF THE LIVER

Primary tumors of the liver are rare in infancy and childhood, and most of those that do occur affect children less than 2 years of age.[50] Unfortunately, the majority of liver tumors are malignant, and optimal management requires thorough preoperative evaluation and considerable skill on the part of the surgeon and anesthesiologist in order to produce the best outcome. Noninvasive imaging, such as ultrasound, contrast-enhanced computerized tomography, and magnetic resonance imaging, has greatly improved the ability to diagnose and stage the tumors.

Surgical excision is the primary therapy for most liver tumors, but, in spite of advances in surgical planning and technique, hepatic resection in childhood carries multiple risks and several anesthetic concerns. These include compromise of ventilation and venous return during upper abdominal manipulation, and sudden and massive hemorrhage accompanying resection. In addition, resection of a hepatic tumor may entail ligation of the hepatic artery, which may lead to further compromise of liver function, coagulopathy, and even renal dysfunction.[21] Finally, as detailed in Table 5-4, the chemotherapeutic agents used in treatment of malignant liver tumors may have side effects that affect anesthetic management.

## Benign Tumors

### Cavernous Hemangioma

The most common of the benign tumors of the liver is cavernous hemangioma; it is usually diagnosed in the older child and adolescent. The tumor is usually discovered as an asymptomatic hepatic mass and is not associated with other visible hemangiomas. Although it may produce abdominal distention and discomfort and may be associated with congestive heart failure, the tumor generally causes no systemic or biochemical abnormalities in older children. In some infants, however, it may consume platelets and produce disseminated intravascular coagulation, a phenomenon referred to as Kasabach-Merritt syndrome. Treatment, which may be necessitated by symptoms such as heart failure, includes steroid therapy and radiation.[51] Surgical resection of a cavernous hemangioma is only rarely indicated (for complications refractory to medical therapy or spontaneous rupture with intraperitoneal hemorrhage). The overall prognosis is excellent.

### Infantile Hemangioendothelioma

A benign tumor affecting infants in the first 6 months of life, infantile hemangioendothelioma may be discovered as an asymptomatic mass but frequently presents in association with heart failure, hepatomegaly, and associated cutaneous hemangiomas. The tumor may enlarge enough to compromise ventilation significantly, and may be accompanied by thrombocytopenia secondary to platelet sequestration. This tumor is difficult to resect, but fortunately it tends to involute spontaneously with time. Therapy is directed toward medical management of congestive failure, and corticosteroid therapy is instituted to promote involution.[52] In cases with heart failure refractory to medical management, radiotherapy may result in improvement; otherwise ligation of the hepatic artery may be necessary.

### Focal Nodular Hyperplasia

Presenting as an asymptomatic hepatic mass, focal nodular hyperplasia occurs in adolescence, usually in girls. A characteristic pattern may be observed on angiography, and, if the diagnosis is certain, no further investigation is indicated. Although biopsy may be necessary to confirm the diagnosis, resection of the mass is not indicated for asymptomatic lesions since there is no evidence that the hyperplasia undergoes malignant change.

### Hepatic Adenoma

An uncommon tumor in children, hepatic adenoma may occur in adolescent girls who are taking oral contraceptives. The adenoma is usually a solitary tumor in the right lobe of the liver, and it presents either as an asymptomatic mass or as the cause of hemoperitoneum from spontaneous rupture. The tumor may regress with cessation of contraceptive administration.[53] Patients with this tumor often require surgical resection because noninvasive imaging is unable to distinguish the lesion from hepatocellular carcinoma, and the risk of spontaneous rupture warrants excision.

**Table 5-4.** Side Effects of Chemotherapeutic Agents Used to Treat Liver Tumors

| *Agent (Trade Name)* | *Side Effects* |
|---|---|
| Bleomycin (Blenoxane) | *Pulmonary:* interstitial pneumonitis (? added effect of $O_2$)<br>*Mucocutaneous:* urticaria, vesiculations, stomatitis |
| Cisplatin (Platinol) | *Renal:* increased serum creatinine and BUN, decreased glomerular filtration rate<br>*Metabolic:* electrolyte imbalance including hypomagnesemia, hypocalcemia, and hypokalemia<br>*Gastrointestinal:* nausea and vomiting<br>*Ototoxicity:* tinnitus, hearing loss<br>*Neurologic:* peripheral neuropathy<br>*Hematologic:* leukopenia, thrombocytopenia, anemia [note: leukocyte and platelet nadirs usually occur at approximately 18–23 days (range, 7–45 days), and return to pretreatment levels within 39 days (range, 13–62 days)] |
| Cyclophosphamide (Cytoxan, Neosar) | *Hematologic:* leukopenia, thrombocytopenia, anemia, and hypothrombinemia (note: leukocyte and platelet nadirs usually occur between 8–15 days after a single dose and recovery usually occurs by 17–28 days)<br>*Gastrointestinal:* nausea, vomiting<br>*Genitourinary:* hemorrhagic cystitis<br>*Pulmonary:* interstitial fibrosis (note: occurs after prolonged high doses)<br>*Metabolic:* hyperuricemia, inappropriate antidiuretic hormone secretion |
| Doxorubicin (Adriamycin, Rubex) | *Hematologic:* leukopenia (principally granuloctyopenia sufficient to produce significant immunocompromise), thrombocytopenia and anemia (nadir occurs during the second week after therapy and recovery by the third week)<br>*Cardiac:* Acute—ST-T wave changes, arrhythmias; chronic—cumulative irreversible dose-related cardiomyopathy producing congestive heart failure and associated complications, especially after cumulative dose of 400–500 mg/m$^2$ (note: many chemotherapy protocols mandate regular assessments of echocardiogram and ejection fraction once an arbitarily cumulative dose of doxorubicin has been administered)<br>*Gastrointestinal:* stomatitis and esophagitis |
| Fluorouracil (Adrucil) | *Hematologic:* granulocytopenia, thrombocytopenia, anemia (nadirs usually occurs 9–17 days and recovery to normal levels by 30 days after treatment)<br>*Gastrointestinal:* anorexia, vomiting, stomatitis, GI ulcer, and bleeding |
| Vincristine (Oncovin, Vincasar) | *Neurologic:* Peripheral neuropathy (including cranial nerve palsy and vocal cord dysfunction), autonomic dysfunction (including orthostatic hypotension)<br>*Mucocutaneous:* alopecia, stomatitis |

## Cystic Disease of the Liver and Biliary Tract

### Choledochal Cysts

Occurring most commonly in infancy and childhood, choledochal cysts[54] may present with isolated cholestasis; with a triad of abdominal pain, jaundice, and mass; or with cholangitis. They are usually not associated with any other abnormalities, except dilatation of the intrahepatic bile ducts. Diagnosis is best made with ultrasonography, and the treatment of choice is surgical excision and choledochojejunostomy.

### Caroli's Disease (Cystic Dilatation of the Intrahepatic Bile Ducts)

Caroli's disease is a nonfamilial congenital disease with saccular dilatation of the intrahepatic bile duct system.[55] It may also be associated with other cystic changes in the liver and biliary system as well as renal tubular ectasia, and usually presents in children and adolescents with a picture of acute cholangitis and/or biliary lithiasis. Treatment is by medical control of cholangitis; surgical intervention may include removal of calculi or partial hepatectomy when the process is confined to a single lobe of the liver.

### Congenital Hepatic Fibrosis

An autosomal recessive disease with fibrotic and cystic changes of the liver that are often accompanied by cystic changes of the kidneys, congenital hepatic fibrosis usually presents in childhood with hepatosplenomegaly, bleeding and other manifestations of portal hypertension, or cholangitis. Treatment is directed toward control of the portal hypertension, including portocaval shunting.

### Solitary Liver Cysts

Cysts may be parasitic or nonparasitic and are rare in childhood. They present with abdominal distention and pain, and occasionally they require surgical treatment due to compression of other organs or internal hemorrhage.

### Polycystic Disease

Polycystic disease involving the liver occurs in two patterns: *adult-type polycystic disease of the kidney* is an autosomal dominant process that may include multiple cysts of the liver, which usually pose no clinical problem; *childhood polycystic disease of the kidneys and liver* is an autosomal recessive disease that is associated with early death due to renal failure or to portal hypertension in those children who survive infancy.

## Malignant Tumors

### Hepatoblastoma

The most common hepatic tumor in childhood, hepatoblastoma usually presents with painless hepatomegaly, nausea, vomiting, and weight loss in children under the age of 3 years. Boys are affected more frequently than girls, and the tumor has been associated with a number of other anomalies, including Beckwith-Wiedemann syndrome and somatic hemihypertrophy. The tumor grows rapidly and may metastasize to the lymph nodes and lungs. Mild anemia, thrombocytosis, leukocytosis, and transaminase elevation are not uncommon, but evidence of significant hepatic dysfunction such as coagulopathy or severe jaundice is unusual. Serum α-FP concentrations are elevated in the majority of patients and may be useful in following the course of therapy. Preoperative evaluation may include radionucleotide scanning, computed tomography, and/or magnetic resonance imaging to delineate the extent of the tumor. Therapy entails surgical excision, which is preceded or followed by aggressive chemotherapy depending upon the resectability of the tumor at presentation. Chemotherapy includes such agents as vincristine, cyclophosphamide, doxorubicin, and 5-fluorouracil, all of which have side effects that may affect anesthetic management (see Table 5-4). Liver transplantation is performed in children whose initial treatment is unsuccessful, although this procedure may be complicated by the toxic effects of the multiple chemotherapeutic agents that have been administered to the children preoperatively.

### Hepatocellular Carcinoma

Occurring in an older age group than hepatoblastoma, hepatocellular carcinoma is rare before the age of 4 years and reaches a peak incidence in late childhood and adolescence. It occurs more frequently in boys, and it is associated with hepatitis B infection and cirrhosis. Jaundice and thrombocytosis are commonly present, and greater than 90 percent of patients have increased serum concentrations of α-FP. Preoperative evaluation is similar to that of hepatoblastoma, and therapy includes a combination of surgical excision and chemotherapy (e.g., vincristine, doxorubicin, cyclophosphamide, 5-fluorouracil, bleomycin, and cisplatin). Prognosis is largely determined by the resectability of the tumor and, despite institution of new therapeutic techniques like continuous infusion of chemotherapeutic agents, prognosis remains poor, most children dying within 2 years of diagnosis.

### Mesenchymoma

A tumor that usually presents as an abdominal mass between 4 and 10 years of age, mesenchymoma is treated by a combination of surgical excision, chemotherapy, and irradiation of the tumor bed.

## METABOLIC DISEASES OF THE LIVER

A large number of metabolic diseases occur in infants and children and involve the liver.[56] Most of these diseases, with the exception of cystic fibrosis, are quite rare. They represent a wide spectrum of disorders in terms of the specific metabolic defect, clinical presentation, treatment, and prognosis. Table 5-5 summarizes information on several specific diseases that may be encountered by the anesthesiologist.[57–64] The description includes the specific considerations for anesthetic management in addition to the general concerns for patients with liver disease, which are detailed above in the section Liver Dysfunction and Anesthesia. Information concerning individual drugs that are used as part of the therapeutic management of each disease is provided in Table 5-6. (Please refer to the Appendix for a more extensive listing of drugs.)

## HEPATIC FAILURE

Hepatic failure is acute liver dysfunction produced by massive necrosis or severe functional impairment of the hepatocytes. When there is associated hepatic encephalopathy, the term *fulminant hepatic failure* is applied.[65]

### Etiology

Hepatic failure may be divided into four broad groups, infectious, toxic, metabolic, and ischemic. Viral hepatitis (es-

**Table 5-5.** Metabolic Diseases Affecting the Liver: Features and Anesthetic Considerations

| *Disease* | *Metabolic Defect* | *Clinical Picture* | *Laboratory Data* | *Treatment* | *Special Considerations for Anesthetic Management* |
|---|---|---|---|---|---|
| Carbohydrate metabolism defects | | | | | |
| Hereditary fructose intolerance | Fructose-1-phosphate aldolase deficiency (autosomal recessive) | Vomiting, jaundice, hypoglycemia, hepatomegaly, ascites, bleeding | ↓ Glucose, ↑ ALT, ↓ $PO_4$, ↓ clotting factors, ↓ albumin; renal tubular dysfunction | Fructose and sucrose restriction | Glucose administration; monitor bleeding; hepatic precautions[a] |
| Galactosemia | Galactose-1-phosphate uridyl transferase deficiency (autosomal recessive) | Vomiting, jaundice, hepatomegaly, ascites, failure to thrive; cataracts; mental retardation | ↓ Glucose, abnormal liver function tests, positive reducing substance in urine | Lactose and galactose restriction | Monitor glucose; hepatic precautions[a] |
| Glycogen storage diseases[57–59] | | | | | |
| Type I, von Gierke's disease | Glucose-6-phosphatase deficiency (autosomal recessive) | Hypoglycemia, hepatomegaly, growth failure; platelet dysfunction; renal enlargement; "doll-like" facies | ↓ Glucose, ↑ lipids, ↑ lactic acid, ↑ uric acid, ↑ transaminases | Frequent feedings; oral bicarbonate | Glucose administration; monitor blood pH, bleeding; hepatic precautions[a] |
| Type III, Forbes disease | Amylo-1,6-glucosidase ("debrancher") deficiency (autosomal recessive) | Hepatomegaly, growth failure; none to moderate hypotonia and cardiomegaly; rare liver or heart failure; milder than type I | ↓ Glucose, ↑ lipids, ↑ transaminases | Frequent feedings of high-protein diet | Monitor glucose, heart function; hepatic precautions[a] |
| Type IV, Andersen's disease | α-1.4-Glucan 6-glycosyl transferase ("brancher") deficiency (autosomal recessive) | Hepatosplenomegaly, cirrhosis; hypotonia; vomiting, diarrhea | Abnormal liver function tests, acidosis | Frequent feedings of high-protein diet | Monitor blood pH; hepatic precautions[a] |

| | | | | | |
|---|---|---|---|---|---|
| Protein metabolism defect | | | | | |
| Hereditary tyrosinemia | Fumaryl acetoacetase deficiency (autosomal recessive) | Acute infantile or chronic forms; failure to thrive, vomiting, diarrhea; jaundice, hepatosplenomegaly, ascites, cirrhosis; hepatomas; rickets; bruising; renal tubular dysfunction | Abnormal liver function tests; ↓ glucose; ↓ clotting factors; proteinuria, glucosuria | Low phenylalanine + tyrosine diet; rickets therapy; liver transplant | Monitor glucose, bleeding; hepatic precautions[a] |
| Lipid metabolism defect | | | | | |
| Wolman's disease | Acid lipase defiency (autosomal recessive) | Vomiting, diarrhea, failure to thrive; hepatosplenomegaly | Abnormal liver function tests; adrenal calcifications | None | Hepatic precautions[a] |
| Bile acid metabolism defects | | | | | |
| Byler syndrome[63] | Unknown: possible defect in bile acid transport, formation or excretion (autosomal recessive) | Pruritus, jaundice, hepatosplenomegaly, heaptic failure, encephalopathy | ↑ Bile acids, ↑ alkaline phosphatase, ↑ bilirubin, ↑ transaminases; normal cholesterol, 5′-NT, GGTP | ? Phenobarbital<br>? Cholestyramine | Hepatic precautions[a] |
| Alagille syndrome-(arteriohepatic dysplasia)[63] | Unknown: possible defect in bile acid formation (autosomal dominant) | Characteristic facies with flat and bulboused tip nose, deep set and widely spaced eyes, small mandible; nonprogressive pruritus, jaundice, hepatomegaly; peripheral pulmonic stenosis, patent ductus arteriosus and other cardiac defects; vertebral anomalies; arthropathy; ophthalmologic changes (embryotoxon); areflexia; xanthomas; rickets | ↑ Bile acids, ↑ alkaline phosphatase, ↑ bilirubin, ↑ 5′-NT, ↑ GGPT, ↑ cholesterol | ? Phenobarbital<br>? Cholestyramine | Monitor cardiac function, subacute bacterial endocarditis prophylaxis; hepatic precautions[a] |

(*Continues*)

**Table 5-5.** *(Continued)*

| *Disease* | *Metabolic Defect* | *Clinical Picture* | *Laboratory Data* | *Treatment* | *Special Considerations for Anesthetic Management* |
|---|---|---|---|---|---|
| Zellweger syndrome (cerebro-hepato-renal syndrome) | Defect in bile acid formation | Distinctive facies with high forehead; hypotonia, seizures; jaundice, hepatomegaly, progressive hepatic failure; renal cortical cysts | ↑ Transaminases, ↑ bilirubin, ↑ prothrombin time; ↑ precursors of cholic and chenodeoxycholic acids | None | Hepatic precautions[a] |
| Bilirubin metabolism defects | | | | | |
| Crigler-Najjar syndrome | | | | | |
| Type I | Absent bilirubin uridine diphosphate glucuronyl transferase (autosomal recessive) | Severe jaundice, kernicterus | ↑ Bilirubin (20–25 mg/dL), mostly unconjugated | Phototherapy; plasmapheresis; exchange transfusion; tin-protoporphyrin; liver transplant | Monitor bilirubin; phototherapy; avoid prolonged fasting; avoid acidosis, hyperosmolarity, and drugs that displace bilirubin from protein (sulfas, cephalosporins, contrast dyes); most anesthetic agents (morphine, muscle relaxants, barbiturates, volatile agents) okay[62] |
| Type II | Deficient glucuronyl transferase (autosomal dominant) | Jaundice, usually milder | ↑ Bilirubin, mostly unconjugated | Phenobarbital, phototherapy | |
| Gilbert syndrome | Deficient glucuronyl transferase activity (autosomal dominant) | Intermitten jaundice, especially with stress | ↑ Bilirubin, mild (mostly unconjugated) | Phenobarbital | Monitor bilirubin, avoid prolonged fasting |
| Dubin-Johnson syndrome<br>Rotor syndrome | Unknown: defects in transfer of bilirubin and other organic acids from liver to bile (autosomal recessive) | Jaundice, mild | ↑ Bilirubin (mostly conjugated | None | Monitor bilirubin |

| | | | | | |
|---|---|---|---|---|---|
| Unclassified | | | | | |
| α-1 antitrypsin deficiency | Unknown (autosomal recessive) (incidence: 1:2,000–4,000) | Neonatal cholestasis or jaundice, hepatomegaly by age 4 y; cirrhosis, portal hypertension, hepatic failure; associated pulmonary disease less common in children than in adults | ↑ Transaminases, ↑ bilirubin; ↓ serum α-1-antitrypsin (10–15% of normal levels in most common subtype, PiZZ) | Liver transplant, smoking avoidance | Monitor pulmonary function; hepatic precautions[a] |
| Wilson's disease (hepatolenticular degeneration) | Unknown: possible defect in biliary excretion of copper (autosomal recessive) (incidence: 1:30,000–50,000) | Acute fulminant hepatitis picture or chronic, indolent hepatic dysfunction, cirrhosis, hepatomegaly; Kayser-Fleischer rings; renal proximal tubular dysfunction; neuropsychiatric signs from teen years (tremor, drooling, rigidity, anxiety, depression, psychosis) | Abnormal liver function tests, ↓ ceruloplasmin, ↑ urine copper, ↑ serum free copper, ↑ hepatic copper | ↓ Cu intake; chelator therapy—dimercaprol (BAL) or D-penicillamine or triethylene tetramine dihyrochloride (trientine); ? zinc therapy; liver transplant | ↓ D-penicillamine dose perioperatively; hepatic precautions[a,60,64] |
| Cystic fibrosis | Unknown: possible α-2-macroglobulin defect (autosomal recessive) (incidence: 1:1,600 | Pancreatic insufficiency; pulmonary infection, fibrosis, obstruction, restriction and hypertension; neonatal cholestasis, jaundice, hepatosplenomegaly, portal hypertension, biliary cirrhosis | ↑ Sweat Cl; arterial hypoxemia, obstruction and restriction by pulmonary function tests; chronic lung changes by chest x-ray; right ventricular hypertrophy by EKG; abnormal liver function tests, ↑ prothrombin time, ↓ albumin | Pancreatic enzyme supplements; antibiotics, bronchodilators, chest physiotherapy; oxygen; diuretics, digoxin | Adequate hydration; monitor cardiopulmonary function; avoid $N_2O$, excessively high airway pressures, antisialagogues; pulmonary therapy and pain control; hepatic precautions[a,1] |

[a] Hepatic precautions: take care with drugs metabolized in the liver, check coagulation, and monitor glucose levels. Halothane may reduce hepatic blood flow; thus, isoflurane is preferred.

(Adapted from Ghishan and Greene,[56] with permission.)

**Table 5-6.** Therapeutic Agents Used in Treatment of Liver Diseases

| *Medication* | *Route* | *Dose* | *Indication* | *Adverse Reactions* |
|---|---|---|---|---|
| Acyclovir (Zovirax) | IV | 250 mg/m$^2$ | Antiviral | Renal insufficiency, rash, headache, nausea |
| Azathioprine (Imuran) | IV<br>Oral | 3–5 mg/kg/d | Immunosuppressive | Myelodepression, nausea, vomiting, diarrhea, hepatotoxicity, rash, fever, arthralgias |
| Captopril (Capoten) | Oral | 0.5–1.5 mg/kg/dose | Antihypertensive | Neutropenia, proteinuria |
| Cholestyramine (Questran) | Oral | 250 mg–1 g/kg/d | Resin for removal of bile acids | Constipation, nausea, interferes with absorption of fat-soluble vitamins |
| Cimetidine (Tagamet) | IV<br>Oral | 5–10 mg/kg/dose | $H_2$-blocker | Inhibits metabolism of many medications |
| Cyclosporine (Sandimmune) | IV<br>Oral | Individualized based on plasma concentrations | Immunosuppressive | Nephrotoxicity, hypertension, hirsutism, nausea, diarrhea |
| Dimercaprol (BAL in Oil) | IM | 2–4 mg/kg/dose | Chelating agent | Hypertension, nephrotoxicity, pain with intramuscular injection |
| Flumazenil (Mazicon) | IV | 5–40 μg/kg/dose | Benzodiazepine antagonist | Seizures in patients habituated to benzodiazepine |
| Methylprednisolone (Solu-Medrol) | IV or oral | 0.1–1.5 mg/kg/dose | Antiinflammatory | Glucose intolerance, hypertension, peptic ulcer, hypokalemia |
| Penicillamine (Cuprimine) | Oral | 250 mg/dose | Chelating agent | Agranulocytosis, proteinuria, interferes with tissue healing |
| Phenobarbital (Luminal) | IV<br>Oral | Load: 10–20 mg/kg; maintenance: 3–5 mg/kg/d | Anticonvulsant; enzyme inducer | Drowsiness, ataxia |
| Propranolol (Inderal) | IV<br>Oral | 0.1–0.2 mg/kg/dose<br>0.2–1.0 mg/kg/dose | Antihypertensive | Bradycardia, hypotension |
| Pyrimethamine (Daraprim) | Oral | 0.5 mg/kg/dose | Antiprotozoal | Myelodepression, ataxia, cutaneous eruptions |
| Pyrimethamine/ sulfadoxine (Fansidar) | Oral | Variable | Antiprotozoal | Myelodepression, ataxia, cutaneous eruptions |
| Ranitidine (Zantac) | IV<br>Oral | 0.25–1 mg/kg/dose<br>1–2 mg/kg/dose | $H_2$-blocker | Dizziness, headache, mental confusion |
| Vidarabine (Vira-A) | IV | 10–15 mg/kg/d (continuous infusion) | Antiviral | Nausea, elevated transaminases, thrombophlebitis |

pecially types A and B) is the most common cause of hepatic failure in children. However, for reasons that are unclear, only 1 to 2 percent of such patients actually develop hepatic failure. Drugs and chemicals may also produce hepatic failure by either a dose-related toxic effect or by an idiosyncratic reaction. Dose-related hepatotoxicity is associated with acetominophen overdose, carbon tetrachloride, or poisoning with *Amanita phalloides.* Idiosyncratic reactions are occasionally seen with sodium valproate administration or (rarely) with exposure to halothane and other volatile anesthetics. Wilson's disease, described in Table 5-5, is the most common metabolic defect producing hepatic failure in the pediatric patient. Ischemic hepatic failure may occur following cardiovascular collapse.

## Clinical and Laboratory Presentation

The clinical manifestations of hepatic failure include fever, vomiting, abdominal pain, progressive jaundice, and encephalopathy, the latter described in detail below. Laboratory evaluation usually reveals an increase in both direct and indirect fractions of bilirubin concentration, although jaundice may be minimal or absent with an acute hepatocellular injury. Serum aminotransferase concentrations are markedly elevated early in the disease process, but these concentrations do not correlate well with the severity of the illness and may, in fact, abruptly decrease preterminally. Serum ammonia is usually elevated, although it should be recognized that ammonia may be simply a marker for disordered metabolism and not an etiologic agent of encephalopathy; in addition, the actual serum concentration of ammonia does not correlate with the presence or stage of hepatic encephalopathy.[66] Prothrombin time is almost always prolonged and does not improve with administration of vitamin K; severe prolongations of prothrombin time are associated with a very poor prognosis. Hypoglycemia may accompany hepatic failure. Other associated abnormalities include hypoxemia secondary to intrapulmonary and extrapulmonary shunting; renal failure; and accompanying electrolyte and metabolic changes (e.g., hypokalemia, hyponatremia, metabolic acidosis, and respiratory alkalosis).

## Hepatic Encephalopathy

The encephalopathy associated with hepatic failure is dramatic but poorly understood, and is characterized by a reversible decrease in level of consciousness. While hepatic encephalopathy is not caused by cerebral edema (described below), it may be associated with cerebral edema in many patients with acute hepatic failure. The encephalopathy results in a constellation of signs and symptoms that include personality change, motor abnormalities, and alterations in consciousness and brainstem responses. In adults, the neurologic condition is commonly graded on a specific four-stage scale (Table 5-7)[67]; in both adults and children in coma, assessment can be graded with the Glasgow Coma Scale, which has also been modified for use in preverbal children (Table 5-8). The etiology of hepatic encephalopathy is unclear, but it may be mediated by multiple synergistic agents, including ammonia, fatty acids, and neurotransmitters. Gamma-aminobutyric acid (GABA) is of particular interest in this regard, first, because the GABA-mediated action of benzodiazepines is exaggerated in patients with encephalopathy, and second, rapid

**Table 5-7.** Grading or Staging of Hepatic Coma

| *Stage* | *Signs* |
|---|---|
| I | Alteration of mood, intellect, and speech; disorientation; personality change, mild confusion, disordered sleep |
| II | Disorientation progressing to lethargic state; inappropriate behavior |
| III | Precoma; stuporous but responsive to stimuli; loss of alpha activity on the electroencephalogram; incoherent and confused |
| IV | Frank coma, poor and inconsistent response to stimuli; decerebrate posture may appear; theta activity on electroencephalogram, moving to diffuse slowing and delta activity; little or no response to painful stimuli |

(From Colon,[67] with permission.)

**Table 5-8.** Coma Scale: Adult Glasgow Coma Scale, Pediatric Modified Glasgow Coma Scale

| *Adult* | | *Pediatric* | |
|---|---|---|---|
| *Parameter* | *Score* | *Parameter* | *Score* |
| Eyes open | | | |
| Spontaneity | 4 | Same | 4 |
| To speech | 3 | Same | 3 |
| To pain | 2 | Same | 2 |
| None | 1 | Same | 1 |
| Verbal response | | | |
| Oriented | 5 | Same | 5 |
| Confused | 4 | Words | 4 |
| Inappropriate | 3 | Vocal sounds | 3 |
| Incomprehensible | 2 | Cries | 2 |
| None | 1 | None | 1 |
| Motor response | | | |
| Obeys commands | 5 | Same | 5 |
| Localizes pain | 4 | Same | 4 |
| Flexion to pain | 3 | Same | 3 |
| Extension to pain | 2 | Same | 2 |
| None | 1 | Same | 1 |
| Normal total scores | | | |
| 0–6 mo | | | 9 |
| 6–12 mo | | | 11 |
| 12–25 mo | | | 12 |
| 24–60 mo | | | 13 |
| > 5 y | | | 14 |

(Modified from Colon,[67] with permission.)

but transient improvement in the level of consciousness of a patient with hepatic encephalopathy can be obtained following administration of the benzodiazepine antagonist flumazenil.[68] This effect of flumazenil can also help to distinguish hepatic encephalopathy from other causes of central nervous system depression in patients with severe liver disease (e.g., cerebral edema or intracranial hemorrhage).

Cerebral edema frequently occurs in children with hepatic failure and may be the cause of death in a significant number.[69,70] This cerebral edema is a separate complication of hepatic failure and is not a cause or result of hepatic encephalopathy. Increased intracranial pressure is a consistent finding in animals with experimentally induced fulminant hepatic failure.[71] Neurologic signs associated with cerebral edema in hepatic failure in children include unequal and abnormally reactive pupils, increased muscle tone, posturing, and seizures. However, the absence of these signs does not necessarily imply normal intracranial pressure since they may not be observed until this is significantly elevated.[72]

## Treatment

The care of children with hepatic failure continues to be limited to supportive measures since there is no known therapy to restore function to the hepatocytes. In advanced cases, intensive care with continuous monitoring is required. Nutrition should be provided, using hypertonic glucose via a central venous catheter, to minimize endogenous protein catabolism and consequent ammonia production. Serum glucose concentrations may fluctuate dramatically and should be monitored frequently. Coagulation status must be assessed and abnormalities treated with vitamin K and fresh-frozen plasma. Prophylactic therapy with antacids and $H_2$-receptor blockers should be instituted since there is a high incidence of gastrointestinal bleeding, which aggravates the production of ammonia. The child's gastrointestinal tract is usually purged, and lactulose is administered by nasogastric tube in an effort to reduce the production of ammonia by intestinal bacteria. Flumazenil may be administered to reverse alteration of consciousness transiently. If airway protection and/or ventilatory support is indicated, endotracheal intubation should be performed in a manner tailored to minimize increases in intracranial pressure.

### Prognosis

The overall mortality with fulminant hepatic failure is about 70 percent, although the prognosis may be better in children than in adults. The individual prognosis may depend on the primary disease, since it appears that the prognosis for full recovery is better for patients whose underlying problem is acetaminophen overdose, viral hepatitis, or Wilson's disease, all of which are relatively common in childhood. Complete recovery with regeneration of normal structure and function of the liver is the usual outcome for those who survive hepatic failure, even those with hepatic necrosis and encephalopathy. Since the overall survival with liver transplantation in children is about 80 percent, it would be optimal to be able to differentiate between those patients who will recover with supportive therapy and those who may benefit from immediate transplantation.

### Anesthetic Considerations

Surgical intervention for patients in hepatic failure is generally limited to emergency procedures (e.g., placement of an intracranial pressure monitoring device, exploration for such complications as hemorrhage and infection, or transplantation). It is apparent from the above discussion that all the anesthetic concerns previously described for patients with hepatic disease are vital for patients in hepatic failure: avoidance of techniques that may reduce hepatic perfusion, and attention to alterations in hepatic, pulmonary, hemostatic, renal, and central nervous system function. The presence of encephalopathy and/or cerebral edema can be expected to compromise significantly the patient's tolerance to sedative and anesthetic agents.

## CHILD WITH A TRANSPLANTED LIVER

### Orthotopic Liver Transplantation in Children

Orthotopic liver transplantation is now an accepted therapeutic option for patients with liver disease. Survival has consistently improved: the 3-year survival rate is now about 70 percent (1992), and 1-year survival rates are as high as 86 percent.[73,74]

Indications for pediatric liver transplantation differ from those for adults. The majority of pediatric transplants (50 to 75 percent) are for cirrhosis caused by obstructive diseases of the biliary system, particularly biliary atresia. Metabolic disorders like α-1 antitrypsin deficiency and Wilson's disease represent a distant second indication. At the same time, experience with transplantation in children with α-1 antitrypsin deficiency has been satisfying because the recipients have developed the phenotype of the donor liver and no other medical complications of the disease.[75] In institutions with a busy transplantation service, the need for retransplantation for allograft dysfunction may increase the number of total transplants to a significant degree. The rate of retransplantation seems to be higher in children than in adults, a finding that may reflect the more technically demanding surgical anastomoses required with small vessels. Transplantation has also been performed with some success as an emergency treatment for children with fulminant hepatic failure, as noted above. Transplant experience for children with primary hepatic tumors has been disappointing, as the rate of tumor recurrence in recipients is high.

## Anesthetic Considerations

The topic of transplantation is broad, and a discussion of the anesthetic management is presented elsewhere.[76] The focus here is on the child with a transplanted liver who presents for surgery (e.g., liver biopsy, any unrelated procedure, even retransplantation). In general, if the transplantation has been successful, the medical and anesthetic concerns that applied to the child before transplantation (e.g., liver dysfunction, portal hypertension, coagulopathy) should not be ongoing. At the same time, other concerns related to the post-transplantation period and to specific complications of transplantation may arise.[77]

In the immediate post-transplantation period, the overriding concern is the possible rejection of the graft, which usually occurs within 1 to 6 weeks. Donor livers are not matched for HLA antigens, only ABO blood group antigens, and patients are therefore maintained on chronic immunosuppressive therapy after transplantation. This therapy (Table 5-4) includes cyclosporin A; azathioprine; prednisone; and, for episodes of rejection, polyclonal antibodies [e.g., antilymphocyte globulin (ALG)], and/or monoclonal antibodies directed specifically against T cells (e.g., OKT3). Cyclosporine, the mainstay of immunosuppressive therapy, may potentiate the anesthetic effects of pentobarbital and fentanyl[78]; in addition, its metabolism is altered by any agent that affects the cytochrome P-450 system. The signs and symptoms of graft rejection are nonspecific (i.e., fever, hepatosplenomegaly, and an elevation of serum transaminases) and cannot be differentiated from other possible complications. Histologic examination of the liver is often the only way to make a specific diagnosis of acute rejection, as well as to follow the course of the child who is apparently doing well; for the uncooperative child, liver biopsy may entail sedation under the supervision of the anesthesiologist.

An additional concern after transplantation is the common occurrence of infections. These may include wound infections, perihepatic abscesses and other infections related to transplantation surgery; bacterial, fungal, and viral infections transmitted by the graft itself or blood administered during the procedure; and any opportunistic infection related to immunosuppressive therapy. These infections pose a potential risk both to the patient and the health-care provider.

Surgical complications other than infection may occur, and may require intervention. Any one of a large number of anastomotic sites may hemorrhage. Thrombosis of the hepatic artery, which may present with fever, abdominal pain, and elevation of serum transaminase concentrations, develops more commonly in children than in adults. Biliary drainage established during transplantation via a cholecystojejunostomy into a Roux en Y loop of bowel may become disrupted and lead to bile leakage and infection. For the anesthesiologist, these surgical complications pose the possible problems of intravascular depletion, abdominal distention, ileus, and renal dysfunction.

## SUMMARY

Liver disease in the infant and child includes a wide array of disorders that may have an infectious, oncologic, metabolic, or developmental origin. These disorders pose a particular challenge to the anesthesiologist because they often involve several systems. The anesthetic management of patients with one of these disorders should include a complete appreciation of the hepatic and systemic effects of the disorder, the side effects of the medications utilized to treat the disorder, and the interaction of the effects of the disorder with individual anesthetic agents and techniques.

## REFERENCES


1. Friedman LS, Maddrey WC. Surgery in the patient with liver disease. Med Clin North Am 71:453, 1987
2. Clark RSJ, Doggart JR, Lavery T. Changes in liver function after different types of surgery. Br J Anaesth 48:119, 1976
3. Brown FH, Shiau Y, Richter GC: Anesthesia and surgery in the patient with liver disease. p. 326. In Goldmann DR, Brown FH, Levy WK et al (eds): Medical Care of the Surgical Patient, Problem-Oriented Approach to Management. JB Lippincott, Philadelphia, 1982
4. Batchelder BM, Cooperman LH: Effects of anesthetics on splanchnic circulation and metabolism. Surg Clin North Am 55: 787, 1975
5. Brown BR, Jr: Adverse effects of volatile anaesthetics. Br J Anaesth 59:14, 1987
6. Conn M: Preoperative evaluation of the patient with liver disease. Mt Siani J Med 58:75, 1991
7. Cooperman LH, Warden MB, Price HL: Splanchnic circulation during nitrous oxide anesthesia and hypocarbia in normal man. Anesthesiology 29:254, 1968
8. Gholson CF, Provenza JM, Bacon BR: Hepatologic considerations in patients with parenchymal liver disease undergoing surgery. Am J Gastroenterol 85:487, 1990
9. Gelman SI: Disturbances in hepatic blood flow during anesthesia and surgery. Arch Surg 111:881, 1976
10. Ngai SH: Effects of anesthetics on various organs. N Engl J Med 302:564, 1980
11. Gelman S: Liver circulation and function during isoflurane and halothane anesthesia. Anesthesiology 61:726, 1984
12. Wark H, O'Halloran M, Overton J: Prospective study of liver function in children following multiple halothane anaesthetics at short intervals. Br J Anaesth 58:1224, 1986
13. Wark H, Earl J, Cooper M, Overton J: Halothane in children with chronic liver disease. Anaesth Intens Care 19:9, 1991
14. Jones RM, Diamond JG, Power SJ et al: A prospective study of liver function in infants and children exposed to daily isoflurane for several weeks. Anaesthesia 46:686, 1991
15. Carrigan TW, Straughen WJ: A report of hepatic necrosis and death following isoflurane anesthesia. Anesthesiology 67: 581, 1987
16. Paull JD, Fortune DW: Hepatotoxicity and death following two enflurane anaesthetics. Anaesthesia 42:1191, 1987
17. Stoelting RK, Blitt CD, Cohen PJ, Merin RG: Hepatic dysfunction after isoflurane anesthesia. Anesth Analg 66:147, 1987
18. Kenna JG, Neuberger J, Mieli-Vergani G et al: Halothane hepatitis in children. Br Med J 294:1209, 1987

19. Strunin L: Anaesthetic management of patients with liver disease. p. 1379. In Wright R, Millward-Sadler GH, Alberti KGMM, Karran S (eds): Liver and Biliary Disease: Pathophysiology, Diagnosis, and Management. WB Saunders, Co: Philadelphia, 1985
20. Farman J: Anaesthesia and periopertive care for patients with liver disease. Br J Hosp Med 36:448, 1986
21. Iwatsuki S, Geis WP: Hepatic complications. Surg Clin North Am 57:1335, 1977
22. McEvedy BA, Shelly MP, Park GR: Anaesthesia and liver disease. Br J Hosp Med 36:26, 1986
23. Kelly DA, Tuddenham EGD: Haemostatic problems in liver disease. Gut 27: 339, 1986
24. Rubin MH, Weston MJ, Langley PG et al: Platelet function in chronic liver disease. Dig Dis Sci 24:197, 1979
25. Bass NM, Williams RL: Hepatic function and pharmacokinetics. p. 235. In Zakim D, Boyer TD (eds): Hepatology: A Textbook of Liver Disease. WB Saunders, Philadelphia, 1990
26. Williams RL: Drug administration in hepatic disease. N Engl J Med 309:1616, 1983
27. Neal EA, Meffin PJ, Gregory PB, Blaschke TF: Enhanced bioavailability and decreased clearance of analgesics in patients with cirrhosis. Gastroenterology 77:96, 1979
28. Chauvin M, Ferrier C, Haberer JP et al: Sufentanil pharmacokinetics in patients with cirrhosis. Anesth Analg 68:1, 1989
29. Ferrier C, Marty J, Bouffard Y et al: Alfentanil pharmacokinetics in patients with cirrhosis. Anesthesiology 62:480, 1985
30. Haberer JP, Schoeffler P, Couderc E, Duvaldestin P: Fentanyl pharmacokinetics in anaesthetized patients with cirrhosis. Br J Anaesth 54:1267, 1982
31. McEvoy GK, Litvak K: American Hospital Formulary Service '91. p. 2342. American Society of Hospital Pharmacists, Bethesda, 1991
32. Meredith CG, Christian CD, Jr, Johnson RF et al: Diphenhydramine disposition in chronic liver disease. Clin Pharmacol Ther 35:474, 1984
33. Pandele G, Chaux F, Salvador C et al: Thiopental pharmacokinetics in patients with cirrhosis. Anesthesiology 59:123, 1983
34. Sebel PS, Lowdon JD: Propofol: a new intravenous anesthetic. Anesthesiology 71:260, 1989
35. Schemel WH: Unexpected hepatic dysfunction found by multiple laboratory screening. Anesth Analg 55:810, 1976
36. Wataneeyawech M, Kelly KA, Jr: Hepatic diseases unsuspected before surgery. NY State J Med 75:1278, 1975
37. Desmet VJ, Callea F: Cholestatic syndromes of infancy and childhood. p. 1355. In Zakim D, Boyer TD (eds): Hepatology: A Textbook of Liver Disease. WB Saunders, Co: Philadelphia, 1990
38. Moyer MS, Balistreri WF: Prolonged neonatal obstructive jaundice. p. 835. In Walker WA, Durie PR, Hamilton JR et al (eds): Pediatric Gastrointestinal Disease: Pathophysiology, Diagnosis, Management. BC Decker, Philadelphia, 1991
39. Thaler MM, Gellis SS: Studies in neonatal hepatitis and biliary atresia. II. The effect of diagnostic laparotomy on long-term prognosis of neonatal hepatitis. Am J Dis Child 116:262, 1968
40. Lawson EE, Boggs JD: Long-term follow-up of neonatal hepatitis: safety and value of surgical exploration. Pediatrics 53:650, 1974
41. Andres JM: Congenital infections of the liver. p. 848. In Walker WA, Durie PR, Hamilton JR et al (eds): Pediatric Gastrointestinal Disease: Pathophysiology, Diagnosis, Management. BC Decker, Philadelphia, 1991
42. Koff RS: Viral hepatitis. p. 857. In Walker WA, Durie PR, Hamilton JR et al (eds): Pediatric Gastrointestinal Disease: Pathophysiology, Diagnosis, Management. BC Decker, Philadelphia, 1991
43. Browne RA: Infectious diseases and the anaesthetist. Can J Anaesth 35:655, 1988
44. Bourke JB, Cannon P, Ritchie HD: Laparotomy for jaundice. Lancet 1:521, 1967
45. Hardy KJ, Hughes ESR: Laparotomy in viral hepatitis. Med J Aust 1:710, 1968
46. Harville DD, Summerskill WHJ: Surgery in acute hepatitis. JAMA 184:257, 1963

47. Powell-Jackson P, Greenway B, Williams R: Adverse effects of exploratory laparotomy in patients with unsuspected liver disease. Br J Surg 69:449, 1982
48. Hargrove MD, Jr: Chronic active hepatitis: possible adverse effect of exploratory laparotomy. Surgery 68:771, 1970
49. Runyon BA: Surgical procedures are well tolerated by patients with asymptomatic chronic hepatitis. J Clin Gastroenterol 8: 542, 1986
50. Randolph JG, Guzzetta PC: Tumors of the liver. p. 302. In Welch KJ, Randolph JG, Ravitch MM et al. (eds): Pediatric Surgery. Year Book Medical Publishers, Chicago, 1986
51. Rotman M, John M, Stowe S, Inamdar S: Radiation treatment of pediatric hepatic hemangiomatosis and coexisting cardiac failure. N Engl J Med 302:852, 1980
52. Rocchini AP, Rosenthal A, Issenberg HJ, Nadas AS: Hepatic hemangioendothelioma: hemodynamic observations and treatment. Pediatrics 57:131, 1976
53. Edmondson HA, Reynolds TB, Henderson B, Benton B: Regression of liver cell adenomas associated with oral contraceptives. Ann Inter Med 86:180, 1977
54. Barlow B, Tabor E, Blome WA: Choledochal cyst: a review of 19 cases. J Pediatr 89:934, 1976
55. Suchy FJ: Cystic diseases of the biliary tract and liver. p. 845. In Behrman RE, Vaughan VC III, Nelson WE (eds): Nelson Textbook of Pediatrics. WB Saunders, Philadelphia, 1987
56. Ghishan FK, Greene HL: Inborn errors of metabolism that lead to permanent liver injury. p. 1300. In Zakim D, Boyer TD (eds): Hepatology: A Textbook of Liver Disease. WB Saunders, Philadelphia, 1990
57. Casson H: Anaesthesia for portocaval bypass in patients with metabolic diseases. Br J Anaesth 47:969, 1975
58. Cox JM: Anesthesia and glycogen-storage disease. Anesthesiology 29:1221, 1963
59. Edelstein G, Hirshman CA: Hyperthermia and ketoacidosis during anesthesia in a child with glycogen-storage disease. Anesthesiology 52:90, 1980
60. Greene MW, King RC, Alley RS: Management of an oroantral fistula in a patient with Wilson's disease: case report and review of the literature. Oral Surg Oral Med Oral Pathol 66:293, 1988
61. Lamberty JM, Rubin BK: The management of anesthesia for patients with cystic fibrosis. Anaesthesia 40:448, 1985
62. Prager MC, Johnson KL, Ascher NL, Roberts JP: Anesthetic care of patients with Crigler-Najjar syndrome. Anesth Analg 74:162, 1992
63. Riely CA: Familial intrahepatic cholestatic syndromes. Semin Liver Dis 7:119, 1987
64. Sternlieb I, Scheinberg IH: Bleeding oesophageal varices in patients with Wilson's disease. Lancet 1:638, 1970
65. Jones EA, Schafer DF: Fulminant hepatic failure. p. 460. In Zakim D, Boyer TD (eds): Hepatology: A Textbook of Liver Disease. WB Saunders, Philadelphia, 1990
66. Sullivan JF, Linder H, Holdener P: Blood ammonia in cerebral dysfunction. Am J Med 30:893, 1961
67. Colon AR: Textbook of Pediatric Hepatology. p. 234. 2nd Ed. Vol. 1. Year Book Medical Publishers, Chicago, 1990
68. Bansky G, Meier PJ, Riederer E et al: Effects of the benzodiazepine receptor antagonist flumazenil in hepatic encephalopathy in humans. Gastroenterology 97: 744, 1989
69. Ware AJ, D'Agostino AN, Combes B: Cerebral edema: a major complication of massive hepatic necrosis. Gastroenterology 61:877, 1971
70. Gazzard BG, Portmann B, Murray-Lyon IM, Williams R: Causes of death in fulminant hepatic failure and relationship to quantitative histological assessment of parenchymal damage. Q J Med 44:615, 1975
71. Hanid MA, Mackenzie RL, Jenner RE et al: Intracranial pressure in pigs with surgically induced acute liver failure. Gastroenterology 61:123, 1979
72. Ede RJ, Williams R: Hepatic encephalopathy and cerebral edema. Semin Liver Dis 6:107, 1986
73. Chin SE, Shepherd RW, Cleghorn GJ et al: Survival, growth and quality of life in

children after orthotopic liver transplantation: a 5 year experience. J Paediatr Child Health 27:380, 1991

74. Salt A, Noble-Jamieson G, Barnes ND et al: Liver transplantation in 100 children: Cambridge and King's College Hospital series. Br Med J 304:416, 1992
75. Esquivel CO, Marino IR, Fioravanti V, Van Thiel DH: Liver transplantation for metabolic disease of the liver. Gastroenterol Clin North Am 17:167, 1988
76. Cook DR: Anesthesia for pediatric orthotopic liver transplantation. p. 74. In Winter PM, Kang YG (eds): Hepatic Transplantation. Praeger, New York, 1986
77. Kang Y: Liver transplantation. p. 59. In Lebowitz PW (eds): International Anesthesiology Clincs: Anesthesia and Organ Transplantation. Little Brown and Co, Boston, 1991
78. Cirella VN, Pantuck CB, Lee YJ, Pantuck EJ: Effects of cyclosporine on anesthetic action. Anesth Analg 66:703, 1987
79. Alpert G, Plotkin SA: A practical guide to the diagnosis of congenital infections in the newborn infant. Pediatr Clin North Am 33:465, 1986

# 6

# Diseases of the Endocrine System

# 6

# Diseases of the Endocrine System

*Gary M. Scott*
*David J. Steward*

Diseases of the endocrine system may produce profound changes in physiology and pharmacology that are of special significance to the anesthesiologist. The infant or young child with endocrine disease may be especially unstable during the perioperative and intraoperative period, a result of the combined effects of endocrine dysfunction and higher metabolic rate. This chapter reviews normal endocrine physiology, as well as the clinical presentation, diagnosis, and treatment of various endocrinopathies in children. Important anesthetic implications of hormonal dysfunction are also discussed.

## PITUITARY GLAND

### Normal Function

The secretions of the pituitary gland modulate many body functions, either directly or by regulating the secretions of other endocrine glands. The pituitary gland is composed of the anterior pituitary (adenohypophysis), derived from a primitive ectodermal outgrowth of the oral cavity (Rathke's pouch), and the posterior pituitary (neurohypophysis), derived from the diencephalon, which essentially is an extension of the hypothalamus. The anterior pituitary secretes growth hormone (GH), prolactin (PRL), thyroid-stimulating hormone (TSH), adrenocorticotropin (ACTH), luteinizing hormone (LH), and follicle-stimulating hormone (FSH), plus other substances suspected as having endocrine function. The posterior pituitary stores and secretes vasopressin [antidiuretic hormone (ADH)]. ADH is synthesized in the hypothalamus and transported to the posterior pituitary as granules via neurosecretory axons. Oxytocin is also released from the posterior pituitary.

Normal anterior pituitary function is influenced by central nervous system signals, hypothalamic releasing and inhibiting factors, and feedback from endocrine organ hormones (Fig. 6-1). Hypothalamic hormones regulating the secretion of pituitary hormones include growth hormone-releasing hormone (GHRH), dopamine, thyrotropin-releasing hormone (TRH), corticotropin-releasing hormone (CRH), luteinizing hor-

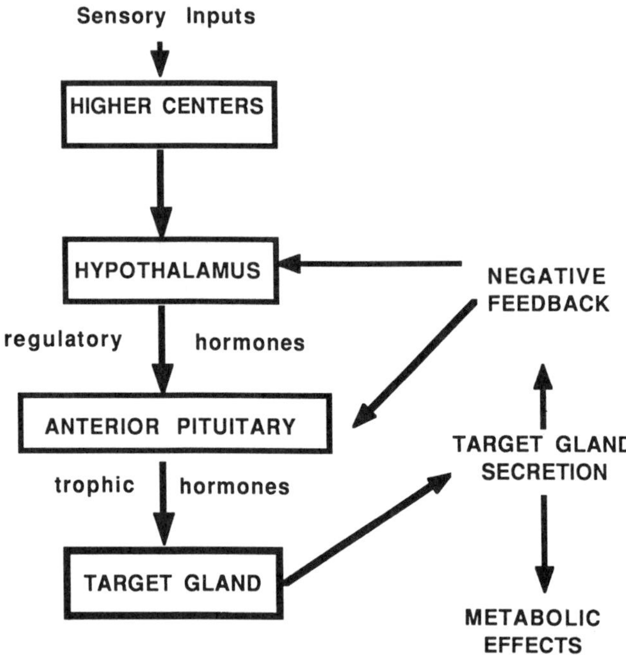


**Fig. 6-1.** Regulatory mechanisms of the endocrine system.

mone-releasing hormone (LHRH), and somatotropin release inhibitory factor (SRIF), which functions as an inhibitor of many other peptides throughout the body.

These regulatory hormones are synthesized in various hypothalamic nuclei and transported from the median eminence to the anterior pituitary via the hypothalamic-pituitary portal circulation. The hormones bind to specific high-affinity receptors on the different pituitary cell types (corticotroph, gonadotroph, lactotroph, somatotroph, thyrotroph), stimulating the release of specific pituitary hormones. Subsequently, the pituitary hormones stimulate target gland hormone production, while peripheral circulating hormones exert a negative feedback on the hypothalamus and pituitary gland.

Disorders of pituitary function in pediatric patients may produce generalized or selective pituitary hormone deficiency or overstimulation of one target gland. Thus a variety of clinical presentations may be encountered by the anesthesiologist. This section reviews disease states associated with deficient and excess production of GH and ADH. Conditions involving dysfunction of other pituitary hormones are discussed elsewhere in this chapter.

## Hypopituitarism

Children rarely have a generalized deficiency of pituitary hormones (panhypopituitarism). However, the term *hypopituitarism* is often used interchangeably with *GH deficiency* in pediatric patients, because a majority of the children will secrete inadequate amounts of GH.

In those patients with true panhypopituitarism, compression of the pituitary gland by a craniopharyngioma is the most common etiology. Other less common causes include hypothalamic tumors, pituitary adenomas, head injury, cranial irradiation, surgical hypophysectomy, infiltrative diseases such as histiocytosis X, infection, and certain congenital malformations.

GH deficiency may be congenital or acquired and will lead to a classical pattern of impaired growth and delayed puberty. In over 50 percent of the children with the diagnosis of hypopituitarism, the precise etiology is unknown, but hypothalmic GHRH dysfunction has been demonstrated.[1] Interestingly, a significant number of these patients have a perinatal history that includes a breech or forceps delivery, intrapartum maternal bleeding, or other form of perinatal insult. It has been suggested that the child's hypothalamic dysfunction may be secondary to the perinatal insult.[2] Craniopharyngioma, septo-optic dysplasia (optic nerve hypoplasia, absence of septum pellucidum, GH deficiency), trauma, cranial irradiation, inflammation, and infection are less frequent causes of GH deficiency.

It is important to realize that impaired growth and other symptoms common to GH deficiency may occur in children without primary pituitary disease, but in association with psychological stress and emotional deprivation. This condition has been referred to as *transient hypopituitrism*, *reversible hyposomatotropism*, and *psychosomatic dwarfism*, but is now generally termed *psychosocial short stature*.[3] Treatment involves modification of the child's social environment, which will often necessitate removal of the child from the home, and a period of hospitalization under the care of a multidisciplinary team. GH levels will usually normalize during the hospital stay. Linear growth eventually accelerates as well.

**Clinical Presentation.** Congenital GH deficiency may present in infancy with episodes of recurrent hypoglycemia associated with fasting or during illnesses, when dietary intake is diminished. Approximately 10 percent of these infants will develop hypoglycemic seizures. Birth weight and length are usually normal, but prolonged direct hyperbilirubinemia may be present. Affected boys often have microphallus and/or cryptorchidism. Failure to achieve normal growth rates may be noted within the first year of life. In older children, GH deficiency manifests as growth retardation and growth velocity deceleration. Usually there is proportional short stature, delayed skeletal maturation, truncal obesity, immature facies, and poor body and facial hair growth. Pubertal onset is delayed.[1]

Craniopharyngioma, a tumor derived from embryonic cell rests of Rathke's pouch, is the most common tumor causing hypopituitarism. The lesion is benign, but may extend above the sella turcica, compressing the hypothalamus and stretching the optic chiasm. The peak incidence occurs at age 7 years, but symptoms may appear at any time during childhood or adolescence. Younger children presenting with craniopharyngiomas often manifest signs and symptoms of increased intracranial pressure, obscuring any endocrine dysfunction. Older patients may present with progressive visual loss, growth failure, and symptoms of increased intracranial pressure (i.e., headache, vomiting). GH deficiency is often the most prominent endocrine abnormality, but a state of panhypopituitarism, evidenced by diabetes insipidus, hypothyroidism, delayed pubertal onset, and (rarely) adrenal insufficiency, may exist.

**Diagnosis.** The biochemical diagnosis of GH deficiency depends upon measurement of GH levels following GH-provocative tests, as the basal level of the hormone varies episodically. Further investigation to exclude tumors in the region of the pituitary gland is essential. Skull radiographs may show suprasellar calcifications, and computed tomography (CT) scan or magnetic resonance imaging (MRI) may reveal a tumor or other abnormality.

**Treatment.** Treatment of GH deficiency is with recombinant DNA-derived GH. Several dosing regimens utilizing thrice-weekly or daily injections have been effective. Potential adverse effects of GH therapy include impaired glucose tolerance, hyperinsulinism, and insulin resistance. Fortunately, these have not proved to be clinically significant.[1]

Surgical resection of the tumor is the treatment of choice in patients with craniopharyngioma. For partially resected or unresectable tumors, cranial irradiation may be indicated.[4] Hormonal supplementation should be initiated in those children with selective or generalized (panhypopituitarism) deficiencies, and perioperative glucocorticoid administration is very important. Diabetes insipidus, if present, can be controlled by intranasal desmopressin (DDAVP) 2.5 to 15 μg/kg every 12 hours. In the immediate postoperative period, diabetes insipidus may be severe; thus meticulous attention to fluid and electrolyte status is essential. Normal serum sodium and osmolality, as well as an appropriate thirst response, are indicative of good control.

## Diabetes Insipidus

Diabetes insipidus is a syndrome of relative or absolute deficiency of ADH referred to as *neurogenic diabetes insipidus,* or an end-organ insensitivity to ADH called *nephrogenic diabetes insipidus.* The diminished action of ADH on the kidney results in hypotonic polyuria despite increases in serum sodium and osmolality.

Finally, some children may demonstrate primary polydipsia, a condition in which compulsive water ingestion produces changes in plasma and urine osmolality similar to those seen in diabetes insipidus. In this disease, which may be due to a defect in the thirst mechanism or may result from psychogenic causes, there is a normal response to water deprivation, and the administration of DDAVP causes an increase in urine specific gravity.

ADH is synthesized in nerve cell bodies in the paraventricular and supraoptic nuclei of the hypothalamus. Granules containing ADH and a carrier protein, neurophysin, are transported down axons that terminate in the posterior pituitary. The hormone is stored in the posterior pituitary and later released in response to various stimuli. The primary function of ADH is osmoregulation and maintenance of blood volume. Once released from the posterior pituitary, ADH is transported via the bloodstream to the kidneys, where it interacts with receptors on the epithelial cells lining the collecting ducts. ADH increases the permeability of the renal tubular epithelium, allowing reabsorption of the relatively hypotonic fluid, and as a result, urine concentrations of 1,200 to 1,400 mOsm/kg $H_2O$ may be reached. Alteration of the renal tubular permeability involves a cyclic adenosine monophosphate (cAMP)-mediated reaction.[5]

Many factors are involved in the control of ADH secretion from the posterior pituitary. The release of ADH is strongly influenced by the hypothalamic osmoreceptors, which sense plasma osmolality. A small increase above the normal plasma osmolality (280 to 285 mOsm/kg $H_2O$) stimulates the osmoreceptors, resulting in ADH release from the posterior pituitary and activation of the thirst mecha-

**Table 6-1.** Nonosmotic Regulators of Antidiuretic Hormone Secretion

| |
|---|
| Facilitate release |
| Prostaglandin $E_2$ |
| Morphine and other narcotics |
| Nicotine |
| β-Adrenergic agents |
| Angiotensin II |
| Anesthetic agents |
| Barbiturates |
| Vincristine |
| Cyclophosphamide |
| Clofibrate |
| Carbamazepine |
| Acetylcholine |
| Histamine |
| Metoclopramide |
| Hypoxia |
| Hypercapnia |
| Suppress release |
| Phenytoin |
| Alcohol |
| α-Adrenergic agents |
| Atrial natriuretic peptide |

nism. Alterations of intravascular volume and blood pressure will also influence the release of ADH, irrespective of the plasma osmolality. Baroreceptors in the wall of the left atrium, carotid sinus, and aortic arch sense changes in blood pressure and stimulate the release of ADH when the pressure is low, or inhibit ADH secretion when the pressure is elevated. Atrial natriuretic factor, secreted principally by the cardiac atria and various regions of the brain, appears to inhibit both the release of ADH and its effect on the renal tubular collecting ducts.[6] A multiplicity of other nonosmotic regulators of ADH secretion exist, including neurotransmitters, catecholamines, drugs, and other chemicals (Table 6-1).

## Neurogenic Diabetes Insipidus

Neurogenic diabetes insipidus is the result of ADH deficiency. This condition may occur as an isolated idiopathic defect or in combination with an anterior pituitary hormone deficiency (see section on GH deficiency). Craniopharyngiomas are a common cause. In addition, the condition may follow surgical procedures involving lesions in the hypothalamic-pituitary region. Less frequent causes include head trauma, central nervous system (CNS) infections, and congenital malformations of the CNS.

**Clinical Presentation.** Infants and children with neurogenic diabetes insipidus classically present with hypotonic polyuria (s.g. 1.001 to 1.005; 30 to 400 ml/kg/d) and polydipsia. Nocturia and enuresis may occur in the previously toilet-trained child. Patients tend to prefer drinking cold water. Decreased caloric intake may result in failure to gain weight. If left untreated, children with neurogenic diabetes insipidus may develop hypernatremia and seizures. Patients with symptoms secondary to a craniopharyngioma may complain of headaches, vomiting, and visual changes. A deceleration in growth may also be noted.

**Diagnosis.** Children presenting with a rapid onset of hypotonic polyuria and polydipsia are likely to have diabetes insipidus. Hypernatremia, increased plasma osmolality, urine specific gravity less than 1.005, and osmolality less than 200 mOsm/kg $H_2O$ are consistent with the diagnosis. Plasma ADH levels may be measured by radioimmunoassay.

A review of the patient's clinical presentation along with results of a water deprivation test utilizing DDAVP will help to differentiate the neurogenic from the nephrogenic form. Following a period of water deprivation and administration of DDAVP, children with the neurogenic form have an almost immediate reduction in urine output and increase in urine osmolality, whereas children with the nephrogenic form show no response to DDAVP. Additional diagnostic studies to rule out a brain tumor or other CNS lesion are essential. These studies include skull films, CT scans, or MRI.

**Treatment.** The goal of therapy is to reduce the daily volume of urine output. The treatment of choice is intranasal DDAVP 2.5 to 15 μg/kg every 12 hours in children 3 months to 12 years of age. With the correct dosing regimen, the child's thirst response should be appropriate and serum sodium and osmolality normal. Patients with evidence of additional anterior pituitary hormone deficiencies require hormonal supplementation.

### Nephrogenic Diabetes Insipidus

Nephrogenic diabetes insipidus is due to renal insensitivity to ADH. This rare condition may occur sporadically, but more often is familial, with an X-linked recessive transmission. Other less common causes of the nephrogenic form include intrinsic renal disease secondary to chronic inflammation or infection, vascular insult, or exposure to toxins (lithium, demeclocycline).[7]

**Clinical Presentation.** Polyuria and polydipsia are also cardinal features of nephrogenic diabetes insipidus. Infants, especially males, will present in the first few weeks of life with irritability, hyperpyrexia, vomiting, and failure to thrive. Severe hypernatremic dehydration with resulting seizures and/or neurologic injury may also be present. Initially, ADH insensitivity is an isolated defect, but renal dysfunction secondary to recurrent episodes of dehydration often develop later. Older children may also have learning impairment from prolonged hypernatremia.[8]

**Diagnosis.** The diagnosis is suggested in patients with a positive family history, onset of polyuria and polydipsia in early infancy, and persistence of symptoms and hypothenuria (s.g. $< 1.005$) unresponsive to ADH administration. Confirmatory laboratory tests include hypernatremia, hyperosmolality, and elevated plasma ADH.

**Treatment.** Children presenting with signs and symptoms of hypernatremic (hypertonic) encephalopathy require emergency treatment, so as to avoid permanent cerebral injury. Seizures, cerebral hemorrhages and thromboses, and subdural effusions may result from severe hyperosmolality. The goal is to replenish body water, thereby restoring osmotic homeostasis and repleting cell volume at a rate that avoids cell swelling and cerebral edema. Ideally, fluids (0.9 percent saline) are administered at a rate that reduces the serum sodium concentration by approximately 1 mmol/L every 2 hours.

Unfortunately, there is no specific treatment. Hydration is essential, and a low-sodium diet to reduce urine volume may help. The most effective therapy involves the use of thiazide diuretics, which may be combined with potassium-sparing diuretics or prostaglandin synthesis inhibitors.[8]

## Hyperpituitarism

GH-producing pituitary tumors are rare in childhood. When present, the pituitary tumor is usually an eosinophilic or chromophobic adenoma. Additionally, increased release of GHRH from the hypothalamus or from an ectopic tumor may result in excessive secretion of GH. Hypersecretion of GH in early childhood before epiphyseal closure leads to gigantism, whereas in older patients with closed epiphyses, features of acromegaly are present.

### Gigantism

Pituitary gigantism is extremely uncommon. The diagnosis is usually established at the time of puberty when clinical features of acromegaly and gigantism are evident.[9]

**Clinical Presentation.** Gigantism is characterized by a proportional increase in growth rate, excessive height, and enlarged hands and feet. Skeletal bone age is normal or advanced. Glucose intolerance and hyperinsulinemia are often present.

**Diagnosis.** An elevated basal GH value in conjunction with a paradoxical increase in GH secretion or lack of suppression during a state of hyperglycemia provides laboratory confirmation of the diagnosis. Radiologic studies utilizing CT and MRI are also of value in localizing pituitary or ectopic tumors.

**Treatment.** GH-secreting pituitary tumors are resected if possible, preferably by the transsphenoidal route. The mainstay of medical management is dopamine agonists (i.e., bromocriptine), which bind to somatotroph dopamine receptors, thereby suppressing GH secretion. Adverse effects include nausea, vomiting, nasal congestion, and transient postural hypotension.[1] Long-acting somatostatin analogs (i.e., octreotide) have also been found to effectively suppress GH secretion from pituitary adenomas. Unfortunately, when octreotide is discontinued, the tumors regrow. Cranial irradiation is best used as an adjunct to surgical and medical therapy. However, long-term complications of irradiation such as hypopituitarism, visual disturbances, and learning impairment have been reported in as many as 50 percent of the patients.

## Acromegaly

Excessive GH secretion in postpubertal patients accounts for the clinical syndrome of acromegaly. A vast majority of these cases are a result of a primary pituitary adenoma. It is of interest that acromegaly may occur as part of the multiple endocrine neoplasia type I syndrome.

**Clinical Presentation.** Patients with acromegaly usually have a gradual progression of signs and symptoms, and body habitus changes often go unnoticed until complications occur. At the time of presentation, the clinical findings may be related to the pituitary tumor itself, hypopituitarism, excessive GH, or a combination of factors.

The patient may complain of excessive growth, or visual defects and headaches due to expansion of the pituitary adenoma. On physical examination, a generalized overgrowth of skeletal, soft, and connective tissue is apparent. Coarse facial features are noted. Prognathism, an enlarged tongue and epiglottis, as well as polypoid masses of pharyngeal tissue make these patients susceptible to upper airway obstruction and obstructive sleep apnea. Endotracheal intubation may also be difficult.[10] Stridor secondary to laryngeal involvement, and subglottic narrowing have been reported.[11] Other manifestations include carpal tunnel syndrome, skeletal muscle weakness, hypertension, and glucose intolerance.

**Diagnosis.** The diagnosis is based on the clinical presentation and biochemical confirmation. Serum GH levels are elevated, but fluctuate widely in patients with acromegaly. However, an elevated serum insulin-like growth factor-I (IGF-I) suggests excessive GH secretion and is thus a good screening test for acromegaly.[12] The definitive investigation is the oral glucose tolerance test, which demonstrates a lack of GH suppression following ingestion of glucose. Skull radiographs may reveal an enlarged sella turcica, and CT or MRI may be used to localize the tumor.

**Treatment.** Treatment for those with acromegaly is similar to that for children with gigantism, mainly surgical resection of the tumor, dopamine agonists, and cranial irradiation.

## Syndrome of Inappropriate ADH Secretion

The syndrome of inappropriate ADH secretion (SIADH) is characterized by euvolemic hyponatremia resulting from excessive secretion of ADH in the absence of either osmotic or nonosmotic stimuli. The excessive antidiuretic effects, coupled with abnormal or mildly increased fluid intake, cause free water accumulation and dilutional hyponatremia. As a compensatory mechanism to extracellular volume expansion, a sodium diuresis (natriuresis) occurs. Increased levels of atrial natriuretic factor also contribute to the natriuresis.[13] Consequently, the hyponatremia of SIADH is associated with increased urinary sodium concentrations.

In children, SIADH is most often associated with CNS injury such as trauma, inflammation, infection, and tumors. Other causes include drugs (cyclophosphamide, vincristine, opioids, carbamazepine, and many others), mechanical ventilation, pulmonary disease, and other malignancies. Surgical stimulation has also been shown to cause a transient increase in ADH secretion, which may be minimized by the administration of opioids.

**Clinical Presentation.** Children with SIADH usually present with nonspecific signs and symptoms of hyponatremia (serum sodium <130 mmol/L) including anorexia, irritability, lethargy, and muscle weakness. With profound hyponatremia (serum sodium <120 mmol/L), nausea, vomiting, disorientation, obtundation, and seizures may be present.

**Diagnosis.** The diagnosis of SIADH is suspected in children with hyponatremia and low serum osmolality, in conjunction with the excretion of small amounts of urine with an inappropriately high osmolality (>100 mOsm/kg $H_2O$). Signs of adrenal, hepatic, renal, or thyroid dysfunction are absent.

**Treatment.** The initial treatment of choice for SIADH is fluid restriction, usually 50 to 60 percent of maintenance volumes. Furosemide has also been advocated. Patients with acute symptomatic hyponatremia (seizures, obtundation) require emergency treatment with 3 percent hypertonic saline to restore serum sodium to 125 mmol/L. Central pontine myelinolysis has been reported in patients who have had rapid correction of hyponatremia.

# THYROID GLAND

## Normal Function

The thyroid gland produces two physiologically active hormones, thyroxine [tetraiodothyronine ($T_4$)] and triiodothyronine ($T_3$). These hormones regulate cellular metabolism and other biochemical reactions in virtually every organ system, and also influence postnatal somatic growth and neurologic development in infants and children. It is the effects of thyroid hormones on the neurologic, respiratory, and cardiovascular systems that are of greatest interest for the anesthesiologist.

The thyroid hormones are iodinated amino acids, and their biosynthesis requires an elaborate series of reactions within the follicular cells of the thyroid. Steps involved include (1) iodide trapping; (2) oxidation of iodide to iodine and iodination of thyroglobulin-bound tyrosyl residues to form monoiodotyrosine (MIT) and diiodotyrosine (DIT); (3) coupling of

MIT and DIT to form $T_4$, $T_3$, and small amounts of reverse $T_3$ ($rT_3$) stored in follicular colloid; (4) proteolysis of colloid thyroglobulin and release of $T_4$, $T_3$, $rT_3$, MIT, and DIT; and (5) deiodination of MIT and DIT with intrathyroidal recycling of the iodotyrosines and iodide. All of the circulating $T_4$ is synthesized and released from the thyroid gland. However, 75 percent or more of $T_3$ and $rT_3$ is formed from the peripheral monodeiodination of $T_4$ to $T_3$, occurring primarily in the liver and kidney. The conversion of $T_4$ to $T_3$ may be impaired by starvation, systemic illness, surgical stress, hepatic or renal dysfunction, glucocorticoid therapy, propranolol, propylthiouracil, and other drugs.[14]

After release from the thyroid, approximately 99 percent of the circulating $T_4$ and $T_3$ is bound to three serum proteins, thyroxine-binding globulin (TBG), thyroxine-binding prealbumin (TBPA), and albumin. Less than 1 percent of the total serum $T_4$ and $T_3$ is in the free or unbound form. Only the unbound fraction is able to cross cellular membranes and therefore is biologically active. The hormonal activity exerted by $T_3$ is more potent than $T_4$, and less $T_3$ is protein bound. $rT_3$ has minimal metabolic activity, but may serve a regulatory role in the intracellular conversion of $T_4$ to $T_3$. The plasma half-life is 6 to 7 days for $T_4$ and approximately 12 to 24 hours for $T_3$.

The precise mode of cellular stimulation by the thyroid hormones has not been completely identified, but appears to be complex and consist of multiple mechanisms. These may include (1) hormonal interaction involving nuclear receptors within the cell and subsequent alteration of gene transcription via mRNA, (2) direct action at the cell membrane, and (3) activation of mitochondrial energy metabolism. Thyroid hormones also potentiate the actions of catecholamines. The increased catecholamine effects observed in hyperthyroidism occur in the presence of normal catecholamine levels. These effects can be diminished by the use of adrenergic blocking agents.

Production and secretion of $T_4$ and $T_3$ are regulated by the hypothalamic-pituitary-thyroid axis. Thyotropin-releasing hormone (TRH), produced in the hypothalamus, is secreted via the hypophyseal portal system to the anterior pituitary gland. There, TRH stimulates the synthesis and release of TSH. TSH acts upon the thyroid gland to regulate production and release of $T_4$ and $T_3$. TSH binds to a specific receptor on the thyroid cell membrane, initiating a cAMP-mediated action.

The regulation of secretion of TRH and TSH is via a classic feedback mechanism involving the circulating concentrations of thyroid hormones. Elevated levels of $T_4$ and $T_3$ inhibit the TRH-induced stimulation of the thyrotropic cells of the anterior pituitary, as well as the synthesis and release of TSH, whereas low levels of circulating hormones stimulate TSH secretion. In addition, other substances are known to stimulate (epinephrine, theophylline) or inhibit (somatostatin, dopamine, glucocorticoids) TSH secretion.

Although TSH is the major regulator of thyroid structure and function, autoregulatory mechanisms involving the thyroid and serum iodine concentrations also play a role. Thyroid autoregulation seeks to maintain constancy of thyroid hormone stores, while TSH feedback regulation attempts to preserve plasma or tissue concentrations of thyroid hormones.[14]

During the first trimester of gestation, the hypothalamic-pituitary-thyroid axis begins to develop, but levels of $T_4$ and TSH remain low. By midgestation, a progressive rise in fetal TSH levels occurs, followed by an increase in fetal $T_4$ and free $T_4$ concentrations. Maturation of hypothalamic and pituitary function and interaction, along with thyroid gland responsiveness, continues through the third trimester. As gestational age advances, an increase in the conversion of $T_4$ to $T_3$ is seen. The fetal pituitary-thyroid axis functions independently of the maternal axis due to limited transplacental passage of TSH, $T_4$, and $T_3$.

At birth, the serum TSH dramatically increases, peaking at 30 minutes of age, but returns to a normal range within several days. This surge of TSH is thought to be a result of the cooling of the neonate that follows emergence into the extrauterine environment. Serum $T_4$ levels increase rapidly from the surge in TSH secretion. TSH elevation also contributes to the increase in $T_3$, as does enhanced extrathyroid conversion of $T_4$ to $T_3$. The increased serum $T_4$ concentrations found in the neonate gradually decrease, reaching the normal adult range by 10 to 15 years of age. Serum $T_3$ remains elevated throughout adolescence, but by the beginning of the third decade of life, adult values have been reached.

Thyroid function is impaired in preterm infants secondary to incomplete maturation of the hypothalamic-pituitary-thyroid axis. The early TSH surge and increase in $T_4$ and $T_3$ levels occur, but are quantitatively reduced. A relative state of transient hypothyroidism thus exists. Levels of $T_4$ and $T_3$ in the preterm infant remain below those values seen in healthy full-term infants for a period of 1 to 4 months. Maturation of the complex regulatory mechanisms of thyroid function is complete by 1 month of age in term infants and an equivalent gestational age in premature infants.[14]

## Hypothyroidism

Hypothyroidism is a clinical state of altered cellular growth and function resulting from a deficiency of the thyroid hormones. The effects of reduced circulating levels of $T_4$ and $T_3$ are manifest in the biologic processes of all the major organs of the body.

**Table 6-2.** Causes of Hypothyroidism

| |
|---|
| Congenital |
| Thyroid dysgenesis (partial or complete) |
| Ectopic thyroid gland |
| Inborn errors of synthesis |
| Hypothalamic-pituitary-thyroid axis abnormalities |
| TRH deficiency, insensitivity |
| TSH deficiency |
| Thyroid gland unresponsiveness to TSH |
| Iodine deficiency (endemic cretinism) |
| Transplacental passage of antithyroid drugs or chemicals |
| Tissue insensitivity to thyroid hormone |
| Acquired |
| Chronic lymphocytic thyroiditis (Hashimoto's disease) |
| Post-thyroidectomy |
| Following $^{131}$I therapy |
| TRH/TSH deficiency |
| Goiter-producing substances (iodine excess, cobalt, propylthiouracil) |
| Infiltration of the thyroid (cystinosis, histiocytosis X) |
| Postradiation therapy |
| Postsuppurative or nonsuppurative thyroiditis |

Multiple etiologies for hypothyroidism have been identified and include (1) maldevelopment (thyroid dysgenesis) or destruction of thyroid gland tissue, (2) defective thyroid hormone biosynthesis (dyshormonogenesis), and (3) hypothalamic or anterior pituitary dysfunction (Table 6-2). Of these three causes, thyroid dysgenesis or destruction and dyshormonogenesis account for upwards of 95 percent of cases of hypothyroidism.[15]

In children hypothyroidism may be congenital or acquired (juvenile hypothyroidism), but the distinction may not always be evident. Patients who become symptomatic following a period of "apparent normal thyroid function" may have an acquired defect or a delayed manifestation of congenital hypothyroidism. The term *cretinism* has been used interchangeably with *congenital hypothyroidism,* but is probably best used when referring to infants with severe growth and neurologic sequelae of congenital hypothyroidism.

Congenital hypothyroidism is most often sporadic, but familial cases have been reported. With the advent of neonatal screening programs, approximately 1 in 4,000 to 5,000 infants have been found to have the disease. Thyroid dysgenesis is the cause in 80 to 90 percent of children with sporadic congenital hypothyroidism. The ratio of affected girls versus boys is 2 to 3:1. This predilection for females and the demonstration of thyroid growth-blocking and cytotoxic antibodies in some infants with thyroid dysgenesis raises the possibility of an autoimmune pathogenesis.[15]

Thyroid dysgenesis includes aplasia, ectopy, and hypoplasia of the thyroid gland. Ectopic thyroid tissue may be present in the lingual, sublingual, or subhyoid regions and be associated with thyroglossal duct cysts. This tissue may provide adequate amounts of thyroid hormones for an extended period of time or may fail in early childhood.

Dyshormonogenesis, or defective thyroid hormone biosynthesis, is the other major cause of congenital hypothyroidism. Due to the autosomal recessive mode of inheritance, the female to male ratio is 1:1. Neonates and young children may have iodide transport or organification defects, thyroglobin synthesis defects, or iodotyrosine deiodinase defects.

Less common causes of congenital hypothyroidism include iodine deficiency (endemic goiter) and hypothalamic-pituitary-thyroid axis abnormalities (TRH deficiency and insensitivity, TSH deficiency, and thyroid gland unresponsiveness to TSH). An increasing number of children are being identified who have peripheral resistance to thyroid hormone. This disorder most often has an autosomal dominant inheritance.

The euthyroid sick syndrome, a transient disorder of thyroid function occurring in newborn infants and children, is of special interest. It is seen in patients with severe acute or chronic nonthyroidal illnesses. Profound alterations in peripheral thyroid hormone metabolism occur. Serum levels of $T_4$ and $T_3$ are decreased, but the infants are euthyroid, as evidenced by normal serum TSH levels and a normal TSH response to TRH. Preterm infants with respiratory distress syndrome may frequently have euthyroid sick syndrome. In older children, the condition has been associated with severe gastroenteritis, acute leukemia, renal failure, severe burns, and untreated insulin-dependent diabetes mellitus. Thyroid function gradually normalizes as the primary illness improves, so thyroid hormone supplementation is not generally required.[16]

Acquired or juvenile hypothyroidism is frequently a result of autoimmune destruction of the thyroid secondary to chronic lymphocytic thyroiditis. Also known as Hashimoto's thyroiditis, it is the most common cause of thyroid disease in children and adolescents, with an incidence as high as 1 percent in school-aged children.[17] Girls are much more often affected. In 30 to 40 percent of patients, a family history of thyroid disease is present. Also, children with autoimmune hypothyroidism are at increased risk for other associated autoimmune diseases, such as insulin-dependent diabetes mellitus, rheumatoid arthritis, and adrenal insufficiency.

Pediatric patients who have undergone a thyroidectomy or $^{131}I$ therapy may also develop hypothyroidism. Other less common causes of acquired hypothyroidism include (1) craniospinal irradiation with direct irradiation to the hypothalamus, anterior pituitary, or thyroid gland; (2) infiltrative diseases of the thyroid (cystinosis or histiocytosis X); (3) ingestion of excess iodide or use of iodide-containing compounds; (4) antithyroid drugs; (5) euthyroid sick syndrome; and (6) rarely, acute suppurative or subacute nonsuppurative thyroiditis.

**Clinical Presentation.** Newborn infants with congenital hypothyroidism seldom present with prominent or specific signs or symptoms, emphasizing the importance of neonatal screening programs. Often the first symptom is prolonged neonatal jaundice. Subtle symptoms of hypothyroidism that may be apparent within the first weeks of life include constipation, feeding problems, failure to gain weight, lethargy, and hypoactivity. Physical findings may include enlarged fontanelles, coarse, puffy facies, large protruding tongue, hoarse cry, abdominal distention and umbilical hernia, cool, dry, mottled skin, and hypotonia. A heart murmur may be present and if associated with cyanosis or cardiovascular instability warrants additional evaluation.

Patients with acquired hypothyroidism may present with a gradual onset of signs and symptoms. The hallmark sign is deceleration of linear growth. In addition, a history of lethargy, cold intolerance, poor appetite, weight gain, constipation, and slow growth of nails and scalp hair may be reported. Sexual maturation is usually delayed, although occasionally may be paradoxically precocious.

On physical examination the facies may appear dull and puffy, with a flattened nasal bridge. The hair is thin, coarse, and brittle. The thyroid gland may be nonpalable, small or enlarged, and firm, as seen often with chronic lymphocytic thyroiditis. Dry, cool skin from cutaneous vasoconstriction and a sallow complexion may be evident. Pleural, pericardial, and abdominal effusions are common. Girls frequently have multicystic ovaries. Neurologic features associated with hypothyroidism include generalized slowing of all intellectual functions and slow, clumsy movements. Possible cardiovascular changes of concern to the anesthesiologist include decreased cardiac output secondary to a reduction in heart rate and decreased stroke volume, reflecting loss of the inotropic and chronotropic effects of thyroid hormones. Peripheral vascular resistance at rest is increased, and blood volume is reduced. Baroreceptor dysfunction has also been demonstrated.[18] A mild normocytic normochromic anemia is often present. It is noteworthy that 5 to 10 percent of patients with chronic lymphocytic thyroiditis, particularly those in adolescence, may present with tachycardia, nervousness, and other signs suggestive of thyrotoxicosis.

Myxedema coma is a severe life-threatening form of hypothyroidism rarely seen in children. This condition is characterized by altered mentation, severe hypometabolism and hypothermia, hypoventilation, bradycardia, and profound hypotension. Adrenal insufficiency is common, and hyponatremia due to SIADH may also be present.

**Diagnosis.** Prompt diagnosis of congenital hypothyroidism is essential so that treatment may be initiated early, in an effort to prevent permanent severe growth and neurologic sequelae. The newborn screening program is the most important tool for establishing the diagnosis. A majority of screening programs utilize filter paper spot $T_4$ testing, with follow-up filter paper spot TSH testing of samples with the lowest 3 to 5 percent of $T_4$ results. In infants with a suspicious or positive screening result, serum determination of $T_4$, TSH, and other laboratory tests as indicated must be obtained to confirm the diagnosis.[16] The classic biochemical signs of primary hypothyroidism are a low serum $T_4$ and an elevated TSH. Additional studies used to differentiate a deficiency of TBG from secondary hypothyroidism (TSH deficiency) include $T_3$ resin uptake, serum thyroid binding proteins, or free thyroxine index. Diagnosing tertiary hypothyroidism (TRH deficiency) requires an evaluation of the hypothalamic-pituitary axis utilizing a TRH provocative test.

Patients with a clinical presentation suggestive of lymphocytic thyroiditis should also have tests to detect autoimmune antibodies, especially antithyroglobin antibody and thyroid antimicrosomal antibody. Other helpful diagnostic studies include bone-age radiographs showing delayed skeletal maturation, and thyroid scintigraphy, which may indicate thyroid agenesis, an ectopic gland, or an alteration of gland function. Ultrasonography of the thyroid may also be useful in those patients with an enlarged thyroid.[19]

**Treatment.** In infants with congenital hypothyroidism, it is imperative that a state of euthyroidism be established as rapidly and safely as possible. Failure to institute therapy by 3 months of age may result in permanent neurologic impairment and severe growth retardation.[15] Synthetic L-thyroxine is the recommended thyroid hormone preparation (Appendix 6-1). As the child grows, the dosage is adjusted in order to normalize serum $T_4$ and TSH levels. During the first few months of therapy, TSH levels may remain elevated, especially in those infants symptomatic at the time of diagnosis. Supplemental thyroid hormone overdosage in young infants may be clinically difficult to detect. Possible indications of hormone excess include tachycardia, profuse sweating, rapid growth, craniosynostosis, and accelerated osseous maturation. Pseudotumor cerebri has also been reported.[16]

Synthetic L-thyroxine is also the treatment of choice in patients with acquired hypothyroidism. Most patients will experience an increase in growth rate and cessation of symptoms within several months of starting therapy. The autoimmune form of hypothyroidism, chronic lymphocytic thyroiditis, occasionally resolves spontaneously; therefore, a trial of hormone supplementation might be considered.[20]

## Hyperthyroidism (Thyrotoxicosis)

Hyperthyroidism is a state of hypermetabolism due to excess production of thyroid hormones. Hyperthyroidism, or thyrotoxicosis, usually presents in late childhood or adolescence as a result of diffuse thyroid hyperplasia. This form of hyperthyroidism is almost always secondary to Graves' disease, an autoimmune thyroid disorder characterized by the autonomous overproduction of $T_4$ and $T_3$. The increased concentration of free $T_4$ suppresses TSH to near undetectable levels; therefore, thyroid hyperfunction is not TSH dependent, and the normal regulatory feedback mechanisms are nonfunctional. Research has shown that Graves' disease has an autoimmune pathogenesis.[21] Thyroid autoantibodies (IgG class immunoglobulin) bind to antigenic regions on thyroid cells, activating a cAMP-mediated reaction that produces thyroid growth, increased vascularity, and hypersecretion of hormone. The antibody responsible for this activity is called long-acting thyroid stimulator or thyroid-stimulating immunoglobulin.

Graves' disease is approximately five times more frequent in females than in males, and family histories are often positive for Graves' disease, goiters, or thyroiditis.

Various other autoimmune disorders may be found in association with Graves' disease. Addison's disease (adrenal insufficiency), insulin-dependent diabetes mellitus, idiopathic hypoparathyroidism, rheumatoid arthritis, lupus erythematosus, and myasthenia gravis have all been identified in patients with Graves' disease.[16] In children, other etiologies for hyperthyroidism are rare, but they include a hyperfunctioning thyroid nodule, chronic lymphocytic thyroiditis, and a TSH-producing pituitary tumor. The other form of this disease is referred to as *congenital hyperthyroidism* or *transient neonatal hyperthyroidism*. Transplacental transfer of thyroid-stimulating immunoglobulin from the mother to the fetus is thought to be the cause in many infants. In other cases, the etiology remains unclear.

**Clinical Presentation.** The onset of symptoms and signs is usually gradual. Emotional lability, nervousness, heat intolerance, excessive sweating, increased appetite with or without weight loss, frequent loose bowel movements, and deterioration of behavior and school performance are the most common symptoms.

Physical examination reveals resting tachycardia, systolic hypertension with widened pulse pressure, warm and moist skin, tremulousness, and proximal muscle weakness. Nearly all patients have a firm, nontender, diffusely enlarged thyroid gland (goiter). Proptosis, lid retraction, and a "bright-eyed stare" are found in a small number of patients.

Infants with neonatal hyperthyroidism may present with poor weight gain, jitteriness, irritability, tachycardia, and congestive heart failure. Thyromegaly, which may compromise the infant's airway, is occasionally noted. Premature craniosynostosis, microcephaly, and neurologic impairment may occur in severely affected infants. The overall mortality may reach 15 to 20 percent.[16]

**Diagnosis.** Hyperthyroidism is diagnosed by documentation of increased serum concentrations of $T_4$ and free $T_4$, $T_3$ and free $T_3$, and $T_3$ resin uptake, as well as an abnormally low TSH. The serum $T_3$ concentration is typically more elevated than the serum $T_4$ concentration, making it a better screening test. TSH receptor antibodies are present in most pediatric patients. Radiographs may indicate advanced bone maturation. If thyroid enlargement is not apparent, a 24-hour $^{131}I$ thyroidal uptake test is helpful. Most children with hyperthyroidism will have an elevated $^{131}I$ thyroidal uptake.

**Treatment.** Conventional therapy includes antithyroid drugs, radioactive iodine, and surgery. Each of these modalities has advantages and disadvantages, and the selection of treatment must be made only after careful consideration. In pediatric patients, medical therapy is the treatment of choice. Remission occurs in 30 to 40 percent of children after 2 to 3 years.[22] Propylthiouracil and methimazole are commonly used antithyroid drugs. Resolution of symptoms and signs, along with periodic measurement of serum $T_4$, $T_3$, and TSH, is important in adjusting the dosage. Potential adverse effects of these drugs include transient leukopenia, headache, skin rash, arthralgias, and arthritis. Agranulocytosis is less common.

In the extremely symptomatic patient (agitation, tremors, tachycardia, or arrhythmias), β-adrenergic antagonists such as propranolol or atenolol are useful. Bradycardia, hypoglycemia, exacerbation of asthma, or complete heart block are potential complications when using β-adrenergic antagonists. Radioactive iodine has been used successfully in the past for treating adults, but its use today in children is controversial.

Surgical intervention (subtotal thyroidectomy) provides rapid control of hyperthyroidism. Indications for surgery include (1) toxicity to antithyroid drugs, (2) failure of medical management, or (3) lack of patient or parent compliance.[16] It is critical that patients scheduled for surgery be rendered euthyroid prior to the operation, so as to avoid precipitating thyroid storm. A common preoperative regimen consists of Lugol's iodine, propylthiouracil, and propranolol or atenolol administered for 10 to 14 days before surgery. Potential risks from surgery include tracheal compression, hypothyroidism, hypoparathyroidism leading to hypocalcemia, and injury to the recurrent laryngeal nerve.

### Thyroid Storm

Thyroid storm is a potentially life-threatening state of severe hypermetabolism caused by sudden excessive release of thyroid hormones into the circulation. This condition is extremely rare in children, but when it does occur, it is usually in patients with partially treated or undiagnosed Graves' disease. Thyroid storm is most often precipitated by infection, emotional stress, trauma, or surgery. Less common precipitating factors include radiation thyroiditis and diabetic ketoacidosis. In adults, thyroid storm usually occurs 6 to 18 hours following surgery.

**Clinical Presentation.** Thyroid storm is a clinical diagnosis that may mimic malignant hyperthermia. Characteristically, patients manifest an abrupt onset of fever, marked tachycardia, vomiting, diaphoresis, and progressive apathy and stupor, leading to coma. Hypotension, pulmonary edema, and congestive heart failure are often present. In severe cases, complete circulatory collapse may occur. If this condition goes unrecognized, it is invariably fatal. Even with prompt and appropriate medical intervention, the mortality rate is still 20 percent.

**Treatment.** Treatment of thyroid storm aims to correct the severe thyrotoxicosis and provide general supportive care. Large doses of propylthiouracil, given by mouth or nasogastric tube, followed several hours later by iodides, will block release of thyroid hormones. In the absence of significant cardiac insufficiency, propranolol or labetalol is titrated to reduce adrenergic symptoms and signs. Large doses of dexamethasone are given to provide glucocorticoid support, as well as to inhibit the release of hormone from the thyroid and the peripheral generation of $T_3$.[23] Supportive therapy including antipyretics, cooling measures, administration of glucose-containing and balanced salt solutions, along with vitamin B, should be given. Patients require close monitoring in an intensive care unit during the initial phases of treatment. When therapy is successful, improvement is usually seen within 1 to 2 days, and recovery occurs in 1 week.

## PARATHYROID GLANDS

### Normal Function

The parathyroid glands serve as the principal regulator of extracellular ionized calcium levels. Calcium is the most abundant cation in the body; the free, ionized form is biologically active. Calcium plays an extremely important role as an enzyme cofactor, in neuronal and neuromuscular transmission, muscular contraction, bone formation, protein synthesis and secretion, blood coagulation, cellular proliferation, and intracellular communication.

Parathyroid hormone (PTH), synthesized and secreted from the chief cell of the parathyroid gland, is the primary hormone responsible for maintaining serum calcium levels. Secretion of PTH is modulated directly by the serum ionized calcium concentration and indirectly by the concentration of phosphorus and magnesium. A decrease in serum calcium stimulates PTH secretion, whereas an increase inhibits the release of PTH. An elevated serum phosphorus level inhibits 1,25-dihydroxyvitamin D [$1,25(OH)_2$ $D_3$] production, thus resulting in a decreased serum calcium concentration. A moderate decline in magnesium concentration enhances PTH secretion, but significant hypomagnesemia suppresses PTH release and decreases the peripheral cell response to PTH.

PTH regulates serum calcium through its direct action on the kidney and skeletal system and its secondary action on the intestinal tract. In the kidney, PTH interacts with specific receptors on cells in the proximal and distal tubules, activating a cAMP-mediated reaction that enhances reabsorption of calcium. Also, PTH promotes the conversion of 25-hydroxyvitamin D to $1,25(OH)_2$ $D_3$, the most active metabolite of vitamin D. Consequently, renal tubular reabsorption of calcium is increased, as well as the excretion of phosphorus.

In the skeletal system, PTH mobilizes calcium by enhancing osteoclastic differentiation and activity. As with cells in the kidney, bone cells have receptors for PTH and respond to hormone-receptor interaction with generation of a cAMP-mediated reaction. Finally, PTH influences the absorption of calcium in the gastrointestinal tract by inducing the synthesis of $1,25(OH)_2$ $D_3$.[24]

Along with PTH, calcitonin also functions as a regulator of calcium homeostasis. Calcitonin, a polypeptide hormone secreted by the parafollicular cells of the thyroid gland, lowers serum calcium concentrations, in contrast to the effect of PTH. In children, calcitonin inhibits PTH and vitamin D-induced osteoclastic resorption of bone. The secretion of calcitonin is stimulated by a rise in serum ionized calcium, β-adrenergic catecholamines, and several peptides including intestinal gastrin, glucagon, secretin, and cholecystokinin.

The parathyroid glands begin to secrete PTH by the 12th week of gestation, but during fetal life calcium concentrations are also dependent upon placental transfer of calcium and vitamin D precursors. Calcium levels are highest in utero and drop rapidly after birth, reaching a nadir at 24 to 48 hours of life. Thereafter, serum calcium increases to a relatively constant level (iCa 4.45 to 5.0 mg/dl or 1.11 to 1.26 mmol/L) as the neonate's own homeostatic mechanisms are activated.[24]

## Neonatal Hypocalcemia

Transient hypocalcemia (iCa $<$ 4.0 mg/dl or 1.0 mmol/L) is very prevalent in the newborn period. Prematurity, difficult delivery, birth asphyxia, and maternal illness such as diabetes, toxemia, or hyperparathyroidism are all predisposing causes (Table 6-3). Neonatal hypocalcemia is probably a result of several factors: (1) loss of placental supply of calcium, (2) a relative state of hypoparathyroidism, (3) immaturity of renal tubular handling of phosphorus, and (4) inadequate intestinal absorption of calcium. Also, it is known that alkalosis (from excessive bicarbonate administration or hyperventilation) decreases ionized calcium levels, as does the administration of citrated blood products.

**Clinical Presentation.** Characteristically, transient neonatal hypocalcemia appears within the first 24 to 48 hours of life. Most healthy neonates will be free of clinical signs. The common manifestations of symptomatic neonates, jitteri-

**Table 6-3.** Causes of Hypocalcemia

Neonatal Hypocalcemia

- Early onset
  - Maternal disease
    - Diabetes mellitus
    - Toxemia of pregnancy
    - Hyperparathyroidism
    - Low birth weight
  - Birth asphyxia
  - Sepsis
  - Alkalosis (respiratory or metabolic)
  - Hypomagnesemia
  - Citrated blood products
- Late onset
  - High phosphorus intake
  - Hypoparathyroidism (transient or permanent)

Hypoparathyroidism

- Congenital
  - Transient neonatal
  - Aplasia or hypoplasia
  - Familial
  - DiGeorge syndrome
  - Dyshormonogenesis
- Acquired
  - Autoimmune
    - Sporadic
    - Familial
  - Postsurgical
  - Postradiation
  - Iron or copper poisoning
  - Idiopathic

Resistance to Parathyroid Hormone

- Pseudohypoparathyroidism
- Pseudopseudohypoparathyroidism
- Vitamin D deficiency

Other

- Calcium deficiency
  - Nutritional
  - Hypercalciuria
- Hypomagnesemia
  - Congenital
    - Malabsorption
  - Acquired
    - Primary
    - Bartter syndrome
    - Renal tubular acidosis
- Miscellaneous
  - Renal failure (acute or chronic)
  - Diuretics
  - Hyperphosphatemia
  - Hypoproteinemia
  - Drugs (calcitonin, mithramycin)
  - Critical illness
  - Pancreatitis
  - Chronic renal failure

ness, increased muscle tone, and seizures, all reflect neuromuscular irritability secondary to reduced ionized calcium levels. Laryngospasm and apnea may occur, and cardiac dysfunction as evidenced by hypotension or (rarely) bradycardia may also be present. Nonspecific symptoms such as poor feeding, vomiting, and lethargy may be noted as well.

**Treatment.** A majority of the healthy full-term infants with asymptomatic hypocalcemia do not require treatment. However, infants with symptomatology or those at high risk receive calcium supplementation via a slow intravenous infusion of 10 percent calcium gluconate, 100 to 200 mg/kg, with careful monitoring of the electrocardiograph (ECG). A follow-up continuous infusion of calcium gluconate 400 to 600 mg/kg/d may be required. Intravenous 10 percent calcium chloride (10 to 20 mg/kg) also effectively increases ionized calcium levels. When administering calcium solutions, care must be taken to avoid extravasation into tissues, or severe necrosis may result.

## Hypoparathyroidism

Hypoparathyroidism is a state of decreased PTH availability or peripheral receptor activity, resulting from inadequate secretion, biologically ineffective hormone, or end-organ insensitivity to PTH. The diminished influence of PTH on the kidney and skeletal system leads to hypocalcemia and hyperphosphatemia. Hypoparathyroidism may be classified as congenital or acquired. Another form of hypoparathyroidism is referred to as pseudohypoparathyroidism (end-organ insensitivity to PTH).

### Congenital Hypoparathyroidism

Persistent neonatal hypoparathyroidism may be due to congenital aplasia or hypoplasia of the parathyroid glands and is often associated with thymic aplasia and anomalies of the great vessels (DiGeorge syndrome).[25] It is of interest that infants with DiGeorge syndrome may also have micrognathia, which can make endotracheal intubation difficult. Congenital hypoparathyroidism may be familial (autosomal dominant and recessive or sex-linked recessive), or due to dyshormonogenesis (Table 6-3).

**Clinical Presentation.** Signs and symptoms of hypocalcemia predominate.

**Diagnosis.** The laboratory diagnosis of congenital hypoparathyroidism is confirmed by low ionized calcium levels and hyperphosphatemia. PTH concentrations are inappropriately low, indicating a lack of PTH response to hypocalcemia. Radiographs of the chest in infants with DiGeorge syndrome reveal the absence of a thymus.

**Treatment.** Emergency treatment for hypocalcemic tetany consists of intravenous 10 percent calcium gluconate or 10 percent calcium chloride. Otherwise, chronic therapy with $1{,}25(OH)_2\ D_3$ is recommended. Calcium supplementation may be required early on, but usually is discontinued later to avoid the complications of hypercalciuria. Serum calcium and phosphorus should be checked frequently. Urinary calcium may also be followed.

### Acquired Hypoparathyroidism

In older children, hypoparathyroidism is usually caused by autoimmune destruction of the parathyroid tissue. These children may have an isolated disorder or part of a polyendocrinopathy.[26] Autoimmune hypoparathyroidism occurs most often in association with adrenal insufficiency (Addison's disease) and chronic mucocutaneous candidiasis. Other less commonly associated disorders include primary hypogonadism, insulin-dependent diabetes mellitus, pernicious anemia, and hypothyroidism. Acquired hypoparathyroidism may also develop following the inadvertent removal of the parathyroid glands during a thyroidectomy, or from radiation therapy (Table 6-3).

**Clinical Presentation.** Young children with acquired hypoparathyroidism may present with signs and symptoms of hypocalcemia, especially seizures. Older patients also exhibit signs of hypocalcemia including muscular pain and cramps, carpopedal spasm, and positive Trousseau and Chovstek signs. Increased intracranial pressure, hyperreflexia, choreiform movements, visual and auditory dysfunction, and metastatic calcification (sclera, lens, basal ganglia) have been reported, and manifestations of other autoimmune-related disorders may be evident. Ectodermal (dry, puffy, yellowish skin, brittle nails, alopecia) and dental abnormalities are prominent.

**Diagnosis.** Classic laboratory findings of hypoparathyroidism include hypocalcemia, hyperphosphatemia, and inappropriately low serum PTH concentrations. However, when hypoparathyroidism occurs in association with Addison's disease, the serum calcium may be normal initially, but will decrease after effective treatment of the adrenal insufficiency.

Specific antiparathyroid antibodies are difficult to isolate; therefore, in the absence of associated autoimmune diseases, the diagnosis of autoimmune hypoparathyroidism may not be obvious.[27] Radiographs of the head or CT scanning may reveal basal ganglia calcifications.

**Treatment.** Mild or partial hypoparathyroidism, such as may be seen after subtotal thyroidectomy, may only require calcium supplementation. In more severe cases, treatment with $1{,}25(OH)_2\ D_3$ and a short course of calcium supplements are required. Serum calcium and phosphorus levels should be closely monitored. Patients with polyendocrinopathies should be under the care of an endocrinologist.

### Pseudohypoparathyroidism

Pseudohypoparathyroidism is an inherited disorder characterized by end-organ insensitivity to PTH. The parathyroids appear to be normal and to synthesize and secrete PTH, but the target organ cells are resistant to PTH stimulation, presumably because of a receptor or postreceptor defect, particularly in the kidney or skeleton. Recent studies have suggested that biologically inactive PTH or an inhibitor of PTH may be secreted in some cases.[28] As with the acquired form of hypoparathyroidism, other associated endocrine abnormalities are common.

**Clinical Presentation.** Children with this type of hypoparathyroidism may also present with symptomatic hypocalcemia, and distinctive skeletal and facial features are usually apparent on examination. These include short stature, round facies, short, thick neck, short metacarpals (first, fourth, fifth), and often short metatarsals (first and fifth). Subcutaneous calcium deposits and metaplastic bone formation are also seen. Mental retardation is common.

**Diagnosis.** As is found in other forms of hypoparathyroidism, serum calcium is low and phosphorus is elevated. Unlike congenital or acquired hypoparathyroidism, PTH levels are very high in these children. When the diagnosis remains in doubt, a PTH responsiveness test may be utilized. Prior to testing, urinary cAMP and phosphate levels are determined. Synthetic human PTH is then administered intravenously; after 1 to 2 hours, postinjection urinary cAMP and phosphate excretion values are measured. Failure to demonstrate an increase in urinary cAMP and phosphate excretion confirms the diagnosis.[29]

**Treatment.** The medical management of pseudohypoparathyroidism is similar to that used for acquired hypoparathyroidism.

## Hyperparathyroidism

The clinical state of excessive PTH production may be attributed to a primary defect of the parathyroid glands (primary hyperparathyroidism) or to a compensatory response by the parathyroids to hypocalcemia, hyperphosphatemia, or hypomagnesemia (secondary hyperparathyroidism). Another form of hyperparathyroidism results from ectopic PTH or PTH-like substance production (pseudohyperparathyroidism); this condition is not discussed here.

With the heightened awareness of hyperparathyroidism and the advent of routine serum calcium analysis, the prevalence rate for this condition has increased. More importantly, patients are being diagnosed and treated early in the course of the disease.

## Primary Hyperparathyroidism

Hypersecretion of PTH with primary hyperparathyroidism may be caused by a single pituitary adenoma, primary chief cell or clear cell hyperplasia of all of the parathyroid glands, or by carcinoma. This form of hyperparathyroidism rarely occurs in children, but when it does, it is usually due to a solitary parathyroid adenoma. Primary hyperparathyroidism may also be familial and a component of both multiple endocrine neoplasia syndromes, types I and II.

In primary hyperparathyroidism the elevated levels of PTH increase renal tubular reabsorption of calcium, while decreasing reabsorption of phosphorus, and stimulate 1,25$(OH)_2$ $D_3$ production with a consequent increase in calcium absorption from the intestinal tract. PTH also enhances mobilization of calcium from bone.

**Clinical Presentation.** The clinical manifestations of hyperparathyroidism are related to hypercalcemia and vary according to the age of the patient. Young infants may present with vomiting, poor feeding, failure to thrive, constipation, dehydration, fever, lethargy, hypotonia, and possibly chest wall abnormalities. Older patients may complain of nausea, anorexia, abdominal pain (occasionally due to a peptic ulcer or acute pancreatitis),[30] polydipsia, polyuria, renal colic and hematuria (secondary to nephrolithiasis), easy fatigability, muscle weakness (proximal muscles of the extremities), poor memory, and depression. Hypertension may be present and an ECG may reveal cardiac conduction disturbances (prolonged P-R interval, wide QRS complexes, shortened Q-T interval).

**Diagnosis.** Hypercalcemia (serum total calcium >11 to 12 mg/dl or >2.75 mmol/L) and hypophosphatemia (<3.0 mg/dl or <0.97 mmol/L) are the laboratory hallmarks of primary hyperparathyroidism. Parathyroid hormone levels, as measured by immunoassay, are elevated relative to the hypercalcemia. Increased alkaline phosphatase and hyperchloremia are also present.

A radiograph of the chest may show subperiosteal bone resorption of the clavicles, while marked periosteal bone erosion in the terminal phalanges is evident on radiographs of the hands. Finally, demineralization of the skull in a "salt and pepper pattern" is frequently seen on skull films. In children suspected of having a pituitary adenoma, preoperative localization may be accomplished by using ultrasonography, CT, MRI, or radiothallium scanning.

**Treatment.** Acute hypercalcemia is treated by intravenous fluid administration with normal saline and loop diuretics (furosemide and ethacrynic acid) to promote calciuresis. A rapid fall of 2 to 3 mg/dl (0.5 to 0.75 mmol/L) in total serum calcium concentration is typical after hydration. Careful monitoring of vital signs, ECG, and electrolyte status is essential because of the significant urinary electrolyte losses. Calcitonin and mithramycin have also been used with variable success. In patients with renal failure, peritoneal dialysis or hemodialysis is effective in reducing serum calcium levels.

In children with diffuse hyperplasia, familial hyperplasia, multiple endocrine neoplasia syndrome, or multiple adenomas, a total parathyroidectomy is often required. Autotransplantation of a part of one parathyroid gland to the forearm has been recommended in some cases. Following a total parathyroidectomy, the possibility of an acute fall in serum calcium levels with resulting neuromuscular irritability or tetany must be anticipated. Serum calcium levels should be monitored and intravenous calcium solutions administered as indicated. Continuing treatment with calcium and vitamin D will be required. In the rare case of a single parathyroid adenoma, selective surgical excision of the lesion may be performed.

### Secondary Hyperparathyroidism

Secondary hyperparathyroidism is a state of compensatory hypersecretion of PTH in response to hypocalcemia, hyperphosphatemia, or hypomagnesemia produced by other diseases. This condition is most commonly seen in children with chronic renal disease, in which hypocalcemia, hyperphosphatemia, decreased production of $1,25(OH)_2 D_3$, reduced intestinal absorption of calcium, and peripheral resistance to the action of PTH all contribute to the pathogenesis of hyperparathyroidism. Renal osteodystrophy (generalized osteopenia, osteitis fibrosa cystica, osteomalacia, and osteosclerosis) may result from the excessive production of PTH and impaired formation of $1,25(OH)_2 D_3$. Other medical conditions associated with secondary hyperparathyroidism include vitamin D deficiency, intestinal malabsorption syndromes, Fanconi syndrome, and renal tubular acidosis.

Transient neonatal hyperparathyroidism has been reported in a few neonates born to mothers with undiagnosed or inadequately treated hypoparathyroidism or pseudohypoparathyroidism. Chronic intrauterine exposure to hypocalcemia led to fetal parathyroid gland hyperplasia. Typically these infants exhibit parathyroid bone disease.

**Treatment.** The mainstay of treatment is correcting the underlying cause of the excessive PTH secretion. Renal transplant may correct secondary hyperparathyroidism of chronic renal failure. There are, however, a few cases of persistent hyperparathyroidism following transplantation that required a parathyroidectomy.

Calcium and vitamin D supplementation, where indicated, are part of the medical management.

## ADRENAL GLANDS

The adrenal glands are composed of two functionally distinct endocrine systems: the cortical system, which synthesizes three groups of steroid hormones (glucocorticoids, mineralocorticoids, and androgens), and the medullary system, responsible for the synthesis of catecholamines (epinephrine, norepinephrine, and dopamine).

## Adrenal Cortex

The adrenal cortex develops from the mesonephros and is subdivided into three functional zones: (1) an outer zona glomerulosa, which produces aldosterone; (2) the zona fasciculata, which primarily synthesizes and secretes glucocorticoids and androgens; and (3) the zona reticularis, which also synthesizes glucocorticoids and androgens (Fig. 6-2).

Steroidogenesis is regulated by hormones released from the hypothalamus and the pituitary gland. CRH from the hypothalamus stimulates pituitary ACTH, which in turn increases synthesis of glucocorticoids in the zona fasciculata and reticularis. Adrenal glucocorticoids regulate the release of CRH and ACTH by a negative feedback mechanism. The hypothalamic-pituitary-adrenal axis is influenced by diurnal variations of plasma ACTH, cortisol, and adrenocortical steroid levels. This diurnal variation is absent in the neonate, but becomes apparent by 6 months of age.[31] Additional regulatory mechanisms involve stress-induced release of these hormones. Trauma, stress related to anesthesia and surgery, infection, sepsis, and hypogly-

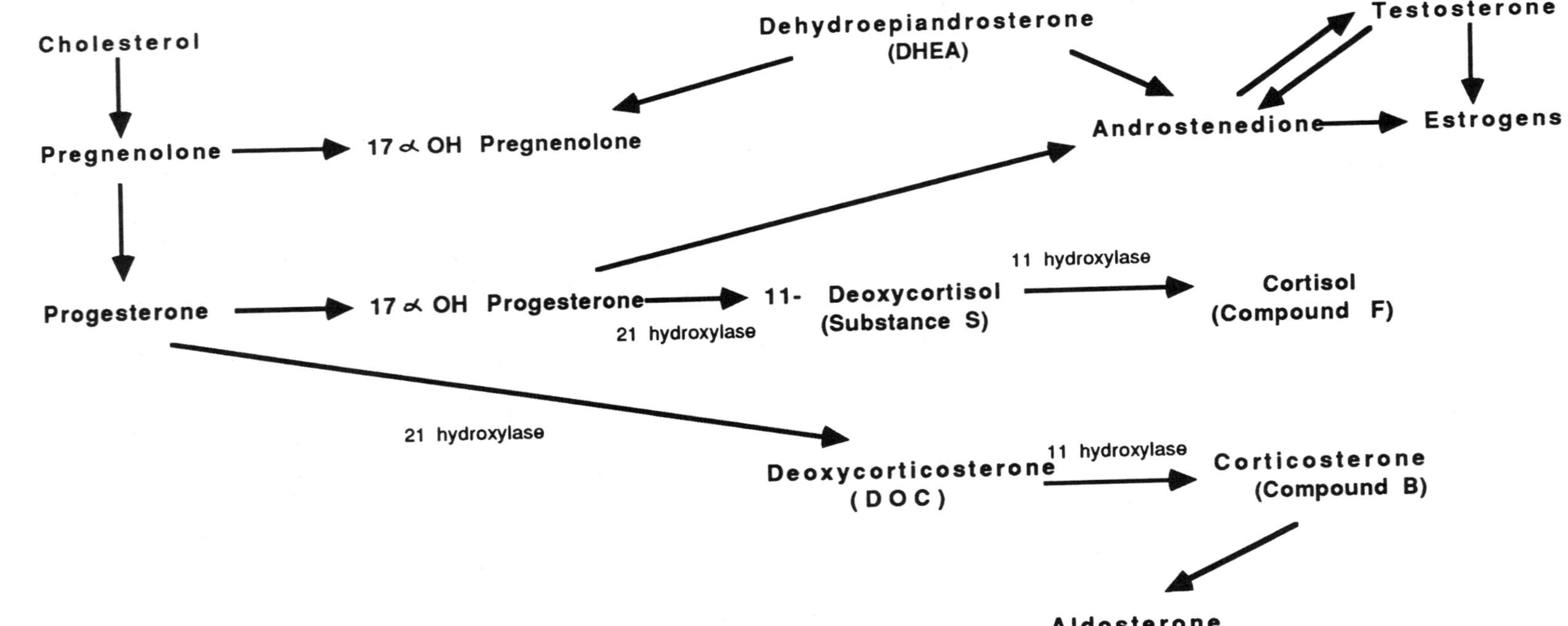


**Fig. 6-2.** Steroid hormone synthesis in the adrenal cortex.

cemia are all known to release ACTH and thus increase plasma levels of adrenal hormones.

Cortisol is the principal glucocorticoid secreted by the adrenal cortex. Once secreted, 70 percent of the cortisol is bound to corticosteroid-binding globulin (CBG), and 20 percent is bound to albumin. The remaining free, unbound cortisol is the active form. Cortisol exerts several important physiologic effects including (1) increased gluconeogenesis and muscle glycogenolysis, (2) inhibition of cellular glucose utilization (antagonizes action of insulin), (3) proteinolysis, (4) fatty acid mobilization, (5) increased catecholamine synthesis in the adrenal medulla and GH secretion from the pituitary, and (6) anti-inflammatory actions.

Aldosterone accounts for about 95 percent of the mineralocorticoid produced by the adrenal cortex. Like cortisol, aldosterone is bound to CBG and albumin. Free aldosterone acts upon the renal tubular epithelial cells in the distal tubules and collecting ducts, resulting in an increase in sodium reabsorption and potassium excretion. Therefore, aldosterone plays an important role in maintaining sodium and water balance in the body.

Control of aldosterone secretion in the zona glomerulosa is regulated by several factors, including extracellular fluid concentrations of potassium ions, the renin-angiotensin system, and total body sodium content.[32] Secretion of aldosterone and other mineralocorticoids is not under the primary control of ACTH. However, dopamine appears to inhibit aldosterone secretion through a direct action on glomerulosa cells.

The primary androgen hormones secreted from the zona fasciculata and reticularis include dehydroepiandrosterone (DHEA), androstenedione, and testosterone. Small amounts of estrogens are also produced. In peripheral tissues, DHEA is converted to the potent androgens testosterone and dihydrotestosterone (DHT). Control of adrenal androgen secretion is not well understood, but ACTH plays a role in the regulatory process. The androgens secreted from the adrenal are metabolized in the liver and excreted by the kidney as 17-ketosteroids. A deficiency or excess of adrenal cortical hormones, or an abnormality in steroid biosynthesis, may produce several significant pathologic conditions.

## Adrenal Insufficiency

The syndrome of adrenal insufficiency results from inadequate adrenocortical function. This may be due to dysfunction or destruction of the adrenal cortex (primary adrenal insufficiency, Addison's disease), deficient pituitary ACTH secretion (secondary adrenal insufficiency), or deficient hypothalamic release of CRH (tertiary adrenal insufficiency).

Primary adrenal insufficiency is extremely rare in pediatric patients. In the newborn, adrenal hypoplasia or adrenal hemorrhage from asphyxia or traumatic delivery may lead to adrenal insufficiency. Infants and young children with overwhelming sepsis, usually from meningococcemia, may present with primary adrenal insufficiency and circulatory collapse (Waterhouse-Friderichsen syndrome). Adrenoleukodystrophy is a X-linked recessive disorder of long-chain fatty acid metabolism associated with progressive central demyelination and adrenal insufficiency.

In older children and adolescents, adrenal insufficiency is usually of autoimmune origin and may occur in association with other autoimmune endocrinopathies (lymphocytic thyroiditis, insulin-dependent diabetes mellitus). Less common causes of adrenal insufficiency include histoplasmosis, various mycoses, amyloid disease, and (rarely) tuberculosis. Primary adrenal insufficiency is associated with both glucocorticoid and mineralocorticoid deficiency. Secondary adrenal insufficiency is characterized by a deficiency of cortisol production due to inadequate pituitary ACTH secretion. Aldosterone secretion, however, is normal. Causes of this condition are similar to those producing hypopituitarism. This condition is often seen in patients after withdrawal from exogenous glucocorticoid therapy. Finally, in tertiary adrenal insufficiency there is a deficiency of normal CRH secretion, resulting in decreased cortisol, but normal mineralocorticoid secretion.

**Clinical Presentation.** Infants with adrenal insufficiency caused by traumatic adrenal hemorrhage or overwhelming infection usually present in acute shock, evidenced by lethargy, tachycardia, and severe hypotension. In those infants with massive adrenal hemorrhage, a hematoma may be palpable in the flank. It is of note that following bilateral adrenal hemorrhage, infants may demonstrate improved adrenal function as they grow, due to regeneration of adrenal tissue.

The manifestations of primary adrenal insufficiency in older children and adolescents are due to deficiencies in glucocorticoids and mineralocorticoids. Symptoms may include fatigue, weakness, nausea and vomiting, diarrhea, failure to gain weight or weight loss, hypotension, salt cravings, and increasing skin pigmentation. On physical examination, postural hypotension and increased pigmentation over joints, scar tissue, lips, and buccal mucosa are commonly seen. In secondary and tertiary adrenal insufficiency, the clinical presentation is solely due to glucocorticoid deficiency and (in females) to loss of adrenal androgen secretion.

**Diagnosis.** The characteristic laboratory findings of primary adrenal insufficiency are hypoglycemia, hyponatremia, hyperkalemia, and mild metabolic acidosis. Anemia with a mild to moderate eosinophilia and leukopenia is common. Urinary sodium is elevated and potassium decreased. Hypoglycemia without electrolyte abnormalities and decreased ACTH levels are present in secondary and tertiary adrenal insufficiency. Confirmatory tests include (1) reduced cortisol levels before and after ACTH stimulation, and (2) the metapyrone test, used to demonstrate cortisol deficiency in patients with a normal pituitary-adrenal responsiveness. Radiographic studies may reveal a small, narrow heart or evidence of adrenal enlargement and hemorrhage.

**Treatment.** In patients with nonacute adrenal insufficiency, the key to therapy is the administration of glucocorticoids and mineralocorticoids. Various glucocorticoids have been used including hydrocortisone 10 to 25 $mg/m^2/d$ in three divided doses, or prednisone 4 to 5 $mg/m^2/d$ in two divided doses (Appendix 6-1). With the initiation of therapy, monitoring for evidence of excessive glucocorticoid replacement is important. Suppressed morning plasma ACTH levels may also indicate excessive replacement.

During acute illness, surgery, or other times of stress, doses of glucocorticoid should be increased three- to fourfold. Patients having surgery should receive intravenous hydrocortisone during the perioperative period to prevent acute adrenal insufficiency. Mineralocorticoid replacement is with fludrocortisone 0.05 to 0.1 mg/d (Appendix 6-1). Serum sodium and potassium levels, along with plasma renin activity, should be monitored. Blood pressure (recumbent and standing) should also be followed to avoid hypertension. Additionally, a liberal salt intake is encouraged. In children with secondary or tertiary adrenal insufficiency, glucocorticoid therapy is similar to that for primary adrenal insufficiency. However, mineralocorticoid supplementation is rarely required, but replacement of other pituitary hormones may be necessary.

**Acute Adrenal Crisis.** Acute adrenal crisis is a life-threatening form of adrenal insufficiency often triggered by intercurrent illness, surgery, or trauma. Clinical manifestations may include nausea and vomiting, dehydration, fever, abdominal pain, weakness, lethargy, confusion or coma, hypotension, cyanosis, or circulatory collapse.

Immediate treatment should include aggressive fluid resuscitation using 0.9 percent saline or 5 percent dextrose and saline, as well as glucocorticoid replacement with hydrocortisone sodium succinate (2 mg/kg diluted in 2 to 10 ml of water, intravenously over 2 to 5 minutes). Thereafter, hydrocortisone sodium succinate is given, 1.5 mg/kg in infants or 12.5 mg/$m^2$ in older children, every 4 to 6 hours until stabilization is achieved and oral therapy tolerated. Suspected infections should be treated with appropriate antibiotics. Additional workup and evaluation are undertaken after stabilization of the patient. Mineralocorticoid therapy may also be instituted when the child is tolerating fluids.

## Congenital Adrenal Hyperplasia

A deficiency of the adrenal steroidogenic enzymes leads to congenital adrenal hyperplasia. The disruption of cortisol synthesis stimulates increased ACTH secretion from the anterior pituitary, with consequent adrenal hyperplasia and accumulation of precursor hormones proximal to the enzymatic defect in the steroid biosynthetic pathway. The clinical characteristics are thus reflective of the specific enzyme defect. These disorders are inherited as autosomal recessive traits. Approximately 95 percent of all cases are due to a deficiency of 21-hydroxylase or 11-hydroxylase.

**21-Hydroxylase Deficiency.** The most common form of congenital adrenal hyperplasia is 21-hydroxylase deficiency, which accounts for 90 percent of all cases and has an incidence of 1 in 5,000 to 1 in 15,000.[33] There are degrees of severity of 21-hydroxylase deficiency (severe, moderate, and mild).

**Clinical Presentation.** In the most severe form (previously referred to as salt-wasting), there is a deficiency of cortisol and aldosterone synthesis and increased ACTH and the precursor 17-hydroxyprogesterone. This precursor is metabolized to the adrenal androgens DHEA and androstenedione. Infants usually present in the first 2 to 4 weeks of life with poor feeding, vomiting, weight loss, dehydration, and potentially life-threatening shock. Hyponatremia, hyperkalemia, hypoglycemia, and acidosis are common. Female infants are born with ambiguous external genitalia (clitoromegaly and labioscrotal fusion) owing to adrenal androgen-induced masculinization. Male infants have normal genitalia.

The moderate form (simple virilizing) is due to excessive production of adrenal androgens. Cortisol levels are near normal, aldosterone levels are either normal or elevated, and hyponatremia is rarely seen. Female infants will have varying degrees of virilization, and both males and females will manifest virilization (penile or clitoral enlargement; premature appearance of pubic hair) in early childhood.

A mild form of 21-hydroxylase deficiency most often occurring in girls or women is associated with an elevated conversion of 17-hydroxyprogesterone to androgens in peripheral tissues. These patients may develop acne, premature sexual hair, hirsutism, and menstrual irregularities.

**Diagnosis.** The clinical presentation, in conjuction with hyponatremia, hyperkalemia, decreased cortisol, and elevated serum 17-hydroxyprogesterone levels, is diagnostic of the severe form of 21-hydroxylase deficiency. In the mild and moderate forms, serum 17-hydroxyprogesterone is mildly elevated. Occasionally, in the milder forms, intravenous ACTH is used to stimulate 17-hydroxyprogesterone; an excessive rise confirms the diagnosis.

**Treatment.** The goals of treatment in children with congenital adrenal hyperplasia include suppression of excessive ACTH stimulation and replacement of the deficient hormones. Oral hydrocortisone is the drug of choice (Appendix 6-1). The adequacy of treatment can be assessed by following the patient's linear growth velocity, skeletal maturation, sexual development, and laboratory tests (hormone levels, plasma renin activity, and urinary 17-ketosteroids).

Additional glucocorticoid supplementation (hydrocortisone) may be required during the perioperative period and other times of stress (fever, systemic illness, trauma). Mineralocorticoid (fludrocortisone) may be given to children with the severe form of 21-hydroxylase deficiency to suppress plasma renin levels. Virilized female infants should also undergo genital reconstructive surgery before the age of 1 year, for optimal results.

**11-Hydroxylase Deficiency.** A deficiency of 11-hydroxylase is characterized by an excessive production of deoxycorticosterone (DOC) and adrenal androgens, as well as a decrease in cortisol secretion. This condition accounts for approximately 5 percent of patients with congenital adrenal hyperplasia.

**Clinical Presentation.** An excess accumulation of DOC, which has mineralocorticoid activity, causes salt and water retention, volume expansion, hypertension, and hyperkalemia. However, hypertension is usually not present before 2 years of age. Female infants are born with masculinized external genitalia. Over time, untreated males and females experience progressive virilization.

**Diagnosis.** Elevated serum concentrations of 11-deoxycortisol and DOC are present, along with increased serum levels of androstenedione and testosterone. Renin and aldosterone levels are suppressed.

**Treatment.** Treatment is based on glucocorticoid administration to suppress ACTH and the accumulation of precursor steroid hormones. Gonadal steroid replacement is initiated at the time of expected puberty.

## Hypercorticism

Hypercorticism, or Cushing syndrome, is a clinical state characterized by chronic excessive endogenous secretion or exogenous administration of glucocorticoid hormones. Cushing syndrome in childhood is rare, but when it does occur, it is usually secondary to iatrogenic exogenous glucocorticoid therapy.

In children who have not received prolonged glucocorticoid therapy, other causes of hypercorticism should be considered. The presence of Cushing syndrome in a child less than 7 years of age is usually indicative of an adrenal adenoma. A young child will rarely have a malignant adrenal carcinoma, but if one is present, excessive cortisol, aldosterone, estrogens, and androgens may be produced. In children older than 7 years, bilateral adrenal hyperplasia due to chronic excess secretion of ACTH by a pituitary tumor (adenoma or microadenoma), is the most common etiology. This condition is referred to as Cushing's disease. Tumors that produce ectopic ACTH or CRH can also cause hypercorticism, but these are very infrequent in children.

**Clinical Presentation.** The clinical features of Cushing syndrome are related to excess cortisol, mineralocorticoids, and androgens. The classic manifestations in childhood are growth retardation, "moon facies," "Buffalo-type" adiposity, easy fatigability, decreased muscle mass and muscle weakness, thin skin and purple striae, impaired carbohydrate metabolism, edema, and hypertension. Hirsutism and amenorrhea may be the presenting complaints in adolescent girls.

**Diagnosis.** The diagnosis of Cushing syndrome is confirmed by increased serum cortisol levels with or without loss of diurnal variation, as well as elevated urinary free cortisol and 17-hydroxycorticoids. If these studies do not show unequivocal elevation of cortisol levels, then an overnight or low-dose dexamethasone suppression test is indicated. Dexamethasone will suppress cortisol production in healthy patients, but not in those with hypercorticism. Additionally, determinations of ACTH levels are helpful in differentiating the location of the lesion. ACTH levels are elevated in patients with a pituitary tumor or ectopic ACTH production, but are suppressed in primary adrenal disease.[34] Adrenocortical lesions may be detected on CT or MRI. Many pituitary microadenomas may not be visualized on CT, but may be detected with MRI.

**Treatment.** The treatment of choice for a child with an adrenal or pituitary tumor is surgical excision. Perioperative glucocorticoid coverage must be provided so as to prevent adrenal insufficiency.

## Adrenal Medulla

The endocrine cell of the adrenal medulla, referred to as the chromaffin cell, is derived from neural crest ectoderm. The chromaffin cells synthesize, store, and secrete catecholamines (epinephrine, norepinephrine, and dopamine) in response to preganglionic sympathetic innervation via the splanchnic nerves. The cell of the adrenal medulla is analogous to a postganglionic neuron and thus is an integral component of the sympathetic nervous system. However, the catecholamines produced by the medulla function as hormones and not as neurotransmitters.

Epinephrine comprises 80 to 85 percent of the adrenomedullary catecholamine store and is synthesized almost exclusively in the medulla by methylation of norepinephrine via the action of phenylethanolamine-*N*-methyl transferase (PNMT) (Fig 6-3). Activity of this enzyme is enhanced by cortisol transported by the intraadrenal portal vascular system from the adrenal cortex. Consequently, any stress that releases glucocorticoids also results in an increase in the synthesis and release of epinephrine.

Norepinephrine is widely distributed throughout the body, functioning primarily as the neurotransmitter for a majority of the postganglionic fibers of the sympathetic nervous system. Only 15 to 20 percent of the adrenomedullary catecholamine output consists of norepinephrine, which functions as a hormone and serves no role as a neurotransmitter. The normal adrenal medulla releases catecholamines by calcium-dependent exocytosis in response to stimulation from preganglionic cholinergic fibers. Plasma half-lives for circulating epinephrine and norepinephrine are less than 30 seconds, reflecting rapid metabolism by the enzyme catechol-*O*-methyltransferase (COMT), located in the liver and kidney (Fig. 6-3). To a lesser degree, monoamine oxidase (MAO), found in all tissues, is involved in the degradation of circulating catecholamines. The major metabolites are vanillylmandelic acid (VMA), ac-

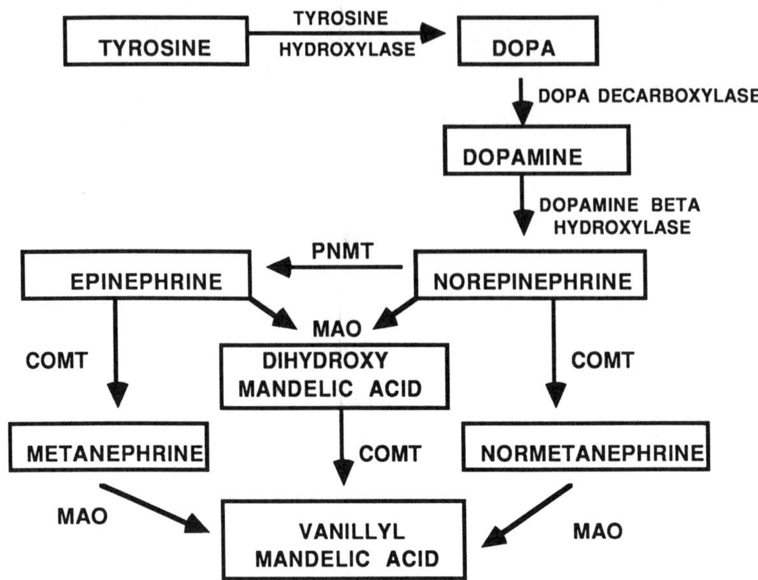


**Fig. 6-3.** Synthesis and metabolism of catecholamines. COMT, catechol-*O*-methyltransferase; MAO, monoamine oxidase; PNMT, phenylethanolamine-*N*-methyltransferase.

counting for approximately 80 percent of the urinary metabolites, and metanephrine, comprising 15 percent. Less than 1 percent of the released epinephrine, norepinephrine, or dopamine appears unchanged in the urine.

Catecholamine activity is mediated via α, β, and dopaminergic receptors located within various organ tissues throughout the body. Epinephrine and norepinephrine exert widespread but variable effects on the cardiovascular, pulmonary, and renal systems, as well as on metabolism. At lower concentrations, dopamine stimulates peripheral dopaminergic receptors, which appear to mediate vasodilatation in renal, mesenteric, coronary, and cerebral vascular beds. At higher concentrations, dopamine directly stimulates β- and α-adrenergic receptors.

In addition to the chromaffin cells localized in the adrenal medulla, small clumps of extra-adrenal chromaffin cells may exist in and around sympathetic ganglia. The most prominent of these is the organ of Zuckerkandl, situated anterior to the aorta and caudal to the inferior mesenteric artery, and a possible site of origin for neuroblastoma. These extra-adrenal chromaffin cells usually regress early in life, but remnants may remain and be the site of subsequent extra-adrenal pheochromocytoma formation.

The two important catecholamine-secreting tumors that occur in pediatric patients and are associated with the adrenal medulla are pheochromocytoma and neuroblastoma. An understanding of the clinical and anesthetic implications is essential for proper management of these patients.

## Pheochromocytoma

Pheochromocytoma is a catecholamine-secreting tumor arising from chromaffin cells of the adrenal medulla or, less frequently, along the paravertebral sympathetic ganglia extending from the pelvis to the base of the skull. These tumors produce increased amounts of norepinephrine and epinephrine, with norepinephrine predominant. Rarely will these tumors secrete epinephrine exclusively. In addition to catecholamines, a pheochromocytoma may also contain various peptides including enkephalins, somatostatin, calcitonin, oxytocin, vasopressin, and vasoactive intestinal peptide.

Pheochromocytoma is a rare tumor in the pediatric age group, with only approximately 30 to 50 cases diagnosed each year in the United States. The tumor may occur at any age, but in children the greatest frequency is at the time of puberty, with nearly 70 percent occurring in boys. In contrast, in adults the tumor typically presents between the ages of 40 to 50 years and demonstrates a mild female preponderance (55 to 60 percent). The majority of pheochromocytomas are solitary tumors originating from a single adrenal gland, most commonly the right. However, in 20 to 25 percent of children, bilateral tumors may be present at the time of diagnosis. The tumor usually arises within the abdomen, but in 5 to 10 percent of cases, may be located in the neck, thorax, or bladder. Fortunately, less than 10 percent are malignant, and metastatic disease, usually to the liver, is rare in the pediatric patient.

Of interest to the anesthesiologist is the fact that pheochromocytoma may occasionally be associated with an autosomal dominant multiglandular neoplastic syndrome known as multiple endocrine neoplasia, types IIA or IIB. Type IIA (Sipple syndrome) consists of pheochromocytoma, medullary carcinoma of the thyroid, and hyperparathyroidism. Type IIB is characterized by pheochromocytoma, medullary carcinoma of the thyroid, multiple mucosal neuromas, and a marfanoid habitus. Neurofibromatosis may occur in approximately 5 percent of patients with pheochromocytoma. In addition, pheochromocytomas have been found in association with von Hippel-Lindau syndrome, tuberous sclerosis, and Sturge-Weber syndrome.[35]

**Clinical Presentation.** The clinical manifestations of pheochromocytoma are related to the physiologic and pharmacologic effects of the catecholamines secreted from the tumor. Signs and symptoms may be paroxysmal and vary from mild (intermittent hypertension, diaphoresis, constipation, weight loss) to life-threatening (malignant hypertension, encephalopathy, cardiomyopathy, and shock). In the child with a pheochromocytoma common clinical features include sustained, or less frequently paraoxysmal, hypertension (often systolic pressures $>$ 200 to 250 mmHg), headache, nausea and vomiting, pallor, anxiety, diaphoresis, weakness, and fatigue. Weight loss, abdominal pain, polyuria, and polydipsia are also frequent findings.

Patients may also experience hypermetabolism and carbohydrate intolerance, as evidenced by elevated plasma glucose concentrations and low plasma insulin levels. A predominance of $\alpha$-receptor-mediated suppression of insulin release and $\beta$-receptor-mediated stimulation of hepatic glycogenolysis and gluconeogenesis contributes to this condition. Symptomatic diabetes is unusual, and indeed, if present, is probably indicative of coexisting diabetes mellitus. Hypercalcemia is an uncommon, but well-recognized complication, particularly in those with familial pheochromocytoma (multiple endocrine neoplasia syndrome).

Regarding the cardiovascular system, a reduced intravascular volume from sustained hypertension may result in orthostatic hypotension, and loss of postural reflexes may also contribute to the hypotension. Another consequence of the diminished intravascular volume is an elevation of the hematocrit. Cardiac arrhythmias and tachycardia are seldom observed in children, and, unlike in adults, the incidence of myocarditis, cardiomyopathies with associated congestive heart failure, myocardial infarction, and noncardiogenic pulmonary edema is low.

In the rare child with a predominantly epinephrine-releasing tumor, the clinical manifestations may differ. Hypotension, tachycardia, cardiac arrhythmias, and noncardiogenic pulmonary edema may be present.[36]

**Diagnosis.** The importance of diagnosing pheochromocytoma preoperatively is emphasized by the very high perioperative mortality rate (45 to 50 percent) in surgical patients with undiagnosed pheochromocytoma. However, in children and adolescents the diagnosis may be delayed for long periods due to the rarity of the condition, the rather vague symptoms, and a low index of suspicion.

The definitive diagnosis of pheochromocytoma is based upon the biochemical documentation of elevated catecholamine production. Laboratory techniques utilized include the measurement of 24-hour urinary catecholamines or their metabolites (VMA or metanephrines) and/or direct plasma concentrations of epinephrine, norepinephrine, and dopamine. Each of these methods has limitations, however. Urinary catecholamine determinations can be time consuming and erratic, and false-negative results from drugs such as β-antagonists and most antihypertensives may occur in up to 50 percent of patients. False positives from increased catecholamine release have been observed in patients consuming foods containing tyramine (e.g., cheese, chocolate, caffeine, amphetamines).

Direct plasma catecholamine measurements are considered to be more reliable in establishing the diagnosis, even in those patients who are normotensive. Most patients with a pheochromocytoma have notably elevated plasma catecholamines, but these levels are also influenced by the effects of drugs and variations in the technique of obtaining, processing, and storing the specimen. If possible, the specimen should be obtained when patients are drug-free and during a symptomatic episode (paroxysm).[37]

Previously, provocative tests using histamine, glucagon, or tyramine were used in the diagnostic process. These tests are no longer used due to the potential hazards associated with induction of a severe paroxysm and the recent advances in radioenzymatic assays. On occasion, the clonidine suppression test has been helpful in differentiating pheochromocytoma from essential hypertension in patients with equivocal plasma catecholamine concentrations (1,000 to 2,000 pg/ml). A single oral dose (0.3 mg) of the $\alpha_2$-adrenergic agonist clonidine suppresses catecholamine secretion and catecholamine plasma concentrations in patients with essential hypertension, but not reliably in those with pheochromocytoma.

Anatomic localization of the tumor should be sought only after biochemical confirmation of a pheochromocytoma. Ultrasonography of the abdomen and adrenal glands is helpful, but there are inherent technical limitations because of the retroperitoneal location of the adrenal glands. Adrenal CT is the most commonly used imaging technique for adrenomedullary pheochromocytoma. For extra-adrenal tumors, MRI is superior. Scintigraphy using $^{131}$I-metaiodobenzylguanidine is effective in localizing recurrent, extra-adrenal or metastatic pheochromocytoma. This guanidine analog is concentrated in sympathomedullary tissue.[38]

Baseline laboratory studies including a complete blood count (CBC), fasting serum glucose, electrolytes, calcium, and creatinine should be obtained. Hypercalcemia in the preoperative period may be indicative of a multiple endocrine neoplasia syndrome. An ECG and echocardiogram are performed to evaluate cardiac function and exclude cardiomyopathy. Renal function may be impaired in some patients.

**Treatment.** The definitive treatment of pheochromocytoma is surgical excision, and the key to successful surgery is appropriate preoperative preparation.

All patients with pheochromocytoma should be started on α-adrenergic blockers a minimum of 10 to 14 days prior to surgery. Preoperative α-adrenergic blockade minimizes the untoward effects of sustained hypertension. Re-expansion of intravascular volume, a reduction in the likelihood of hyperglycemia, and severe intraoperative hypertension may all be achieved with adequate blockade. Significantly, it appears that proper α blockade prior to surgery lowers the perioperative mortality from a high of 45 to between 0 and 3 percent.

Phenoxybenzamine, a long-acting oral $\alpha_1$- and $\alpha_2$-adrenergic antagonist, is commonly used to accomplish alpha blockade. An initial dose of 10 mg bid orally is usually increased over several days until hypertension is controlled, symptomatic paroxysms prevented, and mild postural hypotension occurs. Aside from postural hypotension, other side effects of phenoxybenzamine may include reflex tachycardia, arrhythmias, sedation, nausea, weakness, gastric irritation, and nasal congestion. Daily monitoring of blood pressure (recumbent and seated) and serial determinations of the hematocrit are effective in evaluating the adequacy of alpha blockade.

Prazosin, a relatively selective postsynaptic α-1-receptor antagonist, has also been used to achieve preoperative alpha blockade. However, there is a case report of severe perioperative hypertension in a prazosin-treated patient.[39] Cardiac arrhythmias and tachycardia are rare in children with a pheochromocytoma. If present, effective β-adrenergic blockade can be obtained with propranolol or atenolol. Beta blockade should not be instituted until adequate α blockade is present so as to avoid the possibility of cardiac failure. If the proposed surgery may involve bilateral adrenal exploration, the patient should receive glucocorticoid supplementation preoperatively.

In children with metastatic or unresectable tumors, long-term medical management involves the use of α-methyltyrosine, a tyrosine hydroxylase inhibitor, which reduces catecholamine synthesis. This drug may be used in combination with α-adrenergic blockers. Limited success has been reported with a chemotherapeutic regimen consisting of cyclophosphamide, vincristine, and decarbazine.

Several commonly used anesthetic drugs that should not be administered to patients with pheochromocytoma include sympathetic stimulants (ketamine, pancuronium), halothane (arrhythmogenic), histamine-releasing drugs (d-tubocurarine, metocurine, atracurium, and mivacurium), and droperidol (may provoke hypertensive response).

The persistence of hypertension 48 hours after surgery is suggestive of residual tumor. Postoperative hypoglycemia resulting from decreased plasma catecholamine levels and rebound hyperinsulinemia may be seen; thus, frequent blood glucose estimations are required.

## Neuroblastoma and Ganglioneuroma

Neuroblastoma is a malignant tumor originating from primitive neuroblasts of neural crest ectoderm located in the adrenal medulla or along the sympathetic chain extending from the posterior cranial fossa to the coccyx. Similar to pheochromocytomas, these tumors are associated with an excess production of catecholamines and their metabolites (HVA and VMA). Ganglioneuroblastoma is a tumor composed of neuroblasts and mature sympathetic ganglion cells. It is usually located in the posterior mediastinum, but may be found along the course of the sympathetic chain. This tumor is usually well encapsulated and amenable to surgical resection. The child with a ganglioneuroblastoma may manifest symptoms of increased catecholamine secretion (hypertension, tachycardia, and diaphoresis). Ganglioneuroma is a benign tumor composed of mature ganglion cells, also situated along the sympathetic chain, not usually associated with high urinary catecholamine levels. Ganglioneuroblastoma and ganglioneuroma are considered to represent neuroblastomas that have undergone differentiation toward a more mature cell type. The reason for this maturation is unclear, but this does confer a more favorable prognosis. A syndrome of chronic diarrhea may be associated with ganglioneuroblastoma or ganglioneuroma and is due to a neuropeptide enterohormone, vasoactive intestinal peptide (VIP). The diarrhea may be associated with failure to thrive, abdominal distension, and hypokalemia.

Neuroblastoma is the most common extracranial solid tumor in children, accounting for 8 to 10 percent of all childhood cancers. The occurrence rate is approximately 1 in 10,000 live births. It is a tumor of early childhood, with a median age of 22 months at the time of diagnosis. Over 80 percent of patients are diagnosed by 4 years of age and 97 percent by age 10 years.[40]

The primary tumor site is usually in the abdomen; 50 percent originate in the adrenal glands and the others in pelvic or visceral ganglia or paraganglia. Approximately 15 to 20 percent of neuroblastomas arise along the cervical or thoracic sympathetic chain. Characteristically, these tumors grow rapidly and metastasize to lymph nodes, cortical bone, bone marrow, liver, and skin. However, unlike many solid tumors, neuroblastomas rarely metastasize to the lungs, except as a terminal event. Unfortunately, disseminated disease is found in nearly 66 percent of patients at the time of diagnosis.[40]

**Clinical Presentation.** The signs and symptoms of patients who have neuroblastoma are variable depending on the location of the primary tumor, the extent of metastases, and the presence of paraneoplastic syndromes.

Children may present with a firm nontender abdominal mass or complaints of abdominal pain. Anorexia, vomiting, and weight loss also occur. Hemorrhage into the enlarging tumor may cause pallor, anemia, and, in severe cases, hypotension. Lateral displacement of the kidney by the tumor or compression of the renal vasculature produces hypertension in approximately 1 to 5 percent of patients, while tumors in the pelvis may cause mechanical difficulty with defecation or urination.

Thoracic neuroblastomas, located in the posterior mediastinum, are a common extra-abdominal presentation. These tumors may be associated with dysphagia, a predisposition to respiratory infections, or, less frequently, respiratory distress. On occasion, the tumor may be an incidental finding on a chest radiograph obtained for unrelated symptoms. Neuroblastomas involving the superior, stellate, or cervical ganglion may present with Horner syndrome (unilateral miosis, ptosis, anhidrosis, enophthalmos).

Paraspinal neuroblastomas in the abdomen or chest may invade the spinal canal via intervertebral foramina (dumbbell tumor) and cause symptoms of cord compression including back pain, bowel and bladder dysfunction, and gait disturbances.

Unfortunately, metastatic disease is common at the time of diagnosis and often accounts for the symptoms that lead to the diagnosis. Nonspecific symptoms include fever, weight loss, and failure to thrive. More specific symptoms of metastatic disease that may be present are (1) localized or generalized cortical bone pain that may manifest as a limp if the lower extremities are involved; (2) periorbital ecchymosis and proptosis; (3) liver infiltration leading to massive hepatomegaly and rarely ascites; (4) bone marrow failure as evidenced by anemia, thrombocytopenic purpura and petechia, and leukopenia with infection and fever; (5) skin infiltration appearing as multiple bluish subcutaneous nodules ("blueberry muffin appearance"); and (6) diffuse lymph node enlargement, especially in the supraclavicular, cervical, and inguinal regions.

Other symptoms may include diarrhea (see above); an acute myoclonic encephalopathy characterized by opsoclonus, myoclonus, and cerebellar ataxia is a rare manifestation. The symptoms of both these syndromes usually resolve after resection of the primary tumor.

**Diagnosis.** A specific diagnostic feature of neuroblastoma is an increased urinary excretion of catecholamines and their metabolites (normetanephrine, HVA, VMA). Elevated levels of dopamine and HVA are particularly characteristic of neuroblastoma. In addition to establishing a diagnosis, assays of urinary catecholamine excretion are useful in assessing the response to therapy and detection of recurrence. Neuroblastomas contain relatively small amounts of active catecholamines due to their increased metabolism and release of metabolically inactive compounds. This may explain why hypertension resulting from catecholamine secretion is not frequently present.

Other studies helpful in evaluating the child with a presumed neuroblastoma are determined by the site of tumor origin and evidence of metastases. These include radiographs of the chest and abdomen, abdominal ultrasound, CT scans or MRI, pyelography, myelography, bone scan, and bone marrow aspiration or biopsy. Definitive diagnosis depends on the analysis of tumor tissue obtained at excision or diagnostic biopsy. Each patient diagnosed with neuroblastoma undergoes clinical staging, on which the choice of a therapeutic regimen is based.

**Treatment.** The principle modalities of conventional therapy include surgery, radiation therapy, and chemotherapy. For those patients with localized disease, complete surgical resection carries the best chance for cure. In children with unresectable tumors on initial examination, chemotherapy or radiation therapy may be followed by surgical resection of the primary tumor. Surgery may also serve a palliative role, to relieve compression of vital organs or structures, and surgical placement of a central venous catheter is common practice in children requiring intensive chemotherapy.

Radiation therapy plays a limited role in the management of patients with neuroblastoma. It is used primarily for reduction of tumors that are unresectable and unresponsive to chemotherapy and as palliative treatment of tumor-related pain or organ dysfunction.

Metastatic disease is frequently present at the time of diagnosis; therefore, chemotherapy has become the mainstay of treatment for neuroblastoma. Various single chemotherapeutic agents and recently combinations of drugs have been used to induce remission with some success. Included among the drugs are cyclophosphamide (Cytoxan), doxorubicin (Adriamycin), cisplatin, and VM 26. The drug of special concern to the anesthesiologist is doxorubicin. This drug is known to cause a dose-dependent cardiomyopathy in children who receive a total dose of 250 to 300 mg/m$^2$. In those patients who have also received cyclophosphamide or mediastinal radiation, the risk of doxorubicin-induced cardiomyopathy is enhanced. An echocardiogram to evaluate left ventricular function is important prior to receiving anesthesia.

Currently, autologous or allogenic bone marrow transplantation is being utilized for those children with a poor long-term prognosis (stage 4) who have achieved complete or good partial remission with chemotherapy.

## PANCREAS

### Diabetes Mellitus

Diabetes mellitus is the most common endocrine disorder of childhood and adolescence. It is a chronic systemic disease characterized by impaired carbohydrate metabolism resulting from a relative or absolute deficiency of insulin. Abnormal metabolism of protein and fat is also present. The National Diabetes Data Group classifies diabetes mellitus into two major categories: type 1, or insulin-dependent diabetes mellitus; and type 2, or non-insulin-dependent diabetes mellitus. Type 1 occurs predominantly in childhood, but may present in adulthood. In contrast, type 2 is a disease most commonly seen after the third or fourth decade of life in the obese patient. However, type 2 may occur in children and adolescents, but is usually undiagnosed because the patients are asymptomatic. As the insulin-dependent form of the disease is most commonly seen in children, a thorough discussion of it follows.

The incidence is approximately 1 in every 400 to 500 school-age children; boys and girls are equally affected. The disease is most prevalent among whites, especially those of European descent, and is relatively less common among American blacks, Hispanics, Asians, and American Indians. It most commonly presents at 5 to 7 years of age or at the time of puberty.[41]

**Etiology and Pathogenesis.** The disease is often familial, but the precise mode of inheritance remains unclear. Recent investigations have identified both genetic and environmental factors prominent in the pathogenesis. Susceptibility is linked to the presence of certain human leukocyte antigen (HLA) alleles, specifically the DQ and/or DR loci located on the short arm of chromosome 6.[42] This genetic abnormality appears to be an essential feature, but is not sufficient in itself to cause the disease.

The influence of environmental factors such as viruses (mumps, measles, rubella, Epstein-Barr, cytomegalic, coxsackie) and certain chemicals ($\beta$-cytotoxins), in conjunction with this genetic predisposition, is postulated to induce an autoimmune response. Circulating antibodies directed toward the insulin-producing islet cells of the pancreas have been found in 70 to 80 percent of newly diagnosed patients. Islet cell antibodies may be present years before islet cell dysfunction, suggesting gradual autoimmune destruction.[43] Association with other autoimmune endocrinopathies such as Hashimoto's thyroiditis, Addison's disease, thyrotoxicosis, and myasthenia gravis, as well as the presence of islet cell antibodies and increased numbers of killer T lymphocytes, provides persuasive evidence that insulin-dependent diabetes mellitus is an autoimmune disease.[44]

**Pathophysiology.** The progressive destruction of insulin-producing beta cells results in a deficiency of insulin, the major anabolic hormone. When insulin secretion is reduced to approximately 20 percent or less, diabetes becomes symptomatic. Consequent to the reduction in insulin, glucose utilization in peripheral tissues, especially skeletal muscle and adipose tissue, is impaired. As a result, a complex metabolic interaction involving glucose production and the counterregulatory hormones (glucagon, GH, ACTH, cortisol, and catecholamines) is initiated.

A low plasma insulin level leads to hyperglucagonemia and intensifies the effects of glucagon on hepatic function. The liver increases endogenous glucose production via glycogenolysis and gluconeogenesis. In addition, a deficiency of insulin enhances protein degradation, thus producing elevated levels of amino acids, which are converted to glucose and glycogen in the liver. The combination of impaired glucose utilization, increased glucose production, and continued glucose intake causes hyperglycemia. This, in turn, produces glycosuria when the renal threshold for glucose reabsorption (180 mg/dl) is exceeded. A continuing osmotic diuresis leads to polyuria, urinary losses of electrolytes, dehydration, and compensatory polydipsia. These manifestations precipitate the release of the stress or counterregulatory hormones, which amplify and accelerate the metabolic derangements. The acute stress of trauma, infection, or that associated with the administration of anesthesia and surgery, may also exacerbate the metabolic decompensation, leading to ketoacidosis.

## Diabetic Ketoacidosis

Diabetic ketoacidosis is a common and serious acute metabolic complication among children with diabetes. It accounts for 14 to 31 percent of all diabetes-related hospital admissions, with the highest incidence among adolescents.[45] It carries a morbidity and mortality rate of approximately 1:200, and accounts for more than 50 percent of deaths in diabetic patients under the age of 24 years. Precipitating factors include omitted insulin doses, trauma, infection, physical or emotional stress, hypokalemia, and (rarely) drugs (thiazide diuretics, β-antagonists, dilantin, calcium entry blockers, cortisol).

The metabolic abnormalities of ketoacidosis are secondary to an insulin deficiency, in conjunction with the effects of elevated levels of counterregulatory hormones. Lipolysis and excess release of free fatty acids from adipose tissue occurs as a result of hypoinsulinemia, and excess glucagon increases hepatic ketogenesis (Fig. 6-4). The principle organic acids produced are β-hydroxybutyrate and acetoacetate. Acetone also comprises a small portion of the acid production, but plays no known pathologic role. The rate of formation of these organic acids is greater than their utilization and renal excretion; thus, their accumulation results in metabolic acidosis.[46]

**Clinical Presentation.** The classic presentation is that of a young child with polyuria, polydipsia, and weight loss. Initially, symptoms may wax and wane for several days or weeks, but eventually persist. Children may also have enuresis or complain of fatigue, weakness, and/or abdominal pain. Symptoms in older children and adolescents usually develop over an extended period; thus glucosuria may be detected during routine urinalysis before significant symptoms appear.

Unfortunately, 10 to 20 percent of children will present with diabetic ketoacidosis manifested by vomiting, dehydration, abdominal pain, Kussmaul respirations, and alteration of mental status. These symptoms and signs may evolve over several days. Hyperglycemia (glucose >300 mg/dl), hyperkalemia, ketonemia, acidosis (pH <7.30), leukocytosis, glucosuria, and ketonuria may all be noted.

**Diagnosis.** Diagnosis is confirmed by

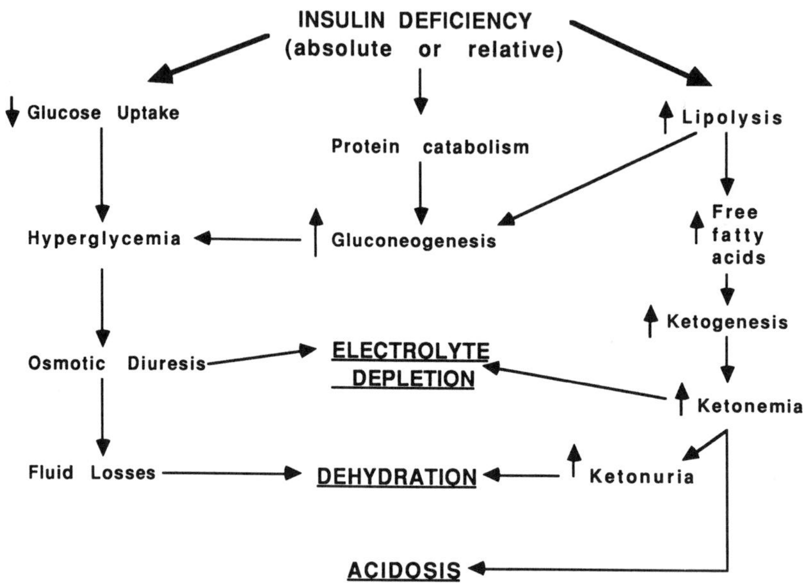


**Fig. 6-4.** Pathophysiology of diabetic ketoacidosis.

documenting hyperglycemia (random glucose > 200 mg/dl; verified on repeat testing). Early in the course of the disease, hyperglycemia and glucosuria may be transient; therefore, a fasting and 2-hour postprandial blood glucose measurement may be helpful in establishing the diagnosis, if the fasting glucose is higher than 140 mg/dl and the 2-hour glucose is greater than 200 mg/dl. An oral glucose tolerance test is rarely indicated. Plasma insulin levels may also be determined. Glucosuria alone is not diagnostic because of the significant individual variation in the renal threshold for glucose reabsorption.

The presence of islet cell antibodies in the serum and increased glycosylated hemoglobin (hemoglobin $A_{1C}$) levels may be present. An evaluation of thyroid function should also be undertaken because of the association with lymphocytic thyroiditis.

**Treatment.** The immediate goal of treatment is to restore fluid and electrolyte losses and reverse the metabolic (catabolic) derangements by administering insulin. Several different approaches to insulin replacement therapy exist, so consultation with an endocrinologist is essential. Long-term management of children with insulin-dependent diabetes mellitus focuses on six major areas: (1) insulin replacement, usually with synthetic insulin; (2) diet, to provide consistent, adequate caloric and protein intake for growth without developing obesity; (3) exercise; (4) patient and family education; (5) stress management; and (6) regular blood glucose and urine ketone monitoring. The goal of insulin therapy and monitoring is to maintain normal glucose levels (glucose <140 mg/dl), thereby delaying or perhaps preventing, long-term complications. Hemoglobin $A_{1C}$ assays provide an objective measure of the average blood glucose levels for the previous 4 to 6 weeks.[47]

Immediate complications include hypoglycemia (glucose level < 50 mg/kg) and diabetic ketoacidosis. Hypoglycemic reactions occur in all children with diabetes. The onset of symptoms (sweating, tremulousness, tachycardia, headache, slurred speech, mental confusion, seizures, and coma) may be sudden. Treatment is aimed at raising the blood glucose level above 100 mg/dl. In children that are awake and cooperative, a drink of fruit juice will often be sufficient to terminate the symptoms. However, in those patients with vomiting, alteration of mental status, or seizures, glucagon 0.5 to 1.0 mg IM should be administered. Additionally, when intravenous access is available, 2 ml/kg of 25 percent dextrose should be given until resolution of symptoms.

Diabetic ketoacidosis in a child is a major emergency that necessitates immediate and aggressive management. Treatment consists of (1) fluid and electrolyte replacement (usually 0.9 percent saline at a rate of 20 to 40 ml/kg over 1 to 2 hours; (2) insulin administration (bolus dose of 0.1 U/kg of regular insulin followed by 0.1 U/kg/h of regular insulin via continuous infusion); (3) frequent clinical monitoring and laboratory determinations of serum glucose, hemoglobin, electrolytes, BUN and creatinine, pH, serum osmolality, and urine ketones. After the initial treatment, the types of intravenous fluids used and possible administration of potassium and bicarbonate are determined by the response of the kidneys and serial glucose and electrolyte determinations.[46]

The late complications, including retinopathy, nephropathy, neuropathy (peripheral and autonomic), and large vessel atherosclerotic complications, are rarely seen in the pediatric age group. These complications normally do not appear clinically for at least 10 years after onset.

**Perioperative Management.** The perioperative management of the child with diabetes should involve close collaboration between the anesthesiologist, surgeon, and endocrinologist. In the past, most children were hospitalized before and after their surgery, but today it has become apparent that the child with well-controlled insulin-dependent diabetes mellitus can be managed safely and effectively on an outpatient basis, if the type of surgery permits. However, a team approach is essential. Management of insulin therapy may vary with the preferences of the endocrinologist; the following are common practices: (1) the patient may be given 50 percent of the normal morning dose of intermediate-acting insulin and an infusion of dextrose may be commenced; (2) on the morning of surgery, a continuous insulin infusion (0.05 to 0.1 U/kg/h of regular insulin) is administered concurrently with a 5 percent dextrose-containing solution at maintenance rates; and (3) insulin and glucose are withheld preoperatively, and no glucose is given during the surgery. This technique should only be used for short, minor procedures (done as the first case on the morning schedule) that allow early postoperative oral intake. When the child tolerates oral intake, 40 to 60 percent of the usual daily insulin dose is administered.

Of the three insulin regimens discussed, the continuous insulin infusion is probably the most rational and physiologic method for perioperative management of the child with diabetes.[48] This technique should be utilized during all major surgical procedures and in children with poorly controlled diabetes. Regardless of the technique chosen, frequent blood glucose levels should be checked throughout the perioperative period and appropriate adjustments in insulin dosing made. The patient should be re-established on a safe regimen prior to discharge.

## REFERENCES


1. Schwartz ID, Bercu BB: Anterior and posterior pituitary gland and pineal gland. p. 55. In Hung W (ed): Clinical Pediatric Endocrinology. Mosby Year Book, St. Louis, 1992
2. Behrman RE, Vaughan VC III: The endocrine system. p. 1397. In: Nelson Textbook of Pediatrics. WB Saunders, Philadelphia, 1992
3. Bacon GE, Spencer ML, Hopwood NJ, Kelch RP: A Practical Approach to Pediatric Endocrinology. p. 107. Year Book Medical Publishers, Chicago, 1990
4. Hoffman HJ, Hendrick EB, Humphreys RP et al: Management of craniopharyngioma in children. J Neurosurg 47:218, 1977
5. Dousa TP: Cyclic nucleotides in the cellular action of neurohypophyseal hormones. Fed Proc 36:1867, 1977
6. Dillingham MA, Anderson RJ: Inhibition of vasopressin action by atrial natriuretic factor. Science 231:1572, 1986
7. Mizrahi EM, Hobbs JF, Goldsmith DI: Nephrogenic diabetes insipidus in transplacental lithium intoxication. J Pediatr 94:493, 1979
8. Schwartz ID, Bercu BB: Anterior and posterior pituitary gland and pineal gland. p. 61. In Hung W (ed): Clinical Pediatric Endocrinology. Mosby Year Book, St. Louis, 1992
9. Costin G, Fefferman RA, Kogut MD: Hypothalamic gigantism. J Pediatr 83:419, 1973
10. Southwick JP, Katz J: Unusual airway difficulty in the acromegalic patient—indication for tracheotomy. Anesthesiology 51:72, 1979
11. Hassan SZ, Matz G, Lawrence AM et al: Laryngeal stenosis in acromegaly. Anesth Anal 55:57, 1976
12. Thorner MO, Vance ML, Horvath E, Kovacs K: The anterior pituitary. p. 273. In Wilson JD, Foster DW (eds): Williams Textbook of Endocrinology. WB Saunders, Philadelphia, 1992
13. Clinkingbeard C, Sessions C, Shenker Y: The physiologic role of atrial natriuretic hormone in the regulation of aldosterone and salt and water metabolism. J Clin Endocrinol Metab 70:582, 1990
14. Wilson JD, Foster DW (eds): Williams Textbook of Endocrinology. p. 360. WB Saunders, Philadelphia, 1992
15. Gruters A: Congenital hypothyroidism. Pediatr Ann 21:1, 1992
16. Hung W: Thyroid gland. p. 140. In: Clinical Pediatric Endocrinology. Mosby Year Book, St. Louis, 1992
17. Rallison ML, Dobyns BM, Keating FR et al: Occurrence and natural history of chronic lymphocytic thyroiditis in childhood. J Pediatr 86:675, 1975
18. Farooki ZQ, Hoffman WH, Perry BL et al: Myocardial dysfunction in hypothyroid children. Am J Dis Child 137:65, 1983
19. Muir A, Daneman D, Daneman A et al: Thyroid scanning, ultrasound, and serum thyroglobulin in determining the origin of congenital hypothyroidism. Am J Dis Child 142:214, 1988
20. Maenpaa J et al: Natural course of juvenile autoimmune thyroiditis. J Pediatr 107:898, 1985
21. DeGroot LJ, Quintans J: The causes of autoimmune thyroid disease. Endocrinol Rev 10:537, 1989
22. Fisher DA, Sack J, Oddie TH et al: Serum T4, TBG, T3 uptake, T3, reverse T3, and TSH concentrations in children 1 to 15 years of age. J Clin Endocrinol Metab 45: 191, 1977
23. Larsen PR, Ingbar SH: The thyroid gland. p. 444. In Wilson JD, Foster DW (eds): Williams Textbook of Endocrinology. WB Saunders, Philadelphia, 1992
24. Root AW: Parathyroid glands, calcium, phosphorus, and vitamin D metabolism. p. 89. In Hung W (ed): Clinical Pediatric Endocrinology. Mosby Year Book, St. Louis, 1992
25. Greenberg F: What defines DiGeorge anomaly? J Pediatr 115:412, 1989
26. Bachrach LK, Foley TP, Jr: Thyroiditis in children. Pediatr Rev 11:184, 1989
27. Salvi M, Fukazawa H, Bernard N et al: Role of autoantibodies in the pathogenesis and association of endocrine autoimmune disorders. Endocrinol Rev 9:450, 1988

28. Aurbach GD, Marx SJ, Spiegal AM: Parathyroid hormone, calcitonin, and the calciferols. p. 1456. In Wilson JD, Foster DW (eds): Williams Textbook of Endocrinology. WB Saunders, Philadelphia, 1992
29. Mallette LE, Kirkland JL, Gagel RF et al: Synthetic human parathyroid hormone (1–34) for the study of pseudohypoparathyroidism. J Clin Endocrinol Metab 67: 964, 1988
30. Daum F, Rosen JF, Boley SJ: Parathyroidadenoma, parathyroid crisis, and acute pancreatitis in an adolescent. J Pediatr 83: 275, 1973
31. McLaughlin B, Barrett P, Finch T et al: Late onset adrenal hyperplasia in a group of Irish females who presented with hirsutism, irregular menses and/or cystic acne. Clin Endocrinol 32:57, 1990
32. Stoelting RK: Endocrine system. p. 747. In: Pharmacology and Physiology in Anesthetic Practice. JB Lippincott, Philadelphia, 1987
33. Pang S, Wallace MA, Hofman L et al: Worldwide experience in newborn screening for classical congenital adrenal hyperplasia due to 21-hydroxylase deficiency. Pediatrics 81:866, 1988
34. Siegel SF, Lee PA: Adrenal cortex and medulla. p. 201. In Hung W (ed): Clinical Pediatric Endocrinology. Mosby Year Book, St. Louis, 1992
35. Cryer PE: Pheochromocytoma. West J Med 156:399, 1992
36. Page LB, Raker JW, Beberich FR: Pheochromocytoma with predominant epinephrine secretion. Am J Med 69:321, 1980
37. Cryer PE: Phaeochromocytoma. Clin Endocrinol Metab 14:203, 1985
38. Shapiro B, Gross MD, Fig L et al: Localization of functioning sympathoadrenal lesions. p. 235. In Biglieri ED, Melby JC (eds): Endocrine Hypertension. Raven Press, New York, 1990
39. Nicholson JP, Vaugh ED, Jr, Pickering TG et al: Pheochromocytoma and prazosin. Am Intern Med 99:477, 1983
40. Behrman RE, Vaughan VC, III: Neoplasms and neoplasm-like structures. p. 1304. In: Nelson Textbook of Pediatrics. WB Saunders, Philadelphia, 1983
41. Sperling MA: Diabetes mellitus. Pediatr Clin North Am 26:149, 1979
42. Segall M: HLA and genetics of IDDM. Holism vs. reductionism? Diabetes 37: 1005, 1988
43. Eisenbarth GS: Type I diabetes. Clinical implications of autoimmunity. Hosp Pract 22:167, 1987
44. Wilson JD, Foster DW (eds): Williams Textbook of Endocrinology. p. 1255. WB Saunders, Philadelphia, 1992
45. Kreisberg RA: Diabetic ketoacidosis: an update. Crit Care Clin 5:817, 1987
46. Siperstein MD: Diabetic ketoacidosis and hyperosmolar coma. Endocrinol Metab Clin North Am 21:415, 1992
47. Nathan DM, Singer DE, Hurxthal K et al: The clinical information value of the glycosylated hemoglobin assay. N Engl J Med 310:341, 1984
48. Gavin LA: Perioperative management of the diabetic patient. Endocrinol Metab Clin North Am 21:457, 1992

# Appendix 6-1

## REPLACEMENT THERAPY FOR PEDIATRIC PATIENTS

| *Drug* | *Dose* |
|---|---|
| Hydrocortisone | 10–25 mg/m²/d PO in 3 divided doses |
| Prednisone | 4–5 mg/m²/d PO in 2 divided doses |
| Desmopressin (DDAVP) | 2.5–15 μg/kg every 12 hours intranasally |
| DOCA | 1.0 mg/d IM |
| Fludrocortisone | 0.05–0.1 mg/d PO |
| Levothyroxine sodium (Synthroid) | Infants: 6–10 μg/kg/d PO |
| | 1–5 years: 5–6 μg/kg/d |
| | 6–12 years: 4–5 μg/kg/d |
| | >12 years: 2–3 μg/kg/d |
| Vasopressin (Pitressin) | 2.5–5 U, 2–4 times daily IM or SC |

## PEDIATRIC ENDOCRINE LEVELS: NORMAL VALUES[a]

| | Pituitary Gland | |
|---|---|---|
| Growth hormone | Basal | Low–undetectable |
| | After stimulation | >15 mU/L |
| ACTH | Basal (0900 hours) | 20–80 ng/L |
| TSH | Basal | <5 mU/L |
| | After TRH | 5–25 mU/L |
| LH | Basal | |
| | Prepubertal | 0.6–1.7 U/L |
| | Pubertal | 0.8–8.7 U/L |
| | After LHRH | |
| | Prepubertal | 1.5–11.9 U/L |
| | Pubertal | 5.9–48.8 U/L |
| FSH | Basal | |
| | Prepubertal | 0.6–3.4 U/L |
| | Pubertal | 0.6–4.9 U/L |
| | After LHRH | |
| | Prepubertal | 3.9–5.6 U/L |
| | Pubertal | 2.2–8.0 U/L |
| ADH | Basal | 1–5 pmol/L |
| | Plasma osmolarity | 275–295 mOsm/L |

| | Thyroid Gland |
|---|---|
| Total $T_4$ | 55–150 nmol/L (4–12 μg/dl) |
| Total $T_3$ | 1.2–3.1 nmol/L (78–200 ng/dl) |
| TSH | <5 mU/L |
| TBG | 12–31 ng/L |
| | Parathyroid Glands |
| PTH | <1.0 ng/ml |
| Calcitonin | <0.08 ng/L |
| Serum calcium | 2.26–2.80 mmol/L (9–11 mg/dl) |
| Serum phosphate | 0.8–1.45 mmol/L (2.5–4.5 mg/dl) |
| Serum magnesium | 0.7–1.2 mmol/L (1.7–2.9 mg/dl) |
| | Adrenal Cortex |
| Cortisol | 140–800 nmol/L (5–29 μg/dl) |
| 17-OHP | <15 nmol/L (<45 ng/dl) |
| 11-Deoxycortisol | <60 nmol/L |

Adrenal Medulla

Urinary excretion of catecholamines and metabolites varies with age, and also shows a diurnal variation. It is usual to take a 24-hour collection for assessment.

| Normal ranges for children: | |
|---|---|
| VMA | <35 μmol/d |
| Metadrenaline | <6.5 μmol/d |
| | Pancreas |
| Plasma insulin | <10 mU/L |
| Plasma glucose (fasting) | 2.8–6.5 mmol/L (50–117 mg/dl) |
| Hemoglobin $A_{1C}$ | 5.7–8.0% |

[a] These values are a guide only—results may vary depending upon individual laboratory standards and techniques.

# 7

# Neurologic and Neuromuscular Diseases

**Trauma**

**Abnormal Development of the Cranial Vault**

- Craniosynostosis
- Apert Syndrome
- Crouzon Syndrome
- Other Syndromes

**Abnormal Development of the Central Nervous System**

- Encephalocele
- Spina Bifida

**Hydrocephalus**

**Brain Tumors**

**Vascular Lesions**

- Arteriovenous Malformations
- Intraventricular Hemorrhage

**Encephalopathies**

- Hypoxic-Ischemic Encephalopathy
- Prenatal Infections
- Viral Infections
- Metabolic and Pharmacologic Conditions
- Reye Syndrome

**Diseases of the Spinal Cord**

**Polyneuropathies**

- Peripheral Polyneuropathies
- Guillain-Barré Syndrome
- Friedreich's Ataxia
- Charcot-Marie-Tooth Disease and Familial Amyloid Polyneuropathy
- Neurofibromatosis
- Cranial Neuropathies

**Movement Disorders**

- Cerebral Palsy
- Tourette Syndrome

**Seizure Disorders**

- Antiseizure Drugs

**Myasthenia Gravis**

**Muscular Dystrophies**

- Duchenne's Muscular Dystrophy
- Facioscapulohumeral and Myotonic Dystrophies
- Leukodystrophies

**Congenital and Metabolic Myopathies**

**Down Syndrome**

7

# Neurologic and Neuromuscular Diseases

*Mark Harris*

Children with neurologic and neuromuscular disease have specific anatomic and physiologic abnormalities that set them apart from the general surgical population. Important physiologic variables such as intracranial hypertension, attenuated airway reflexes, abnormal cardiopulmonary drive, generalized autonomic nervous system dysfunction, and altered responses to neuromuscular relaxants may accompany congenital or acquired disorders of the brainstem, upper cervical spinal cord, cranial nerves, and peripheral neuromusculature.

Intracranial hypertension is the single most important physiological variable in children with diseases of the central nervous system (CNS). Any increase in the intracranial compartments [brain, blood cerebrospinal fluid (CSF)] or premature closure of the cranial vault (craniosynostosis) can decrease intracranial compliance and increase intracranial pressure (ICP). In these situations any acute rise in intracranial volume (trauma, spontaneous hemorrhage, or obstructive hydrocephalus) is poorly tolerated because normal physiologic compensatory mechanisms are bypassed. In contrast, slow changes in intracranial volume may be well tolerated because compensatory mechanisms (displacement of CSF or compression of tissue) have not been exhausted. The goal of this chapter is to assist the anesthesiologist in evaluating the child with neurologic or neuromuscular disease who is scheduled for surgery.

## TRAUMA

Trauma is the most common neurologic abnormality in childhood. Head, spinal, and peripheral neurologic injury are common sequelae of vehicular accidents, child abuse, and peer-directed violence. The altered physiology in neurologic trauma, the emergency management of elevated ICP, hypoxia, hemorrhagic shock, the unstable cervical spine, crush injury, and a review of outcome following trauma are all beyond the scope of this chapter. Traumatic neurologic injury is an extremely important public health issue costing more than all of the other disease processes described in this chapter. Injury prevention is essential. Automobile airbags and passive restraints have made a significant impact upon traumatic head injury in adults and similar safety design engineering is now being applied to children (rear-facing infant's seats, bicycle helmets). Crisis intervention, family counseling, and efforts to reduce community violence are other strategies designed to prevent pediatric trauma.

## ABNORMAL DEVELOPMENT OF THE CRANIAL VAULT

### Craniosynostosis

Craniosynostosis is a relatively common cranial vault abnormality defined as the premature closure of some or all of the cranial sutures. Craniosynostosis may represent an isolated defect or may exist as part of many complex craniofacial syndromes. The incidence of isolated craniosynostosis varies between 25 and 60 in 10,000 live births and usually involves the sagittal and metopic sutures.[1,2] According to Tessier,[3] the father of craniofacial surgery, craniosynostosis results in diminished cranial volume, intracranial hypertension, constraint of further brain growth, and compensatory cranial deformity. The primary preoperative consideration in craniosynostosis is the presence of intracranial hypertension, which, according to Shillito and Matson,[1] occurs in 19 percent of isolated metopic, 13 percent of sagittal, and 41 percent of multiple synostoses. Intracranial hypertension may be difficult to diagnose in craniosynostosis, and as many as 65 percent of children without radiographic or clinical evidence of intracranial hypertension may have either persistent or episodic periods of elevated ICP during direct measurement.[4]

Craniosynostosis may coexist with a variety of complex pediatric craniofacial syndromes that may also include respiratory, neurologic, systemic, skeletal, and soft tissue abnormalities. The preoperative considerations of these syndromes include intracranial hypertension, airway difficulty, and additional specific systemic abnormalities unique to each syndrome.

### Apert Syndrome

Apert syndrome is a rare autosomal dominant defect characterized by multiple craniosynostosis, ocular proptosis, midfacial hypoplasia, and symmetrical syndactyly. Associated cardiovascular anomalies such as pulmonic stenosis, overriding aorta, ventricular septal defects, and endocardial fibroelastosis have been reported. Significant developmental abnormalities can occur in both the upper and lower airways. According to one report, 4 of 19 patients with Apert syndrome required preoperative bronchoscopic intubation.[5] Temporomandibular joint dysfunction, cleft palate, choanal atresia, and severe laryngo-, tracheo-, or bronchomalacia may be present.[6]

### Crouzon Syndrome

The most common craniofacial abnormality is Crouzon syndrome, an autosomal dominant disorder associated with craniosynostosis, altered intracranial compliance, midface hypoplasia, and ocular proptosis. Unlike Apert syndrome, a characteristic "parrot-beaked" nasal defect and inverted V-shaped palate are seen. Airway obstruction occurs commonly, and mild adenoid hypertrophy or airway edema can lead to increased obstruction and critical respiratory distress. As with Apert syndrome, lower airway abnormalities may be present,[7] and endotracheal intubation may be difficult. According to one study, 4 of 25 children with Couzon syndrome required bronchoscopic intubation during induction of anesthesia.[5]

### Other Syndromes

Other rare craniofacial syndromes include *Pfeiffer* (tracheo- and bronchomalacia, mental retardation, seizures, Arnold-Chiari malformation), Carpenters, Saethre-Chotzen, Greig cephalopolysyndactyly, Antley-Bixler and Baller-Gerold syndromes. In general, all craniofacial syndromes are at risk for intracranial hypertension and airway difficulty should always be anticipated.

## ABNORMAL DEVELOPMENT OF THE CENTRAL NERVOUS SYSTEM

Congenital malformations of the CNS occur as a result of agenesis or dysgenesis of nearly all of the recognized structures of the brain and spinal cord. Agenesis of the cranial vault, cerebral cortex, basal ganglia, and brainstem is referred to as anencephaly, and children with this disorder usually die shortly after birth. In contrast hydranencephaly and its many variants are characterized by varying degrees of cystic degeneration of cerebral structures. Infants can live for years if the degeneration is relatively mild. Porencephaly is characterized by multiple cystic cavitations of the cerebral cortex and leads to variable neurologic dysfunction including mental retardation, seizures, and cerebral palsy. Cystic dilatation of ventricle IV in association with cerebellar hypoplasia is known as the Dandy-Walker syndrome, while dilatation of the central canal of the spinal cord is syringomyelia (or hydromyelia). Children with Dandy-Walker syndrome occasionally present with neonatal apnea, posterior fossa mass effect, brainstem compression, or upward brain herniation and death (Figure 7-1). Careful preoperative radiographic evaluation can usually diagnose fatal upward herniation.[8] Surviving infants with cystic CNS disease usually require palliative shunting, and most are at risk for intracranial hypertension.

Other common congenital central nervous system anomalies include Arnold-Chiari malformation, encephalocele, and meningomyelocele. The Arnold-Chiari (or type II Chiari) malformation is an abnormality of the neural tube characterized by caudal displacement of posterior fossa structures, kinking of the cervicomedullary junction, and disruption of the brainstem vascular supply and lower cranial nerves (Fig. 7-2). It is often found in association with meningomyelocele, hydrocephalus, and syringomyelia. Brainstem dysfunction is relatively rare, but can result in decreased airway protection,[9,10] abnormal respiratory drive,[11] and cardiovascular instability.[12] Swallowing difficulty, stridor, apnea, and opisthotonos may respond to posterior fossa decompression.[13] Seventy-five percent of these children will develop hydrocephalus, and a unknown percentage will present with cervical syringomyelia (dilatation of the central canal) that can lead to progressive muscle wasting and gait disturbances.

### Encephalocele

Encephalocele is an abnormality characterized by protrusion of the brain and its coverings through midline defects. The incidence ranges from 1 in 5,000 to 10,000 live births. Seizures, abnormalities in respiratory drive and temperature regulation, and hydrocephalus and cerebral dysgenesis may be associated findings. Small nasal encephaloceles may be

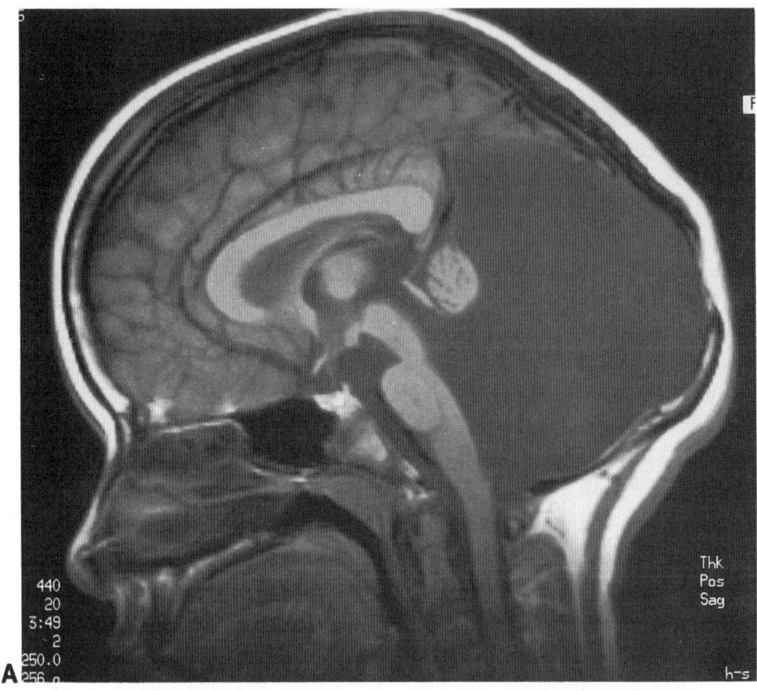


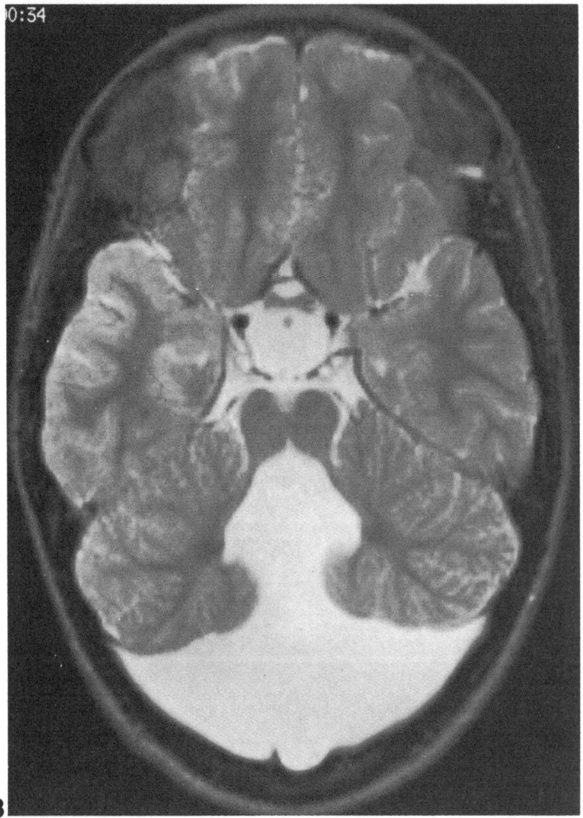


**Fig. 7-1.** **(A & B)** Massive posterior fossa cystic dilatation in a child with Dandy-Walker syndrome. Displacement of the cerebellar hemispheres and cerebral structures is apparent.

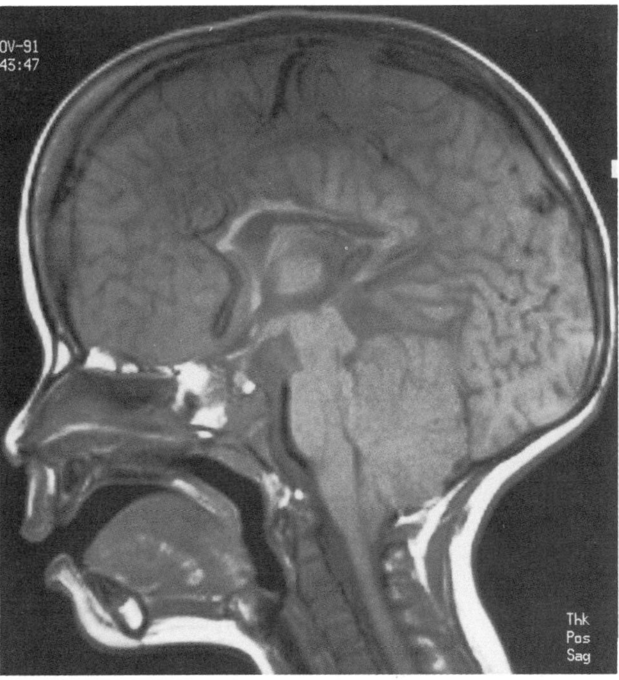


**Fig. 7-2.** Arnold-Chiari malformation showing characteristic caudal displacement of the hindbrain and inferior cerebellar lobes into the cervical canal.

relatively asymptomatic; however, larger lesions can cause recurrent meningitis, frequent nasal drainage, and respiratory obstruction. Airway difficulty should be anticipated with large nasopharyngeal lesions. Large posterior occipital lesions will affect head positioning for endotracheal intubation.

## Spina Bifida

Spina bifida occulta is a heterogeneous collection of different neural tube disorders characterized by radiographic abnormalities of the spinal vertebrae. These findings occur in 20 to 30 percent of the general population. Meningomyelocele is a common subtype and is characterized by a posterior thoracolumbar defect containing CSF, meninges, caudal equina, or residual spinal cord in association with vertebrae anomalies and the Arnold-Chiari malformation. Meningomyelocele shows significant regional variation[14] and appears to be decreasing in frequency.[15] When the prenatal diagnosis is known and the dorsal lesion is large, efforts may be taken to deliver the infant by cesarean section since rupture of the meninges can lead to significant fluid and electrolyte loss and contribute to infection. As a general rule, the newborn with this condition is transferred to a constant temperature environment and rehydrated with intravenous fluids; the lesion is covered with moistened sterile dressings. Severe associated gastrointestinal, pulmonary, cardiovascular, or genitourinary anomalies should be diagnosed prior to repair because they may preclude a successful long-term outcome and may complicate anesthetic management. Airway management is a potential problem only if the defect is so large that the child cannot be positioned supine prior to induction of general anesthesia.

Children with meningomyelocele are "regulars" in the pediatric wards and operating rooms. Older children frequently appear knowledgeable about medical care and will voice strong feelings about their anesthetic management. Generally, the anesthetic considerations for these children are not different from other children. Once rapport has been established, anesthesia can be induced in the healthy child with meningomyelocele using standard pediatric induction techniques followed by intubation using either depolarizing or nondepolarizing neuromuscular relaxants. (Nondepolarizing neuromuscular relaxants can be administered without a hyperkalemic response.[16])

The preoperative assessment should always include an assessment of allergic history. Many of these children are at increased risk for IgE-mediated latex anaphylaxis.[17] Periorbital edema, erythema and lip-tingling after blowing up balloons, and papular lesions after contact with rubber gloves are important findings in the history. This reaction is believed to result from repeated exposure to latex gloves or catheters.

Children with meningomyelocele and other congenital anomalies of the spine may suffer gradual deterioration of lumbar sacral neurologic function caused by a tethered cord. Deterioration results from mechanical stretching of the cord in a cephalocaudal plane, and the patient may present with localized dilatation of the central canal (hydromyelia) on radiographic examination. These children have clinical evidence of cord involvement and display gait abnormalities and bowel or bladder dysfunction. Lumbar laminectomy and release of the cord is sufficient to restore function to baseline in many. Preoperative considerations in tethered cord are related to concurrent medical conditions (e.g., hydrocephalus), altered airway function, abnormal respiratory drive, or cardiovascular instability. Depolarizing neuromuscular relaxants appear to be safe in patients with symptomatic tethered cord.

## HYDROCEPHALUS

Hydrocephalus is defined as the accumulation of excessive CSF and, in general, may either result from anatomic blockage (noncommunicating), excessive production, or insufficient reabsorption (communicating) (Fig. 7-3). Excessive accumulation of CSF may also occur in hydrocephalus ex vacuo conditions, in which CSF replaces atrophic or absent cerebral structures. (Porencephaly and hydranencephaly are examples.) Other disorders such as supratentorial cysts, isolated ventricle IV, and Dandy-Walker syndrome represent examples of compartmentalized hydrocephalus of the noncommunicating variety. Ventricular shunts or reservoirs are palliative procedures for most types of hydrocephalus, and they drain into a variety of anatomic sties including the peritoneum, the right atrium, and external reservoirs. Valve-regulated ventriculoperitoneal shunt procedures are probably the most common neurosurgical operation performed today. Shunt infection or occlusion are common sequelae in shunted children, and the reader is referred to other excellent sources for more detailed discussion of hydrocephalus.[18]

The anesthetic implications in hydrocephalus include those related to the underlying medical, neurologic, or anatomic condition of the child and depend upon the presence of intracranial hypertension, meningitis, seizure disorders, altered re-

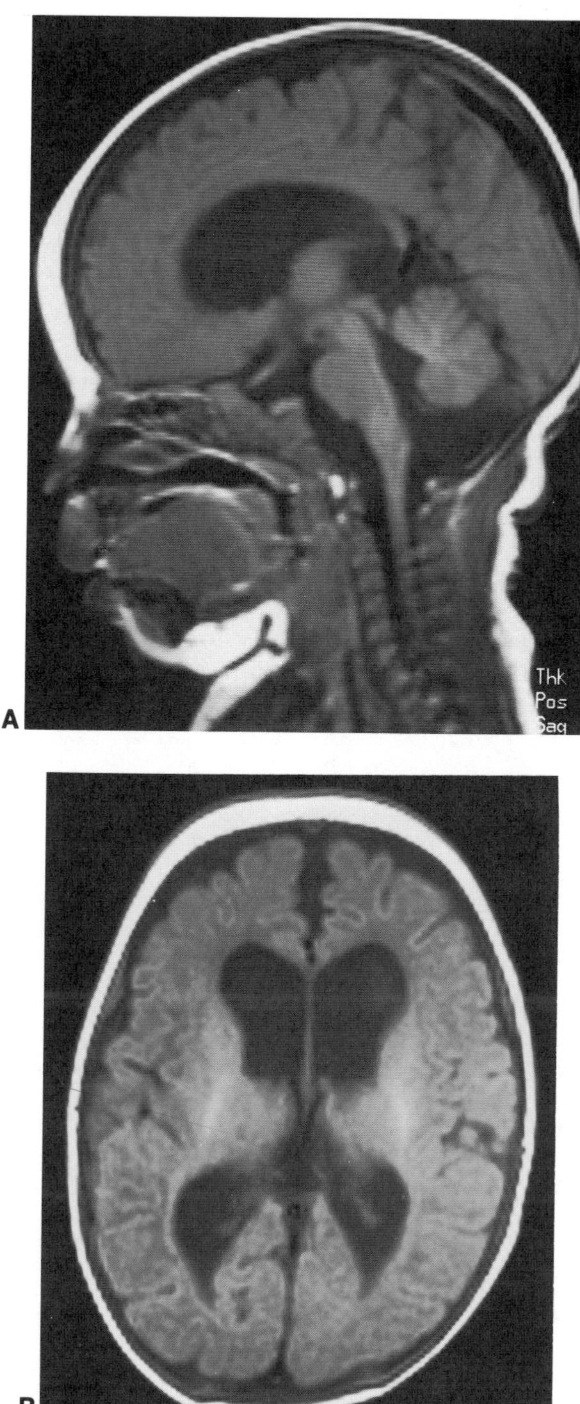


**Fig. 7-3.** (**A & B**) Childhood communicating hydrocephalus. Note that the entire ventricular system is dilated.

spiratory drive, mental retardation, airway difficulty, cerebral palsy, and volume status. Volume deficiency and electrolyte imbalance occur when excessive CSF drains into an external shunt. (The composition of cerebrospinal fluid is similar to that of plasma: Na, 130 to 150 mEq/L; K, 2.7 to 3.9 mEq/L; Cl, 115 to 132 mEq/L). Hypothalamic-pituitary dysfunction leading to hypothermia, obesity, precocious or delayed puberty, amenorrhea, impotence, diabetes insipidus, and deficient anterior pituitary hormones have also been reported in hydrocephalus and should be considered in the preoperative assessment.[19]

Infants, toddlers, and older children with hydrocephalus are at increased risk of intracranial hypertension during initial shunt placement and later during subsequent shunt revisions. Bulging fontanels, reports of abnormal feeding behavior, apnea, bradycardia, decreased level of consciousness, nausea, vomiting, headache, diplopia, gaze paralysis, and increased head circumference are signs and symptoms of intracranial hypertension. Computed tomography (CT) scans and magnetic resonance imaging (MRI) may reveal dilated ventricles, or skull series films may reveal a "copper beaten" presentation when chronic intracranial hypertension exists (Table 7-1). When the signs and symptoms are confusing, radiographic examination will differentiate intracranial hypertension with ventricular dilatation from symptomatic low intracranial pressure due to overshunting in slit ventricle syndromes.[20] (Fig. 7-4). When directly measuring ICP, the anesthesiologist must be aware that "normal" adult pressures may be abnormally high for infants and toddlers who have lower "normal" ICPs.[21]

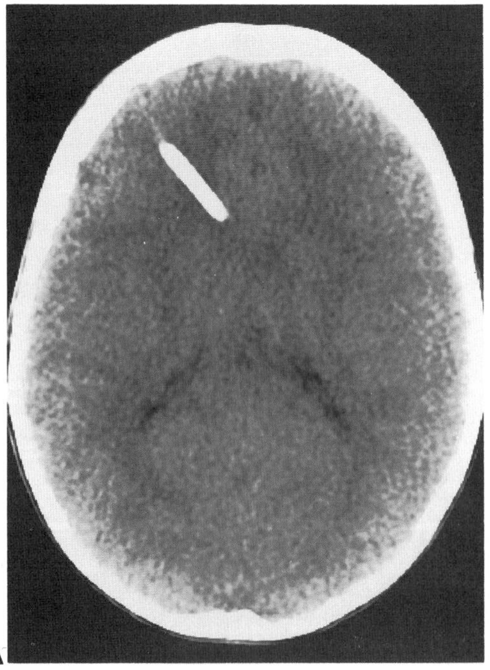


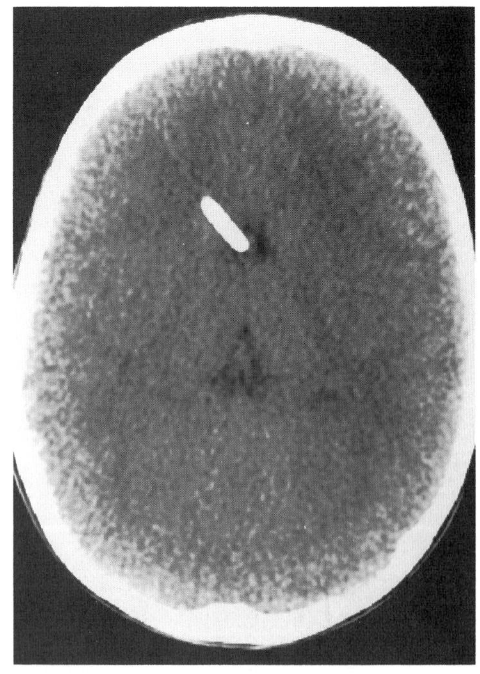


**Fig. 7-4.** (**A & B**) Overdrainage following placement of a ventricular shunt leads to the slitlike appearance of the lateral ventricles.

**Table 7-1.** Signs and Symptoms of Intracranial Hypotension

| *Acute Intracranial Hypertension* | *Chronic Intracranial Hypertension* |
|---|---|
| Physical appearance | |
| Bulging fontanel | Increased head circumference and compensatory skull growth |
| Sunset eyes | |
| Small, irregular pupil, dilated pupil, abnormal papillary reflexes | May have papillary abnormalities |
| Decreased level of consciousness, leading to abnormal posturing, seizures, altered respiratory pattern, Cushing response, brain herniation and death | May have normal rentation, mental retardation, or seizure disorder |
| Episodic feeding disorders or behavioral changes | |
| Nausea, headache, vomiting | May have nausea, headache or vomiting |
| Radiographic | |
| Dilated ventricles | Dilated ventricles |
| Flattening of quadrigeminal plate cistern; flattening the posterior 3rd ventricle (ascending transtentorial herniation) | "Copper beaten" skull |

## BRAIN TUMORS

Brain tumors are the second most common malignancy in childhood and occur with a frequency of 2 to 5 cases/100,000/year.[22] Most are found above the tentorium (54 percent),[23] and astrocytomas are the most common cell type (36 to 57 percent). The vast majority are low grade with little malignant potential. Cerebellar astrocytomas, representing 15 percent of brain tumors in children less than 15 years, usually present with signs and symptoms of intracranial hypertension and have 5-year survivals of 91 percent.[22] Supratentorial astrocytomas account for 25 percent of tumors and usually present with signs and symptoms of direct hemispheric growth: headaches, visual field abnormalities, weakness, seizures, and elevated intracranial pressure. A combination of radiation and local excision results in an approximate 50 percent 5-year survival.[24] Deep axial astrocytomas (thalamic, optic pathways, hypothalamic) usually present with signs and symptoms referable to local involvement such as autonomic nervous system and endocrine dysfunction, visual disturbances, emotional lability, and confusion.[24] Medulloblastomas are the second most common histopathologic grouping in childhood (20 to 23 percent) and are thought to be derived from fetal tissue remnants in the posterior fossa. These usually present with intracranial hypertension, and 5-year survival is 50 to 70 percent[24] (Fig. 7-5).

The preoperative considerations for children with brain tumors include residual neurologic function, altered intracranial compliance, and increased intracranial pressure. Alteration of respiratory drive or airway protection, severe alterations of consciousness, and disruption of vital structures may follow direct tumor invasion. Chemotherapy, radiation therapy, high-dose steroids, and mannitol are valuable for reducing tumor edema, decreasing intracranial hypertension, and improving symptoms. Steroid therapy af-

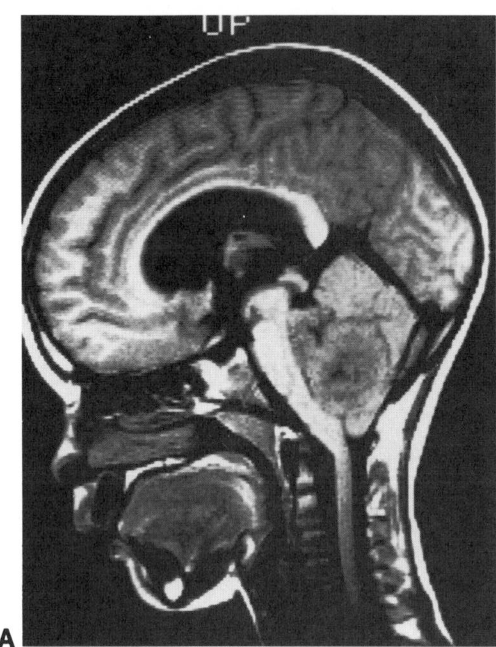


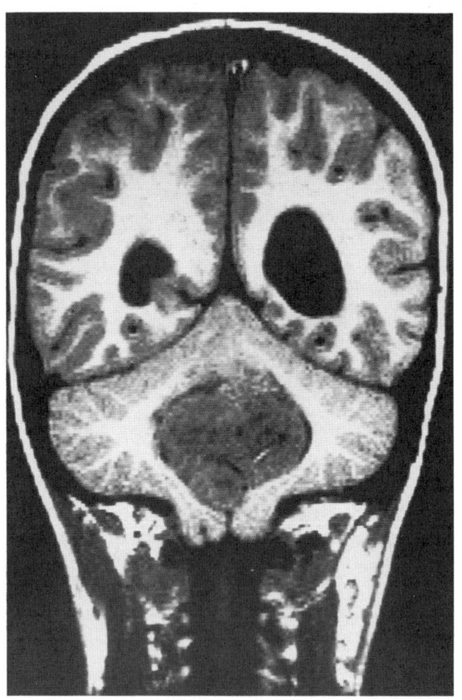


**Fig. 7-5.** **(A & B)** Large posterior fossa medulloblastoma compressing the brainstem and displacing the tentorium.

fects glucose homeostasis and endogenous steroid synthesis and can produce the Cushing syndrome; mannitol can result in dehydration, electrolyte imbalances, and hyperosmotic states.

## VASCULAR LESIONS

Intracranial vascular disease is very rare in childhood. Among children less than 15 years, strokes and subarachnoid and intracerebral hemorrhage occur with a total incidence of 2.52/100,000.[25] Ischemic cerebrovascular disease in childhood may result from a variety of preconditions including perinatal asphyxia and trauma, accelerated atherosclerosis (hyperlipidemia), cerebral arteritis, fibromuscular dysplasia, sickle cell anemia, migraine headaches, and moya-moya disease. The principal anesthetic considerations in these disorders center on the underlying medical conditions (e.g., steroid therapy in arteritis; normoxia, hydration, and normothermia for sickle cell disease; avoiding hyperventilation in moya-moya disease[26]), the presence of intracranial hypertension, and residual neurologic functions.

### Arteriovenous Malformations

Arteriovenous malformations are a frequent cause of catastrophic cerebrovascular events in childhood. They may present with hemorrhage, seizures, ischemic stroke, or congestive heart failure.[27] Therapy includes surgical excision and irradiation using the Leksell gamma knife or a comparable source of radiation.

Symptomatic intracranial arterial aneurysms are very rare in childhood, although intracranial hemorrhage can result from rupture. Definitive treatment for pediatric aneurysms, as for adult lesions, is surgical excision.[27]

### Intraventricular Hemorrhage

Neonatal intraventricular hemorrhage occurs in about 40 percent of preterm infants in neonatal intensive care units and is associated with fluctuating cerebral blood flow velocity, hypoxia-ischemia, polycythemia, and birth trauma.[28,29] Many of these infants have seizure disorders and are neurologically impaired. There is no evidence to suggest that the stress of general anesthesia is likely to worsen preexisting intraventricular hemorrhage.[30]

## ENCEPHALOPATHIES

The term *encephalopathy* refers to any alteration of cerebral function and includes such diverse etiologies as hypoxic-ischemic, bacterial and nonbacterial infection, metabolic and pharmacologic, Reye syndrome, hypertension, demyelinating, familiar, and others. The sequelae of encephalopathy are diverse and include alterations of muscle tone, irritability, seizures, coma, and mental retardation.

### Hypoxic-Ischemic Encephalopathy

There has been a significant decrease in the hypoxic-ischemic encephalopathy syndrome of the newborn over the last 25 years due, in part, to the increased use of fetal monitoring, lumbar epidural analgesia, and cesarean section.[31] This condition presents in the first 12 hours of life with deep stupor, periodic breathing, and hypotonia to be followed by fluctuating levels of consciousness, increased motor tone, seizure-like activity, and often death within 24 to 72 hours. Perioperative considerations include providing normoxia, avoiding hypertension, treating brain swelling, maintaining cerebral perfusion pressure, and supporting blood glucose. (Although optimal blood glucose in this condition is unknown, current practice is to maintain blood glucose between 75 and 100 mg/dl.)[32]

### Prenatal Infections

Prenatal CNS infections (toxoplasmosis, rubella, cytomegalovirus, and herpes) have a devastating effect upon patient outcome but little direct impact upon anesthetic management. Congenital rubella may lead to hearing loss, congenital heart disease, cataracts, mental retardation, and intrauterine growth retardation. Cytomegalovirus (CMV) may result in microcephaly, retardation, seizures, and visual or hearing impairment. Herpes infection causes a septic picture in the immediate neonatal period; herpetic encephalitis is frequently fatal. Under the age of 5 years, the incidence of bacterial meningitis is approximately 87/100,000/year, and 60 to 85 percent is caused by *Haemophilus influenzae* type b.[33] Anesthetic considerations for acute bacterial meningitis include raised ICP, seizures, and hematologic abnormalities resulting from disseminated intravascular coagulation (especially from *Neisseria meningitidis*).

### Viral Infections

Viral infection of the CNS can produce a clinical picture of aseptic meningitis, meningoencephalitis, or isolated encephalitis. The latter is most commonly seen in neonatal herpes simplex type 2 infection. Viral encephalitides often present with alterations in consciousness, convulsions, behavioral disturbances, and seizures. Roseola may cause common febrile seizure.[34] As with acute bacterial meningitis, acute viral encephalitis may result in alterations of intracranial compliance, brain swelling, and hydrocephalus. Anesthesia services are occasionally required for brain biopsy, ventriculoperitoneal shunt placement, or radiographic imaging.

Subacute viral neurologic disorders such as rabies, hemorrhagic leukoencephalitis, and chronic encephalopathies such as subacute sclerosing panencephalitis, acquired immunodeficiency syndrome (AIDS) encephalitis, Kuru, and Creutzfeldt-Jakob disease represent a heterogeneous collection of infectious encephalopathies without specific anesthetic considerations other than intracranial hypertension and abnormal cardiopulmonary reflexes.

### Metabolic and Pharmacologic Conditions

Metabolic and pharmacologic encephalopathies may result from alterations in common physiologic substances such as sodium, calcium, magnesium, and glucose. In utero exposure to alcohol (fetal alcohol syndrome), cocaine, narcotics, and a variety of other substances will present as alterations in behavior. Toxins such as heavy metals, solvents, pesticides, biologic toxins, and hallucinogens, along with many household plants and substances, can also result in encephalopathy.

### Reye Syndrome

Reye syndrome is a unique acute encephalopathy first described in 1963 and characterized by a prodromal viral syndrome, protracted vomiting, stupor or coma, intracranial hypertension, fatty infiltration of the liver, and abnormal glucose homeostasis. Although the etiology is unknown, a close relationship exists between salicylate ingestion and subsequent development of Reye syndrome.[35] Decrease in the use of salicylates during pediatric illness is thought to be responsible for the declining incidence of the disorder. Intensive management of intracranial hypertension and metabolic abnormalities have reduced mortality in severe encephalopathy to between 10 and 20 percent.[35] Operating room and radiology requirements for anesthesia services are infrequent; however, management of elevated intracranial pressure, frequent monitoring of serum glucose for hypoglycemia, and general supportive care are the common issues confronting the consultant anesthesiologist.

## DISEASES OF THE SPINAL CORD

Infectious diseases of the spinal cord include acute viral infection of the gray matter and the anterior horn cells known as poliomyelitis. This is caused by one of three viral agents, and produces a flacid paralysis. Hyperkalemia has been implicated in severe adverse reactions following administration of succinylcholine to such patients.[36] Transverse myelitis is a less discriminate inflammatory condition of the entire spinal cord at a single level and is often the result of host immune reaction to viral pathogens such as mumps, measles, mononucleosis, echovirus, herpes, poliovirus, and others.[34] A disease of unknown etiology, juvenile amyotropic lateral sclerosis is a slowly progressive degenerative disease of the corticospinal tracts, as well as upper and lower motor units, that presents during the first two decades of life with weakness, atrophy, and lower extremity spasticity.[37] The anesthetic considerations include altered airway reflexes due to cranial nerve involvement and abnormal responses to neuromuscular relaxants. The latter are characterized by relative insensitivity to nondepolarizing relaxants,[38] myotonia following depolarizing relaxants,[39] and no risk of hyperkalemia. Polyradiculitis is a lower CNS disorder involving the spinal meninges, proximal and posterior roots, and ganglion cells occasionally accompanied by a peripheral polyneuropathy and myelopathy. It is often caused by Epstein-Barr viral infection, and hyperkalemia may follow administration of succinylcholine.

Spinal cord function may be compromised by several congenital defects and degenerative disease processes. The tethered cord syndrome has been discussed and may be seen in meningomyelocele, diastematomyelia (anteroposterior septae dividing the cord into two or three "hemicords"), and the tight filum terminale syndrome (abnormally short and thick filum terminale). Laminectomy and release of the cord is usually curative. General spinal muscular atrophies such as Werdnig-Hoffmann disease and Kugelberg-Welander syndrome and numerous other focal spinal atrophies (distal spinal muscular atrophy, progressive juvenile bulbar palsy, and Möbius syndrome) are examples of rare disease processes that many predispose to abnormal responses to succinylcholine, may display cardiac involvement (Kugelberg-Welander syndrome),[40] and may include brainstem abnormalities (apnea and abnormal respiratory drive in Möbius syndrome).[41]

## POLYNEUROPATHIES

Polyneuropathies are generalized disease processes characterized by variable muscle weakness, sensory loss, hyporeflexia, and automatic dysfunction. They result from such diverse causes as toxins (heavy metals), inflammation (Guillain-Barré syndrome), myelin abnormalities (Fabry's disease), hereditary demyelinating (Charcot-Marie-Tooth disease), and metabolic conditions (vitamin deficiencies), vasculopathies (lupus and rheumatoid arthritis), hereditary degenerative conditions (Friedreich's ataxia), systemic disease (diabetes mellitus), entrapment, trauma, and so forth. The term *polyneuropathy* includes disease processes that involve solely peripheral or cranial nerves and others that cause a mixed pattern. Because of the variable nature of the term *neuropathy,* there are few unifying anesthetic considerations other than the potential for abnormal responses to neuromuscular relaxants and the unique systemic features of each underlying disease process.

### Peripheral Polyneuropathies

Patients with long-standing peripheral polyneuropathies who have had significant muscle denervation and weakness are at risk for hyperkalemia following intravenous succinylcholine and tend to be relatively insensitive to nondepolarizing relaxants.[42,43] This is thought to result from proliferation of acetylcholine receptors.[44]

### Guillain-Barré Syndrome

Guillain-Barré syndrome is an ascending paralysis of unknown etiology that can involve both peripheral and cranial nerves. Autonomic dysfunction and respiratory compromise are important components. Hyperkalemic cardiac arrest has been reported following intravenous succinylcholine.[45] Preoperative considerations should include careful assessment of postoperative ventilatory need.

## Friedreich's Ataxia

Friedreich's ataxia is an autosomal recessive disorder characterized by ataxia, dysarthria, weakness, diabetes mellitus (40 percent), scoliosis, and cardiomyopathy (90 percent). It is an example of a disease process with severe multisystem involvement and associated polyneuropathy (cranial and peripheral). The primary anesthetic considerations relate to cardiac function[46] and abnormal responses to neuromuscular relaxants.[47] The functional cardiac status is usually obvious, but the response to neuromuscular relaxants is difficult to predict. Normal responses, sensitivity to nondepolarizing relaxants, and hyperkalemia following succinylcholine have all been noted.[47]

## Charcot-Marie-Tooth Disease and Familial Amyloid Polyneuropathy

Charcot-Marie-Tooth disease is a collection of degenerative conditions affecting a variety of sensory, motor, and autonomic nerves. The most common finding is peroneal muscle wasting. Pes cavus and peroneal muscle atrophy are common; cardiac rhythm disturbances and respiratory insufficiency may also occur. Regional anesthesia and depolarizing neuromuscular relaxants are both reported to be safe.[48] Familial amyloid polyneuropathy is an inherited, progressive sensory and motor polyneuropathy usually involving the legs and arms. Like other polyneuropathies, it may present with significant autonomic dysfunction; patients may display abnormal responses to neuromuscular relaxants.[49,50]

## Neurofibromatosis

Neurofibromatosis is a relatively common autosomal dominant disorder with variable clinical expression characterized by cutaneous café-au-lait spots and Schwann cell growth throughout the nervous system. Neurofibromas can affect anesthetic management in many ways: airway neurofibromas can lead to obstruction,[51] intracranial lesions can alter intracranial compliance, vertebral lesions may cause scoliosis and restrictive pulmonary disease, and renal artery neurofibromas can produce hypertension. (Although very rare, hypertension in the child with neurofibromatosis should alert the physician to the possibility of an associated pheochromocytoma.) Although the neurofibromatosis can be described as a mixed polyperipheral and polycranial neuropathy, the response to neuromuscular relaxants differs from that seen with other neuropathies. Instead of a denervation (lower motor neuron-type disorder), the response has been variously characterized as "myasthenic" (resistance to succinylcholine and increased sensitivity to nondepolarizing relaxants)[52] or "normal".[53,54]

## Cranial Neuropathies

Cranial neuropathies occur in a variety of other conditions including exposure to toxins, brain tumors, neurofibromatosis, Friedreich's ataxia, and following cervical epidural blockade.[55] Impaired laryngeal function should be considered in the preoperative assessment.

# MOVEMENT DISORDERS

## Cerebral Palsy

Cerebral palsy is a relatively common movement disorder (20 to 40/10,000) of diverse etiology resulting from inherited and acquired causes (asphyxia, infection, injury, and metabolic conditions).[56] Spastic cerebral palsy is the most common type; it presents with hyperreflexia and abnormal reflexes in one or more extremities. Extrapyramidal cerebral palsy (9 to 22 percent) involves defects of posture, involuntary movement, and hypertonus. Mixed cerebral palsy has characteristics of both types. Mental retardation, seizures, deafness, and learning difficulties are common; many children receive drugs such as baclofen, diazepam, and dantrolene to control spasticity. The implications of medical therapy include the potential for seizures following acute withdrawal of baclofen, altered benzodiazepine requirements due to chronic therapy, and potentiation of nondepolarizing neuromuscular relaxants by dantrolene. There are few specific anesthetic complications aside from one report of transient excitement during emergence from sevoflurane.[57]

### Tourette Syndrome

Tourette syndrome is an inherited movement disorder characterized by ticlike movements of the face, partial vocalizations (grunts, barks, etc.), repetitive touching, and normal mentation. The disorder may be exacerbated by a variety of stimuli found in the perioperative setting such as unusual smells and stress. The anesthesiologist should review these triggers with the patient and consider preoperative sedation to minimize such attacks.[58] The primary anesthetic considerations in Tourette syndrome are the side effects of standard medical therapy: haloperidol, clonidine, and pimozide. The former two are well known to anesthesiologists; pimozide is an antipsychotic implicated in sudden death, prolonged QT interval syndromes, and the neuroleptic malignant syndrome.[58]

## SEIZURE DISORDERS

Epileptic seizures represent acute changes in neurologic behavior due to paroxysmal electrical discharge in the brain. These may be generalized (tonic, clonic, grand mal, atonic, myoclonic, or petit mal), partial (simple, complex, or Jacksonian), or unclassifiable. The etiologies of seizure disorders are diverse and include metabolic abnormalities [e.g., calcium, sodium, maple syrup urine disease, phenylketonuria (PKU)], dysplastic development (e.g., tuberous sclerosis, Down syndrome, Sturge-Weber syndrome), infection (e.g., syphilis, cytomegalovirus, toxoplasmosis, encephalitis), acquired encephalopathy (e.g., ischemic-hypoxic, traumatic), vascular malformations, brain tumors and many others.

There are few unifying rules for the anesthesiologist to consider in the child with epilepsy except that emotional stress, alkalosis, ketamine, enflurane, low-dose methohexital, normeperidine, and laudanosine have proconvulsant potential and may worsen underlying seizures.

### Antiseizure Drugs

#### Phenytoin

Antiseizure medications may be an important element in the preoperative anesthetic evaluation. Phenytoin (Dilantin) is structurally related to barbiturates, is effective against many different seizure disorders, and has a wide variety of physiologic functions. It is administered in doses of 5 to 10 mg/kg/d and preferentially acts at the motor cortex to diminish after discharges and limit posttetanic potentiation. It is 70 to 95 percent protein bound and is effective in the treatment of cardiac arrhythmias, hypertension, movement disorders, pain syndromes, and other conditions. (The reader is referred elsewhere for a more complete discussion of the drug.[59]) Because phenytoin is dependent upon hepatic metabolism, medications or disease processes that alter hepatic function will affect phenytoin pharmacokinetics: benzodiazepines, cimetidine, salicylates, and halothane decrease phenytoin metabolism and increase serum phenytoin concentrations while carbamazepine and chronic alcoholism tend to accelerate elimination and lower serum concentration. Chronic valproic acid therapy is reported to have a variable effect upon phenytoin concentration. Phenytoin is also known to stimulate the microsomal enzyme system and accelerate hepatic metabolism of other drugs.

Phenytoin has important clinical implications in general anesthesia because of its effects on cardiac conduction, neuromuscular function, hepatic metabolism, and central nervous activity. Rapid IV administration (greater than 1 to 3 mg/kg/min in children or in excess of 50 mg/min in adults) may lead to cardiac conduction defects, ventricular fibrillation, and death. Intravenous administration (10 mg/kg given at rates less than 50 mg/min) causes a clinically slight but statistically significant increase in vecuronium-induced neuromuscular blockade.[60] In contrast, chronic phenytoin therapy will antagonize pancuronium, metocurine, (perhaps D-tubocurine),[61,62] doxacurium,[63] and probably vecuronium-induced neuromuscular blockade. Chronic phenytoin therapy is reported to have either no effect upon atracurium duration of action[61] or to reduce duration.[64] Phenytoin has been studied in models of acute halothane-mediated liver injury and there is no evidence that it increases toxic halothane intermediates and causes injury.[65] Decreased duration of fentanyl action has been observed in chronic phenytoin therapy, due in part to increases in narcotic metabolism.[66]

## Phenobarbital

Phenobarbital is administered in doses of 3 to 5 mg/kg/day for a variety of generalized and partial seizure disorders. It acts upon multisynaptic and spinal monosynaptic circuitry to suppress posttetanic potentiation. Primidone (Mysoline) is a phenobarbital precursor and has a similar spectrum of action; the dose of primidone is 10 to 20 mg/kg/d. Phenobarbital induces hepatic enzyme activity and chronic therapy has been implicated in both accelerated neuromuscular relaxant and narcotic metabolism.[64,66] The combination of phenobarbital pretreatment, hypoxemia, and halothane increases the risk of halothane-induced liver damage in specific animal models.[65,67]

## Valproic Acid

Valproic acid (Depakene) is highly effective against generalized, myoclonic, and absence seizures. The dose is 30 to 60 mg/kg/d, and the principle side effects are hepatotoxicity, pancreatitis, and bone marrow suppression. Valproic acid is conjugated in the liver and is 90 percent protein bound. It can displace other drugs from binding sites and increase free drug concentration. For example, the unbound fraction of thiopental increases from 15 to 22 percent and recovery time doubles (17 versus 37 minutes) when administered after valproic acid.[68]

## Carbamazepine

Carbamazepine (Tegretol) is effective in a variety of seizure disorders and can cause bone marrow suppression and impair hepatic function. It is 76 percent protein bound and is metabolized in the liver. Chronic administration has been reported to antagonize doxacurium-induced neuromuscular blockade[63] and may also antagonize vecuronium, metocurine, and D-tubocurine.

### Ethosuximide and Clonazepam

Ethosuximide (Zarontin) is highly effective for petit mal seizures. Its side effects include hepatic and renal dysfunction, aplastic anemia, and systemic lupus erythematosis. The daily dose is 20 to 30 mg/kg. Clonazepam (Clonopin) is a benzodiazepine metabolized by the liver and is useful for minor motor and generalized motor seizures. There are no specific anesthetic implications for either ethosuximide or clonaxepam.

## MYASTHENIA GRAVIS

Myasthenia gravis is a neuromuscular disease affecting voluntary muscle; it is characterized by weakness, easy fatigability, and improvement with rest or anticholinesterase therapy. It is thought to be caused by a circulating antiacetylcholine receptor immunoglobulin, although as many as 30 percent of patients do not possess such as antibody. The disease may be limited to ocular and cranial nerves or may be generalized. Respiratory involvement occurs commonly in generalized disease. Patients display decreased inspiratory force, decreased vital capacity, and chronic obstructive pulmonary disease.[69] Although autonomic dysfunction is generally thought to be uncommon in myasthenia, 16 percent of 108 patients ranging in age from 2 to 91 years displayed cardiac arrhythmias, sudden death, or focal myocarditis.[70]

Childhood myasthenia is extremely rare and has a variety of clinical expressions: a transient weakness is seen in neonates born to myasthenic mothers; a variety of congenital syndromes occur with and without antireceptor antibodies, and an adult type of the disease affects young teenage girls (juvenile myasthenia gravis).[71,72] In the latter, treatment includes anticholinesterases, thymectomy, immunosuppression, steroids, plasmapheresis, and cyclosporine. These patients have a 20-year life expectancy in excess of 80 percent.[72]

The anesthetic considerations in childhood myasthenia include underlying cardiopulmonary disease, concurrent medical therapy, and abnormal response to neuromuscular relaxants. The characteristic "myasthenic" response includes resistance to succinylcholine and relative sensitivity to nondepolarizing neuromuscular relaxants and reversal agents. Doses of succinylcholine may have to be increased to 10 mg/kg for complete neuromuscular relaxation, while small doses of short-acting nondepolarizing and reversal agents should be titrated carefully for full effect—even to asymptomatic, seronegative patients.[73] The presence of severe pulmonary symptoms can be predicted from history and from pulmonary function tests. A careful history should rule out underlying cardiac disease. Chronic therapy with oral pyridostigmine (Mestinon) and neostigmine (Prostigmin) inhibits plasmacholinesterase and prolongs the action of drugs such as succinylcholine and ester local anesthetics.

## MUSCULAR DYSTROPHIES

Muscular dystrophies represent groups of hereditary myopathies characterized by progressive weakness and loss of striated musculature. The specific biochemical defect(s) underlying the dystrophies are unknown but are thought to involve structural proteins (such as dystrophin and nebulin). The usual taxonomy of muscular dystrophies includes Duchenne's, Becker's, limb-girdle, facioscapulohumeral, scapuloperoneal, myotonic, oculopharyngeal, congenital, and a distal type.

## Duchenne's Muscular Dystrophy

Duchenne's muscular dystrophy is an X-linked recessive disorder with a reported incidence of 3/10,000 live births. The disease is usually diagnosed around 3 years of age when the child presents with gait disturbances, proximal muscle weakness, pseudohypertrophy of the muscles, and difficulty standing (Gowers sign). Progressive muscle weakness, kyphoscoliosis, restrictive pulmonary disease, cardiomyopathy, gastrointestinal abnormalities, pharyngeal dysfunction, pneumonia, and finally death by the third decade are the predictable sequelae.

The principal anesthetic considerations in muscular dystrophy include cardiopulmonary dysfunction and abnormal responses to neuromuscular relaxants. Clinical evidence of cardiac dysfunction is difficult to detect in wheelchair-bound patients, but in one study 11 of 17 children had global left ventricular dysfunction.[74] Occult cardiac disease is probably responsible for the majority of intraoperative cardiac arrhythmias and arrests reported.[75] Myocardial depressants such as halothane and thiopental should be used cautiously, and prolonged postoperative ventilatory management may be required in advanced disease states.

Several abnormal responses to neuromuscular relaxants have been characterized. Prolonged apnea,[76] generalized myotonia,[77] hyperkalemic cardiac arrest,[78] rhabdomyolysis,[79] abdominal pain, hypermetabolism, and a syndrome similar to malignant hyperthermia[80] have been reported following intravenous succinylcholine. In general, succinylcholine should be avoided in Duchenne's muscular dystrophy because of the risk of potassium flux and hyperkalemic cardiac arrest. (Such atypical responses following succinylcholine, however, may lead to a diagnosis of this condition previously unsuspected patients.) Direct evidence linking it with the syndrome of malignant hyperthermia is suggested in halothane-caffeine contracture testing,[81] but whether the structural protein abnormalities found in the disorder are equivalent to those of malignant hyperthermia is, as yet, unproved.

## Facioscapulohumeral and Myotonic Dystrophies

Facioscapulohumeral dystrophy is a muscular dystrophy with a reported incidence of 5/1,000,000. It presents in the second decade of life with facial and shoulder weakness. Cardiomyopathy and restrictive pulmonary disease are not common, although severe bradyarrhythmias are reported.[82] The response to neuromuscular relaxants is uncertain: succinylcholine has not been extensively studied. For nondepolarizing relaxants such as atracurium, the duration of action is reported to be significantly reduced.[83] Myotonic dystrophy is inherited as an autosomal dominant disorder with an incidence of 5/100,000. It is a relentless condition characterized by abnormal muscle relaxation, progressive muscle atrophy, cardiac conduction defects, diminished ventilatory capacity, gastrointestinal dysfunction, impaired laryngeal reflexes, and altered respiratory drive.[84,85] The response to succinylcholine is characterized by a rise in baseline tension (myotonic contracture) and a slight decrease in the twitch height.[86] An acute rise in serum potassium has been reported. Positive halothane-contracture tests have also been reported,[81] but these may represent artifact.[87] In general, patients are not believed to be at increased risk for malignant hyperthermia. The response to atracurium and curare appears to be normal.[86,88]

### Leukodystrophies

The leukodystrophies are a heterogeneous collection of autosomal recessive disorders characterized by abnormal myelin formation resulting in sensory and motor involvement with progressive dementia. Generalized hypotonia, spasticity, airway dysfunction, gastroesophageal reflux, seizures, and adrenal insufficiency (in adrenoleukodystrophy) can complicate the perioperative management. The leukodystrophies include Pelizaeus-Merzbacher, Krabbe's, Canavan's and Alexander's diseases, metachromatic leukodystrophy, and adrenoleukodystrophy. The safety of succinylcholine is unclear in this group of patients and until further study should be avoided.[89]

## CONGENITAL AND METABOLIC MYOPATHIES

The myopathies present with hypotonia and proximal muscle weakness during infancy and are caused by defects of lipid metabolism, glycogen storage, endocrine status, mitochondrial function, and muscle fiber composition. Central core disease is well known among anesthesiologists because of its reported association with malignant hyperthermia.[90] Abnormal type 1 fibers and reduced phosphorylase and ATPase activity are characteristic. The clinical presentation includes multiple skeletal abnormalities, restrictive pulmonary disease, and normal mentation. Nemaline myopathy is named for the rodlike structures found in muscle and has for four clinical presentations ranging from minimal involvement to progressive hypotonia and rapid death within the first year of life. In one case report, an 18-year-old with a benign variant displayed slight resistance to succinylcholine and a normal response to pancuronium.[91] There are few other specific principles to define anesthetic considerations in the these myopathies aside from postoperative weakness and the need for prolonged ventilatory support.

Periodic paralyses are syndromes and primary disease entities characterized by potassium flux and episodic weakness. The response to succinylcholine is normal,[92] and there is no association with malignant hyperthermia,[87] although halothane-caffeine contracture tests may be positive.[81]

Dermatomyositis is a common childhood inflammatory myopathy and usually presents during the first decade of life. It can progress to generalized hypotonia, pharyngeal weakness, respiratory failure, gastrointestinal infarction, joint deformities, and a scleroderma-like picture. The anesthetic considerations include reports of abnormal responses to neuromuscular relaxants. A myotonic type of response has been described following succinylcholine,[93] and prolonged vecuronium-induced neuromuscular relaxation is reported in a similar disorder, polymyositis.[94] Polymyositis may occur in infancy and is associated with collagen vascular diseases or immunoglobulin deficiencies. Corticosteroid and immunosuppression therapy are effective in both inflammatory myopathies.

## DOWN SYNDROME

Down syndrome is the most common chromosomal abnormality (trisomy 21) and occurs with an incidence of 1/700 to 1/1,100 live births. Mental retardation is a constant feature of the disorder (100 percent IQ < 65), and seizure disorders are common (2 to 9 percent). Cardiac disease is reported in 7 to 70 percent of patients. Ventricular septal defects (32 to 49 percent), endocardial cushion defects (32 percent), and pulmonary hypertension (32 to 100 percent) are the most common congenital cardiac lesions.[95] Intracardiac shunts, pulmonary disease, paradoxical emboli, and Eisenmenger syndrome should also be anticipated.[95,96] Early reports suggested hyperreactivity following atropine, but subsequent work has documented the safety of anticholinergics.[97,98]

Major cervical spine abnormalities are relatively common in Down syndrome. Between 10 and 31 percent will have radiographic evidence of cervical stenosis or atlantoxial subluxation, but a much smaller percentage (1 to 2 percent) become symptomatic.[99] Nonetheless, the American Academy of Pediatrics and the Special Olympics have recommended careful cervical spine evaluation and restriction of activities in children with radiographic evidence of instability.[100] Do these findings have any impact upon the preoperative considerations of the child with Down syndrome? In one study, Davidson[101] noted that dislocation was preceded by weeks of readily detectable physical signs such as neck pain, torticollis, hyperreflexia, weakness, abnormal gait, and bilateral clonus. Among the anesthesia literature, Williams et al.[102] reported symptomatic atlantoaxial subluxation in a previously healthy 6-year-old Down syndrome child following cardiac surgery. Whether physical signs were present before surgery in this report is unclear, but it is wise to follow the authors' recommendation "to avoid forceful flexion of the neck."[102]

Other preoperative considerations in Down syndrome include an increased incidence of subglottic stenosis, moyamoya disease, thyroid disease, and hematologic cancer. Decreased ventilatory drive and decreased cortical choline acetyltransferase and neurotransmitter concentration (dopamine, serotonin, norepinephrine) are reported. An enlarged tongue and increased secretions are clinically important in the airway management of these children.[103]

## ACKNOWLEDGMENTS

Special appreciation is extended to Wayne Cail, M.D., who supplied the radiographs, and to Kim Jenner, who typed the manuscript.

## REFERENCES

1. Shillito J, Matson DD: Craniosynostosis: a review of 519 surgical patients. Pediatrics 41:829, 1968
2. Shuper A, Merlob P, Grunebaum M et al: The incidence of isolated craniosynostosis in the newborn infant. Am J Dis Child 139:85, 1985
3. Tessier P: Relationship of craniostenoses to craniofacial dysostoses, and to faciostenoses: a study with therapeutic implications. Plast Reconstr Surg 48:224, 1971
4. Whittle IR, Johnston IH, Besser M: Intracranial pressure changes in craniostenosis. Surg Neruol 21:367, 1984
5. Crysdale WS, Kohli-Dang N, Mullins GC et al: Airway management in craniofacial surgery: experience in 542 patients. J Otolaryngol 16:207, 1987
6. Mixter RC, David DJ, Perloff WH et al: Obstructive sleep apnea in Apert's and Pfeiffer's syndromes: more than a craniofacial abnormality. Plast Reconstr Surg 86:457, 1990
7. Devine P, Bhan I, Feingold M et al: Complete cartilaginous trachea in a

child with Crouzon's syndrome. Am J Dis Child 138:40, 1984
8. Osborn AG, Heaston DK, Wing SD: Diagnosis of ascending transtentorial herniation by cranial computed tomography. AJR 130:755, 1978
9. Holinger PC, Holinger LD, Reichert TJ et al: Respiratory obstruction and apnea in infants with bilateral abductor vocal cord paralysis, meningomyelocele, hydrocephalus, and Arnold-Chirai malformation. J Pediatr 92:368, 1978
10. Oren J, Kelly DH, Todres ID et al: Respiratory complications in patients with myelodysplasia and Arnold-Chiari malformation. Am J Dis Child 140:221, 1986
11. Davidson Ward SL, Nickerson BG, van der Hal A et al: Absent hypoxic and hypercapneic arousal responses in children with myelomeningocele and apnea. Pediatrics 78:44, 1986
12. Ishak BA, McLone D, Seleny FL: Intraoperative autonomic dysfunction associated with Arnold-Chiari malformation. Child's Brain 7:146, 1980
13. Park TS, Hoffman HJ, Hendrick EB et al: Experience with surgical decompression of the Arnold-Chiari malformation in young infants with myelomeningocele. Neurosurgery 13:147, 1983
14. Greenberg F, James LM, Oakley GP: Estimates of birth prevalence rates of spina bifida in the United States from computer-generated maps. Am J Obstet Gynecol 145:570, 1983
15. Stein SC, Feldman JG, Friendlander M et al: Is myelomeningocele a disappearing disease? Pediatrics 69:511, 1982
16. Dierdorf SF, McNiece WL, Rao CC et al: Failure of succinylcholine to alter plasma potassium in children with myelomeningocoele. Anesthesiology 64:272, 1986
17. Slater JE, Mostello LA, Shaer C: Rubber-specific IgE in children with spina bifida. J Urol 146:578, 1991
18. McLaurin RL, Schut L, Venes JL, Epstein F: Pediatric Neurosurgery. 2nd Ed. WB Saunders, Philadelphia, 1989
19. Jacobson RI, Abrams GM: Disorders of the hypothalamus and pituitary gland in adolescence and childhood. In Swainman KF (ed): Pediatric Neurology. CV Mosby, St. Louis, 1989
20. Oi S, Matsumoto S: Infantile hydrocephalus and the slit ventricle syndrome in early infancy. Childs Nerv Syst 3:145, 1987
21. Newton RW: Intracranial pressure and its monitoring in childhood: a review. J R Soc Med 80:566, 1987
22. Duffner PK, Cohen ME, Myers MH et al: Survival of children with brain tumors: SEER Program, 1973–1980. Neurology 36:597, 1986
23. Rorke LB, Schut L: Introductory survey of pediatric brain tumors. p. 335. In McLaurin RL, Schut L, Venes JL, Epstein F (eds): Pediatric Neruosurgery. 2nd Ed. WB Saunders, Philadelphia, 1989
24. Cohen ME, Duffner PK: Tumors of the brain and spinal cord including leukemic involvement. p. 661. In Swainman KF (ed): Pediatric Neurology. CV Mosby, St. Louis, 1989
25. Schoenberg BS, Mellinger JF, Schoenberg DG: Cerebrovascular disease in infants and children: a study of incidence, clinical features, and survival. Neurology 28:763, 1978
26. Bingham RM, Wilkinson DJ: Anaesthetic management in Moya-moya disease. Anaesthesia 40:1198, 1985
27. Humphreys RP: Arteriovenous malformations of the brain. p. 508. In McLaurin RL, Schut L, Venes JL, Epstein F (eds): Pediatric Neurosurgery. 2nd Ed. WB Saunders, Philadelphia, 1989
28. Meidell R, Marinelli P, Pettett G: Perinatal factors associated with early-onset intracranial hemorrhage in premature infants. Am J Dis Child 139:160, 1985
29. Perlman JM, Goodman S, Kreusser KL et al: Reduction in intraventricular hemorrhage by fluctuating cerebral bloodflow velocity in preterm infants with respiratory distress syndrome. N Engl J Med 312:1353, 1985
30. Friesen RH, Honda AT, Thieme RE: Perianesthetic intracranial hemorrhage in preterm neonates. Anesthesiology 67: 814, 1987
31. Cyr RM, Usher RH, McLean FH:

Changing patterns of birth asphyxia and trauma over 20 years. Am J Obstet Gynecol 148:490, 1984
32. Hill A, Volpe JJ: Hypoxic-ischemic encephalopathy of the newborn. p. 372. In Swainman KF (ed): Pediatric Neurology. CV Mosby, St. Louis, 1988
33. Snyder RD: Bacterial infections of the nervous system. p. 447. In Swainman KF (ed): Pediatric Neruology. CV Mosby, St. Louis, 1988
34. Dyken PR: Viral diseases of the nervous system. p. 475. In Swainman KF (ed): Pediatric Neurology. CV Mosby, St. Louis, 1988
35. Hurwitz ES, Barnett MJ, Bergman D et al: Public health service study of Reye's syndrome and medications. JAMA 257: 1905, 1987
36. Beach TP, Stone WA, Hamelberg W: Circulatory collapse following succinylcholine: report of a patient with diffuse lower motor neuron disease. Anesth Analg 50:431, 1971
37. Swainman KF: Anterior horn cell and cranial motor neuron disease. p. 1083. In Swainman KF (ed): Pediatric Neruology. CV Mosby, St. Louis, 1988
38. Rosenbaum KJ, Neigh JL, Strobel GE: Sensitivity to non-depolarizing muscle relaxants in amyotrophic lateral sclerosis: report of two cases. Anesthesiology 35:638, 1971
39. Orndahl G, Stenberg K: Myotonic human musculature: stimulation with depolarizing agents. Mechanical registration of the succinylcholine, succinylmonocholine, and decamethonium. Acta Med Scand 172:389:S3, 1962
40. Tanaka H, Uemura N, Noyama Y: Cardiac involvement in the Kugelberg-Welander syndrome. Am J Cardiol 38: 528, 1976
41. Brazy JE, Kinney HC, Oakes WJ: Central nervous system structural lesions causing apnea at birth. J Pediatr 111:163, 1987
42. Fergusson RJ, Wright DJ, Willey RF et al: Suxamethonium is dangerous in polyneuropathy. Br Med J 282:298, 1981
43. Hagley SR, Griggs WM: Succinylcholine and polyneuropathy. Anesthesiology 63:225, 1985
44. Hogue CW, Itani MS, Martyn JAJ: Resistance to D-tubocurarine in lower motor neuron injury is related to increased acetylcholine receptors at the neuromotor junction. Anesthesiology 73: 703, 1990
45. Feldman JM: Cardiac arrest after succinylcholine administration in a pregnant patient recovered from Guillain-Barré syndrome. Anesthesiology 72:942, 1990
46. Campbell AM, Finley GA: Anaesthesia for a patient with Friedreich's ataxia and cardiomyopathy. Can J Anaesth 36:89, 1989
47. Bell CF, Kelly JM, Jones RS: Anaesthesia for Friedreich's ataxia. Anaesthesia 41:296, 1986
48. Antognini JF: Anaesthesia for Charcot-Marie-Tooth disease: a review of 86 cases. Can J Anaesth 39:398, 1992
49. Tavares JC, Maciel L: Anaesthetic management of a patient with familial amyloid polyneuropathy of the Portuguese type. Can J Anaesth 36:209, 1989
50. Eriksson P, Boman K, Jacobsson B et al: Cardiac arrhythmias in familial amyloid polyneuropathy during anaesthesia. Acta Anaesthesiol Scand 30:317, 1986
51. Dodge TL, Mahaffey JE, Thomas JD: The anesthetic management of a patient with an obstructing intratracheal mass: a case report. Anesth Analg 56:295, 1977
52. Baraka A: Myasthenic response to muscle relaxants in von Recklinghausen's disease. Br J Anaesth 46:701, 1974
53. Mitterschiffthaler G, Maurhard U, Huter O et al: Prolonged action of vecuronium in neurofibromatosis (von Recklinghausen's disease). Anaesthesiol Reanim 14: 175, 1989
54. Naguib M, Al-Rajeh SM, Abdulatif M et al: The response of a patient with von Recklinghausen's disease to succinylcholine and atracurium. Middle East J Anesthesiol 9:429, 1988
55. Hankey GJ, Perlman D: Polyneuropathy cranialis following cervical epidural anaesthesia. J Neurol Neurosurg Psychiatry 51:1106, 1988
56. Nelson KB; Cerebral palsy. p. 363. In Swainman KF (ed): Pediatric Neurology. CV Mosby, St. Louis, 1989

57. Ogasawara H, Shimodate Y, Isozaki K et al: Sevoflurane anesthesia for a patient with cerebral palsy. Masui 39:500, 1990
58. Morrison JE, Lockhart CH: Tourette syndrome: anesthetic implications. Anesth Analg 65:200, 1986
59. Smith BH, Bogoch S, Dreyfus J: The Broad Range of Clinical Use of Phenytoin. Dreyfus Medical Foundation, New York, 1988
60. Gray HSJ, Slater RM, Pollard BJ: The effect of acutely administered phenytoin on vecuronium-induced neuromuscular blockade. Anaesthesia 44:379, 1989
61. Ornstein E, Matteo RS, Young WL et al: Resistance to metocurine-induced neuromuscular blockade in patients receiving phenytoin. Anesthesiology 63:294, 1985
62. Liberman BA, Norman P, Hardy BG: Pancuronium-phenytoin interaction: a case of decreased duration of neuromuscular blockade. Int J Clin Pharm Ther Tox 26:371, 1988
63. Ornstein E, Matteo RS, Weinstein JA et al: Accelerated recovery from doxacurium-induced neuromuscular blockade in patients receiving chronic anticonvulsant therapy. J Clin Anesth 3:108, 1991
64. Tempelhoff R, Modica PA, Jellish WS et al: Resistance to atracurium-induced neuromuscular blockade in patients with intractable seizure disorders treated with anticonvulsants. Anesth Analg 71: 665, 1990
65. Nomura F, Hatano H, Ohnishi K et al: Effects of anticonvulsant agents on halothane-induced liver injury in human subjects and experimental animals. Hepatology 6:952, 1986
66. Tempelhoff R, Modica PA, Spitznagel EL: Anticonvulsant therapy increases fentanyl requirements during anaesthesia for craniotomy. Can J Anaesth 37:327, 1990
67. Schieble TM, Costa AK, Heffel DF et al: Comparative toxicity of halothane, isoflurane, hypoxia, and phenobarbital induction in monolayer cultures of rat hepatocytes. Anesthesiology 68:485, 1988
68. Aguilera L, Calvo R, Garcia RC: Interaction between thiopentone and sodium valproate. Br J Anaesth 58:1380, 1986
69. Leventhal SR, Orkin FK, Hirsh RA: Prediction of the need for postoperative mechanical ventilation in myasthenia gravis. Anesthesiology 53:26, 1980
70. Hofstad H, Ohm OJ, Mork SJ et al: Heart disease in myasthenia gravis. Acta Neurol Scand 70:176, 1984
71. Roach ES, Buono G, McLean WT et al: Early-onset myasthenia gravis. J Pediatr 108:193, 1986
72. Brown TCK, Gebert R, Meretoja OA et al: Myasthenia gravis in children and its anesthetic implications. Anaesth Intens Care 18:466, 1990
73. Kim JM, Mangold J: Sensitivity to both vecuronium and neostigmine in a seronegative myasthenic patient. Br J Anaesth 63:497, 1989
74. Sanyal SK, Tierney RC, Rao PS et al: Systolic time interval characteristics in children with Duchenne's progressive muscular dystrophy. Pediatrics 70:958, 1982
75. Sethna NF, Rockoff MA: Cardiac arrest following inhalation induction of anaesthesia in a child with Duchenne's muscular dystrophy. Can Anaesth Soc J 33: 799, 1986
76. Copbham IG, Davis HS; Anesthesia for muscle dystrophy patients. Anesth Analg 43:22, 1964
77. Paterson IS: Generalized myotonia following suxamethonium. Br J Anaesth 34: 340, 1962
78. Sethna NF, Rockoff MA, Worthen HM et al: Anesthesia-related complication in children with Duchenne muscular dystrophy. Anesthesiology 68:462, 1988
79. Miller ED, Sanders DB, Rowlingson JC et al: Anesthesia-induced rhabdomyolysis in a patient with Duchenne's muscular dystrophy. Anesthesiology 48:146, 1978
80. Larsen UT, Juhl B, Hein-Sorensen O et al: Complications during anaesthesia in patients with Duchenne's muscular dystrophy (a retrospective study). Can J Anaesth 36:418, 1989
81. Heiman-Patterson TD, Rosenberg H, Fletcher JE et al: Halothane-caffeine

contracture testing in neuromuscular diseases. Muscle Nerve 11:453, 1988
82. Duncan PG: Neuromuscular disease. In Katz H and Steward DJ (eds): Anesthesia and Uncommon Pediatric Diseases. WB Saunders, Philadelphia, 1987
83. Dresner DL, Ali HH: Anaesthetic management of a patient with facioscapulohumeral muscular dystrophy. Br J Anaesth 62:331, 1989
84. Aldridge LM: Anaesthetic problems in myotonic dystrophy. Br J Anaesth 57: 1119, 1985
85. Ishizawa Y, Yamaguchi H, Dohi S et al: A serious complication due to gastrointestinal malfunction in a patient with myotonic dystrophy. Anesth Analg 65: 1066, 1986
86. Mitchell MM, Ali HH, Savarese JJ: Myotonia and neuromuscular blocking agents. Anesthesiology 49:44, 1978
87. Lehmann-Horn F, Iaizzo PA: Are myotonias and periodic paralyses associated with susceptibility to malignant hyperthermia? Br J Anaesth 65:692, 1990
88. Nightingale P, Healy TEJ, McGuinness K: Dystrophia myotonica and atracurium. Br J Anaesth 57:1131, 1985
89. Tobias JD: Anaesthesia considerations for the child with leukodystrophy. Can J Anaesth 39:394, 1992
90. Eng GD, Epstein BS, Engel WK et al: Malignant hyperthermia and central core disease in a child with congenital dislocating hips. Arch Neurol 35:189, 1978
91. Heard SO, Kaplan RF: Neuromuscular blockade in a patient with nemaline myopathy. Anesthesiology 59:588, 1983
92. Melnick B, Chang JL, Larson CE et al: Hypokalemic familial periodic paralysis. Anesthesiology 58:263, 1983
93. Johns RA, Finholt DA, Stirt JA: Anaesthetic management of a child with dermatomyositis. Can Anaesth Soc J 33:71, 1986
94. Flusche G, Unger-Sargon J, Lambert DH: Prolonged neuromuscular paralysis with vecuronium in a patient with polymyositis. Anesth Analg 66:188, 1987
95. Laursen HB: Congenital heart disease in Down's syndrome. Br Heart J 38:32, 1976
96. Park SC, Mathews RA, Zuberbuhler JR et al: Down syndrome with congenital heart malformation. Am J Dis Child 131: 29, 1977
97. Harris WS, Goodman RM: Hyper-reactivity to atropine in Down's syndrome. N Engl J Med 279:407, 1968
98. Wark HJ, Overton JH, Marian P: The safety of atropine premedication in children with Down's syndrome. Anaesthesia 38:871, 1983
99. Pueschel SM, Scola FH: Atlantoaxial instability in individuals with Down syndrome: epidemiologic, radiographic, and clinical studies. Pediatrics 80:555, 1987
100. Committee on Sports Medicine: Atlantoaxial instability in Down syndrome. Pediatrics 74:152, 1984
101. Davidson RG: Atlantoaxial instability in individuals with Down syndrome: a fresh look at the evidence. Pediatrics 81: 857, 1988
102. Williams JP, Somerville GM, Miner ME et al: Atlanto-axial subluxation and trisomy-21: another perioperative complication. Anesthesiology 67:253, 1987
103. Kobel M, Creighton RE, Steward DJ: Anaesthetic considerations in Down's syndrome: experience with 100 patients and a review of the literature. Can J Anaesth 29:593, 1982

# 8
# Infectious Diseases

**Bacterial Infections**
- Gram-Positive Aerobic Pathogens
- *Clostridium* (Gram-Positive Anaerobic Bacteria)
- Gram-Negative Bacteria

**Antibiotics**
- β-Lactam Antibiotics
- Aminoglycosides
- Vancomycin
- Erythromycin
- Choramphenicol

**Viral Infections**
- Enterovirus Family
- Herpesvirus Family
- Other Common Exanthematous Viral Pathogens

**Other Organisms**
- Spirochaetacea
  - *Treponema pallidum* (Syphilis)
- Rickettsia
- *Borrelia*
- *Candida*

**Syndromes Associated with Infection**
- Mucocutaneous Lymph Node Syndrome
- Reye Syndrome
- Guillain-Barré Syndrome

# 8

# Infectious Diseases

*Kathleen R. Rosen*
*David A. Rosen*

Infectious disease, a major source of morbidity in the pediatric population, accounts for more than one-half of pediatric office visits. In previously healthy children it is seldom a primary cause of death. Infection does, however, contribute significantly to the mortality (and morbidity) associated with trauma, malignancy, and surgery. Although widespread community vaccination has reduced the occurrence of many common childhood illnesses (Table 8-1) and vaccines are available for use in specific high-risk populations, infection is still present uniformly, especially in certain populations (Table 8-2).[1] For example, the population of children with congenital and acquired immune deficiencies is expanding as therapy for many of the primary diseases progresses. These immune-compromised children are at increased risk for an infectious disease (Table 8-3).[2] Normal pediatric pathogens may yield fulminant disease, and there is also risk of infection by unusual pathogens.

Neonates and infants are another group at risk because of the developmental immaturity of their immune system. In spite of the initial immunity afforded by the passive transplacental antibodies, response to vaccination or infectious challenge may be inadequate for the first 18 to 24 months of life.[3]

While fever or temperature instability is a key feature of the inflammatory response, the signs and symptoms of infection are nonspecific.[4] Although many anesthesiologists focus on the rash, there is a considerable overlap in causative agents and the specific type of rash (Table 8-4). Furthermore, the rash may change significantly over the course of the disease. The concurrent appearances of a skin rash, fever, and malaise are subtle indicators of septicemia. The clinical presentation for serious infections in childhood is often not specific for any single agent. Many bacteria, viruses, or other unusual organisms may produce a similar disruption of organ function.

When infectious disease is suspected there are three objectives for care: to support organ function, to obtain samples of body fluids for pathogen identification, and to begin antimicrobial treatment. Antimicrobial therapy is often started before the etiology is determined. Selection of drugs is based on the most common pathogens in a specific age group for the organ systems involved. Other modifying factors include vaccination history, geography, known exposure to infectious disease, socioeconomic variables, and

**Table 8-1.** Recommended Schedule for Routine Childhood Immunizations

| *Organism* | *Vaccine Abbreviation* | *Number* | *Ages* |
|---|---|---|---|
| *Corynebacterium diphtheriae*<br>*Clostridium tetani*<br>*Bordetella pertussis* | DPT | 5 | 2, 4, 6, 18 months; 4–6 years |
| Polio (trivalent, oral) | TOPV | 5 | 2, 4, 18 months |
| Rubella<br>Rubeola (measles)<br>Mumps | MMR | 2 | |
| *Haemophilus influenzae* type b | HIB | 1 | 18 months |
| *Corynebacterium diphtheriae*<br>*Clostridium tetani* | TD | | Every 5–10 years after last DPT |

immune function. Diagnosis may be facilitated by rapid diagnostic tests (e.g., the gold standard Gram stain) or newer, more rapid identification techniques (e.g., latex agglutinization or counterimmunoelectrophoresis).

Surgery and anesthesia may be necessary for the diagnosis or treatment of infection or may be performed coincidentally in a child with infectious disease. Consequently, potential exposure to infected body fluid is a real risk to healthcare personnel in procedure-oriented environments (e.g., operating room, emergency room, and intensive care unit). Appropriate precautions must be used consistently if the nosocomial spread of infection is to be controlled. Simple barrier methods of protection, such as the routine use of gloves, face masks, and foot covers during procedures, are quite effective. In addition, early education of medical trainees about the safe handling of contaminated needles is essential.

This chapter focuses on the common pathogens responsible for infectious disease in normal children; the information is presented from the perspective of the infectious agent. A review of septic shock is included. The antimicrobial drugs are listed in the Appendix. Other chapters cover infections that relate to specific organ systems.

**Table 8-2.** Available Vaccines

| *Vaccine* | *Indication* |
|---|---|
| Hepatitis B | High-risk exposure to hepatitis carrier or blood products |
| *Streptococcus pneumoniae* | Impaired splenic function |
| Varicella | Leukemia |
| Influenza | Immunocompromised patients |
| *Neisseria meningitidis* | Meningococcal epidemics, type specific |
| *Salmonella typhi* | Extended travel to endemic regions |

## BACTERIAL INFECTIONS

Bacterial organisms are responsible for a wide variety of local and generalized illness in children. Localized disease is the most common clinical presentation for most organisms. Adjacent tissues may become involved secondarily. Occasionally hematogenous or lymphatic spread of the organisms results in infection at a distant site. Primary septicemia with multisystem organ compromise is rare in nor-

**Table 8-3.** Conditions Associated with Diminished Resistance to Infection

| *Onset* | *General Description* | *Specific Examples* |
|---|---|---|
| Congenital | Defects of humoral immunity | Hypogammaglobulinemia<br>Agammaglobulinemia<br>Selective immunoglobulin deficiency |
| | Defects of cellular immunity | Di-George syndrome |
| | Combined cellular and humoral defect | Wiskott-Aldrich syndrome<br>Ataxia telangiectasia<br>Severe combined immune deficiency |
| | Defects of leukocyte function or number | Chédiak-Higashi syndrome<br>Glucose-6-phosphate dehydrogenase deficiency (G6PD)<br>Lazy leukocyte |
| Acquired | Physical status | Age: Neonates and prematures<br>Malnutrition<br>Prolonged hospitalization<br>Trauma<br>Surgery and anesthesia<br>Burns<br>Other infections |
| | Chronic disease | Malignancy<br>Splenic insufficiency<br>Inflammatory bowel disease<br>Renal dysfunction<br>Cirrhosis<br>Diabetes<br>Cystic fibrosis<br>Sickle cell disease/hemoglobinopathy |
| | Immunosuppressive therapy | Chemotherapy<br>Radiation<br>Steroids |

mal children, but is a significant risk in the compromised host.

In addition to local tissue disruption, many bacterial exotoxins and endotoxins can cause widespread nonsuppurative tissue damage. Endotoxins are lipopolysaccharides found within the cell walls of gram-negative bacteria. Endotoxin release into the circulation occurs during cell wall growth or as a result of bacterial cell death. Endotoxins affect all organ systems and are the foundation for septic shock. Exotoxins, which are proteins excreted by many gram-positive and a few gram-negative bacteria, act through a variety of mechanisms. Some produce tissue damage through lysis of cell membranes or connective tissue (such as staphylococcal and streptococcal toxins). Other exotoxins interfere with cellular metabolism or protein synthesis (such as diphtheria and *Pseudomonas* toxins). Table 8-5 summarizes the organ systems at risk for compromise as a function of specific bacteria.

In general, health-care personnel are at lower risk for nosocomial infection from bacterial pathogens than from viral or other infectious agents. Transmission does not occur over long distances or by means of fomites unless the organism is capable of forming spores, and spore forms are of minimal risk in the person with normal immune function and intact

**Table 8-4.** Infectious Rashes and Possible Etiologies

| *Erythematous Rash (Scarlet Fever-like)* | *Maculopapular Rash* | *Petechial or Purpuric Rash* | *Vesicular Rash* | *Bullous Rash* | *Erythema Multiform* | *Curvilinear Rash* | *Urticarial Rash* |
|---|---|---|---|---|---|---|---|
| Group A *Streptococcus* | Measles | Meningococcemia | Chickenpox | Herpesvirus | Herpesvirus | Lyme disease | Herpesvirus |
| *Staphylococcus* infection | Rubella | *Haemophilus influenzae* | Herpes zoster | Syphilis | Enterovirus | Rheumatic fever | Coxsackievirus |
| Kawasaki disease | Adenovirus | Rocky Mountain spotted fever | Herpes simplex | *Staphylococcus* | Kawasaki disease | | Echovirus |
| Toxic shock | Syphilis | *Streptococcus* | Coxsackievirus | Chickenpox | Atypical measles | | Hepatitis B |
| Atypical measles | Coxsackievirus | Toxic shock | Echovirus | *Streptococcus* | *Vibrio parahaemolyticus* | | Mycoplasma |
| *Corynebacterium haemolyticum* | Echovirus | *Staphylococcus aureus* | *Mycoplasma pneumoniae* | *Pseudomonas* | | | Giardiasis |
| | Pityriasis rosea | *Pseudomonas* | Atypical measles | *Escherichia coli* | | | Syphilis |
| | Typhoid fever | *Gonococcus* | Scabies | *Aeromonas* | | | |
| | Shigellosis | Epstein-Barr virus | | *Yersinia* | | | |
| | Enterovirus | Atypical measles | | | | | |
| | *Pseudomonas aeruginosa* | Adenovirus | | | | | |
| | | Cytomegalovirus | | | | | |
| | | Rubella | | | | | |
| | | Murine typhus | | | | | |
| | | Histoplasmosis | | | | | |
| | | *Escherichia coli* | | | | | |
| | | *Mycoplasma pneumoniae* | | | | | |
| | | Congenital toxoplasmosis | | | | | |
| | | Congenital cytomegalovirus | | | | | |
| | | Congenital rubella | | | | | |

**Table 8-5.** Organs and Systems at Risk in Pediatric Infectious Disease

| *Organism or Syndrome* | *Organ or System Affected* |
|---|---|
| Group A beta-hemolytic *Streptococcus* (GABHS) | Skin, pharynx, kidneys, heart |
| Group B beta-hemolytic *Streptococcus* (GBBHS) | Lungs, central nervous system |
| *Streptococcus viridans* | Heart |
| *Streptococcus pneumoniae* | Ears, lungs, central nervous system |
| *Staphylococcus aureus* | Skin, bones, gastrointestinal system; toxic shock |
| *Corynebacterium diphtheriae* | Pharynx, heart, peripheral nervous system, kidneys |
| *Clostridium perfringens* | Gastrointestinal system, skin, muscles |
| *Clostridium botulinum* | Nervous system |
| *Clostridium tetani* | Nervous system |
| *Clostridium difficile* | Gastrointestinal system |
| *Salmonella* | Gastrointestinal system |
| *Shigella* | Nervous system, gastrointestinal system, kidneys |
| *Escherichia coli* | Gastrointestinal system, central nervous system, kidneys |
| *Haemophilus influenzae* | Pharynx, respiratory system, central nervous system, bones and joints, skin |
| *Neisseria meningitidis* | Pharynx, respiratory system, central nervous system, heart, bones and joints, blood |
| *Bordetella pertussis* | Respiratory system |
| Herpesvirus | Skin, mucous membranes, pharynx, central nervous system |
| Enterovirus | Respiratory system, gastrointestinal system |
| Rubeola | Ears, respiratory system, central nervous system |
| Rubella | Bones and joints, central nervous system |
| Mumps | Central nervous system, genitourinary system |
| Mucocutaneous lymph node syndrome | Heart |
| Reye syndrome | Central nervous system, liver |
| Guillain-Barré syndrome | Central nervous system |
| Syphilis | Skin, genitourinary system, central nervous system, heart, bones |
| Rickettsia | Skin, heart, lungs, muscles |
| *Borrelia* | Bones and joints, central nervous system, heart |
| *Candida* | Eyes, lungs, kidneys, liver, heart |

epithelium. Transmission occurs through direct contact with an infected site, blood, or respiratory secretions; thus, in persons with intact skin, infection can readily be prevented by hand-washing or the use of protective barriers. In healthy individuals, even the introduction of bacteria onto a mucous membrane surface is likely to result in only an asymptomatic carrier state.

Bacterial infectivity is usually coincident with the onset of symptoms, in contrast to viral shedding, which may occur for several days preceding the clinical presentation.

## Gram-Positive Aerobic Pathogens

The most common organisms causing gram-positive bacterial infections in children are *Streptococcus* and *Staphylococcus*. These organisms most commonly produce infections of the skin or respiratory tract. They are less frequently associated with infection at distant sites or disseminated sepsis. Several recognized syndromes describe multisystem disease caused by these gram-positive organisms through exotoxin production.

### *Streptococcus pyogenes* (Group A Beta-Hemolytic *Streptococcus*)

One of the most frequent sources of bacterial diseases of childhood is group A beta-hemolytic streptococcal (GABHS) organisms. In 15 to 20 percent of the population, GABHS organisms are part of the normal flora of the nasopharynx. Anal carriage or transmission via contaminated food (especially milk and eggs) is also possible.[5] The spread of disease is facilitated by crowded living or working conditions (e.g., urban low socioeconomic status or military recruit camps). The period of greatest risk of transmission is during the acute phase of the infection, while most of the secondary spread occurs within the first 2 weeks after acquisition.[6] Spread from the acute disease is usually not a problem after 3 days of penicillin therapy. The common infections that result are impetigo and isolated pharyngitis.

**Impetigo.** A highly contagious infection of the superficial layers of the skin, impetigo occurs most commonly in preschool children during warm weather. Streptococcal impetigo requires a prior disruption of the skin to establish an infection. Patients have no fever or systemic symptoms. Painless vesicles with a halo of erythema are initially seen at the site of skin trauma. These lesions progress to pustules and eventually develop a honey-colored crust. This infection is found most often on the lower extremities but may also be found on the arms or the face. Staphylococcal organisms are often grown concurrently in cultures. Mild cases require only superficial cleansing with or without topical antibiotics. In more severe cases there may be widespread lesions, superficial cellulitis, or lymphadenitis, and systemic antibiotics are indicated. Late hypersensitivity-type reactions are possible after GABHS infections. Glomerulonephritis, but not rheumatic fever, is a nonsuppurative complication of GABHS impetigo occurring 1 to 4 weeks later.

**Pharyngitis.** The predominate GABHS infection in temperate climates during the winter is pharyngitis. Up to 50 percent of all cases of isolated pharyngitis in school-age children are due to GABHS. This organism produces an acute self-limited illness that lasts for an average of 4 days with or without antibiotic treatment.[7] Onset of the exudative pharyngitis may be accompanied clinically by fever, headache, vomiting, abdominal pain, and anterior cervical adenopathy. Symptoms of a general upper respiratory tract infection (URTI) are absent. The presence of rhinitis, conjunctivitis, stomatitis, cough, hoarseness, or diarrhea suggests a viral etiology. The clinical course in preschool children is not as clearly defined,[8] but the disease frequently presents as an URTI or pharyngitis. Cultures of both the nares and throat are recommended. In children under 3 years a positive nasal culture correlates with an infection; in older children it correlates with the carrier state. Identification of GABHS as the pharyngeal pathogen by throat culture necessitates antibiotic therapy. Antibiotic prophylaxis of household contacts, especially other school-age children, is also recommended.

Although the initial infection may be relatively benign, multiple serious suppurative and nonsuppurative complications are possible. GABHS infection may extend locally to produce otitis media, mastoiditis, sinusitis, cervical adenitis, pneumonia, or pharyngeal or retropharyngeal abscesses. Septicemia with

GABHS can result in meningitis, endocarditis, osteomyelitis, or septic arthritis. Both glomerulonephritis and rheumatic fever are potential late nonsuppurative complications. Adequate eradication of streptococcal organisms from the pharynx is effective in the prevention of all of these complications except glomerulonephritis. Certain nephrogenic strains can produce glomerulonephritis in up to 15 percent of patients.

**Scarlet Fever.** Scarlet fever is the term for a classic exanthem that may accompany either GABHS impetigo or GABHS pharyngitis. Certain strains of GABHS produce an erythrogenic toxin. Hypersensitivity to this toxin yields the typical (scarlatiniform) scarlet fever rash within the first 24 hours of infection. A red, finely punctate rash with the texture of coarse sandpaper begins on the trunk and spreads peripherally to become generalized. The red color disappears with pressure except in skin folds at joints, where petechiae or hyperpigmentation may occur (pastia lines). A white or red mottled, swollen strawberry tongue is frequently present. Desquamation of the rash in fine flakes occurs at the end of one week.

**Rheumatic Fever.** Rheumatic fever, a serious late nonsuppurative sequela of GABHS, occurs after 0.3 to 3.0 percent of untreated GABHS infections[9]; it is rare in children under 3 years. It can be prevented by adequate antibiotic therapy of the acute GABHS infection. To remove GABHS from the pharynx completely, oral antibiotics such as penicillin or erythromycin are necessary for a full 10 days. Tetracycline or sulfonamides should not be used.[10] Intramuscular benzathine penicillin is an alternative therapy recommended when patient compliance is doubtful. This regimen is effective in the prevention of rheumatic fever even when it is delayed for several days pending culture results.[11] Although the occurrence of rheumatic fever has been declining since the 1970s, it has not been eliminated.

The clinical manifestations of rheumatic fever are variable. The common major manifestations include arthritis, carditis, and Sydenham's chorea, which by itself is specific for rheumatic fever. Less frequent major manifestations include painless subcutaneous nodules and erythema marginatum. Minor manifestations include fever, arthralgia, prior history of rheumatic fever, elevation of acute phase parameters erythrocyte sedimentation rate (ESR), and prolonged P-R interval. Diagnosis of rheumatic fever requires documentation of a GABHS infection by positive culture during the earlier acute illness (approximately 2 to 4 weeks prior) or elevation of antistreptolysin or other antistreptococcal antibody titers and fulfillment of Jones clinical criteria.[12] The presence of two major manifestations or one major and two minor manifestations satisfy Jones criteria. All of the major and minor manifestations of rheumatic fever resolve spontaneously without sequelae except for moderate to severe carditis. Structural damage to the mitral or aortic valve is a frequent residual effect.

Patients with a history of rheumatic fever are at an increased risk for acquiring subsequent GABHS infections, and the risk of recurrence of rheumatic fever after GABHS increases to 15 percent.[9] Carditis will recur with each episode of rheumatic fever. Therefore, it is recommended that patients with a history of rheumatic fever continue antibiotic prophylaxis until the third decade of life or until free from recurrence for 5 years. Patients with a history of carditis or those with frequent contact with school-age children are considered high risk and may require antibiotic prophylaxis indefinitely.

It is uncommon for the child who has

had rheumatic fever to develop significant cardiac symptomatology until late adolescence or early adulthood. Echocardiographic evaluation within 12 months before the planned anesthetic will allow the anesthesiologist to adjust the anesthetic plan to account for any cardiac disease.

### *Streptococcus agalactiae* (Group B Beta-Hemolytic *Streptococcus*)

Group B beta-hemolytic streptococcal (GBBHS) organisms are the most frequent source of sepsis in neonates. Neonatal sepsis has a high mortality rate (50 to 80 percent) due to the inability of the neonate to mount an adequate immune response to localize or limit the spread of infectious disease. Accordingly, the signs of sepsis in the neonate are nonspecific, and antibiotic therapy must be started before an infectious etiology can be ascertained. Respiratory distress with or without apnea, vomiting, diarrhea, jaundice, lethargy, seizures, unstable body temperature, and decreased peripheral perfusion are general distress signs that may be associated with sepsis. The presence of a skin rash in a neonate with nonspecific signs of distress strongly suggests an infectious etiology. Pneumonia and meningitis are the primary clinical manifestations.

The occurrence of GBBHS sepsis is bimodal. Most cases (75 percent) present within the first week of life and are usually evident less than 24 hours after birth. Up to 0.4 percent of live births may be complicated by early GBBHS infections.[13] Several maternal risk factors are associated with an increased incidence of neonatal sepsis: positive GBBHS cervical culture, fever, prolonged rupture of membranes, premature labor, and chorioamnionitis. In mothers who harbor GBBHS, strategies to avoid neonatal sepsis include expedient delivery after rupture of membranes, and penicillin prophylaxis 2 weeks prior to and during delivery.

Late-onset neonatal sepsis has a much lower mortality rate (< 20 percent). Infants are better able to localize infection by 1 month of age, and signs of GBBHS infection will be related to the organ systems involved. Meningitis is the primary late clinical manifestation in 75 percent of patients. The long-term morbidity is quite high and is related to the presence of residual neurologic defects.

### *Streptococcus viridans* (Group D, Gamma Hemolysis)

The penicillin-resistant organism *S. viridans* is associated with surgical wound infections and peritonitis. It is also the most common cause of bacterial endocarditis.

### *Streptococcus pneumoniae* (*Pneumococcus,* Alpha Hemolysis)

*S. pneumoniae* is the most common source of bacterial infection in children aged 6 to 24 months. While nasopharyngeal carriage is unusual in adults, 25 to 50 percent of normal children are colonized.[14] This frequency may increase to 97 percent in institutional environments. Upper respiratory infections facilitate the spread of this organism via large respiratory droplets. Otitis media is the most frequent pneumococcal infection in children, occurring in one-half of all children by 3 years of age.[15] Pneumococcus is also a frequent pathogen in pediatric sepsis, pneumonia, and meningitis.

*S. pneumoniae* is distinguished from other streptococcal organisms by the presence of a thick polysaccharide polymer capsule. Virulence is related to capsule size. The quellung reaction (capsular swelling) allows rapid identification of pneumococci in body fluids. The capsule allows the bacterium to resist elimination by the normal mechanism of phagocytosis. Patients with diminished or absent splenic function are at risk for overwhelming pneumococcal infection. Medical conditions at risk include sickle cell disease (and other hemoglobinopathies), Hodgkin's disease, chronic cardiopulmonary disease, nephrosis, cirrhosis, and asplenia, whether medical or surgical. Vaccination is recommended for high-risk patients under 2 years of age. Inadequate immune response is seen in younger patients and when chronic antibiotic prophylaxis (e.g., ampicillin, sulfisoxazole) is utilized.

### *Staphylococcus aureus*

*S. aureus* is a ubiquitous organism, which 35 percent of adults carry in the nasopharynx or on the skin.[16,17] Direct contact with pus or nasal secretions is necessary for transmission of the infection. Intact skin and respiratory mucosa make up excellent barriers against staphylococcal invasion, but when those barries are broken, the organisms can gain access to deep and distant tissues. Abscess formation is the hallmark of staphylococcal infections. Purulent superficial infections (e.g., impetigo, cellulitis, furuncles, carbuncles, paronychia) are the most common. Impetigo lesions are clinically indistinguishable from those of GABHS, and both organisms frequently coexist. Respiratory infections and local extension of respiratory infections (see GABHS section) are often preceded by a viral URTI. Hematogenous or lymphatic spread may produce abscess formation in distant organs such as muscle, bone, brain, joint, heart, lung, and kidney. *S. aureus* is the organism most commonly associated with osteomyelitis or septic arthritis. Patients at increased risk for staph infection include those with disruption of skin (e.g., by trauma, surgery, intravascular catheter, or medical disease), intrathecal catheters, poor nutrition (e.g., starvation, azotemia), acidosis, or altered immune resistance (e.g., newborn infants, or persons who have taken staph-resistant antibiotics or steroids). Effective treatment requires both drainage of abscesses and use of antibiotics.

**Ritter's Disease.** Scalded skin syndrome (Ritter's disease) is an extensive superficial skin disease in which the disruption of tissue is enhanced by the production of an exotoxin (exfoliatoxin). The syndrome is preceded by a local staph infection of the skin, pharynx, conjunctiva, or gastrointestinal tract. Prodromal symptoms include fever, malaise, irritability, and skin tenderness. Mild cases are similar to scarlet fever. In more severe cases, macular erythema of face, neck, axilla, and groin extend and develop into flaccid, sterile bullae that desquamate in large sections with simple stroking of the skin (Nikolsky sign).

Staphylococci are also common sources of acute food poisoning. Improper storage of previously cooked protein-containing foods allows for elaboration of exotoxin. The organisms can be introduced into the food source through skin contaminants and poor hygiene of the food handlers and are most common in salads with mayonnaise and potatoes or eggs, in ham, and in custard-containing pastries. Acute onset of abdominal pain, nausea, vomiting, and diarrhea occurs within hours of ingestion. The gastroenteritis usually resolves without treatment within 48 hours. A primary anesthetic concern for the child presenting with this problem is adequate hydrational status.

**Toxic Shock Syndrome.** The most severe manifestation of disease produced by staphylococcal exotoxin is toxic shock syndrome (TSS). A clinically indistinguishable form of TSS is less frequently associated with streptococcal exotoxin. TSS was first recognized in 1978 in a group of pediatric patients. This multisystem disease is now most often associated with tampon usage but may accompany any type of staph infection.[18] Staphylococcal colonization of the cervix or vagina is present in approximately 10 percent of females and is an important precedent for TSS associated with menstruation. Important precedents of nonmenstrual TSS are use of nasal packing, tracheitis, and sinusitis.[18–20]

The four major criteria of TSS are fever, hypotension (at rest or postural), rash (macular erythroderma or scarlatinaform), and subsequent generalized desquamation of skin, hair, and nails (telogen effluvium). The rash can be accompanied by erythema and edema of the palms and soles, strawberry tongue, conjunctival hyperemia, and generalized nonpitting edema. Multisystem organ dysfunction at a minimum of three sites ensues [(i.e., gastrointestinal distress, erythema of mucous membranes, arthralgia, myalgia or increased creatine phosphokinase (CPK), altered mental status, thrombocytopenia, acute respiratory distress syndrome (ARDS), shock, or renal or hepatic dysfunction]. Recently several cases have been reported in children with atypical clinical courses.[21] Atypical TSS may follow food poisoning or influenza, and cardiac dysfunction may manifest as impaired conduction rather than hypotension.[4,19,20,22]

The treatment in TSS is mainly supportive. Much of the support is involved with maintenance of intravascular volume.[21] The use of antibiotics is controversial since exotoxin is responsible for TSS. Antibiotics are indicated if there is any evidence of residual infection or to eliminate staph colonization and prevent recurrence of menstrual-associated cases.

### *Corynebacterium diphtheriae*

The incidence of diphtheria in this country has been minimized with routine toxoid immunization. Transmission of infection occurs by means of respiratory droplets. The *C. diphtheriae* bacterium, a pleomorphic, nonmotile bacillus, classically produces an invasive infection of respiratory mucosa; some strains elaborate an exotoxin. Infections of the skin, conjunctiva, and genital mucosa are possible. Severe tissue necrosis with an adherent exudate are characteristic of diphtheria. Attempts to dislodge the membrane will result in bleeding because host tissue is an integral part of the membrane. This membrane sloughs spontaneously during the second week of infection.

Nasal infection is most common in those infants in whom local extension of infection and toxin absorption are minimal. The symptoms are similar to a mild URTI, with coryza, low-grade fever, malaise, and anorexia early in the clinical course. A purulent nasal discharge with excoriation of the nares and upper lip develops later. Pharyngeal and tonsillar infection also begins unimpressively. Within 1 to 2 days the characteristic exudate develops and extends to cover the palate. Downward extension to the larynx and tracheobronchial tree is a potential and serious problem. Isolated laryngeal diphtheria is rare and is clinically indistinct from croup. Progressive pharyngeal involvement can include cervical adenitis, brawny erasure edema (bull neck), palatal paralysis, difficulty in swallowing, and acute airway obstruction. GABHS secondary infection is common.[12] Exotoxin release is associated with some strains of diphtheria but only with pharyngeal infection. Diphtheria toxin may harm any organ; however, the myocardium, peripheral nerves, and kidneys are most frequently affected. Acute myocarditis is the most frequent cause of death. Disorders of the regulation of the peripheral circulation and cardiac conduction system may also be present. Palatal paralysis is the initial focus of the neuritis. This motor dysfunction is manifest as a change in voice and difficulty in swallowing. The bilateral limb weakness is indistinguishable from Guillain-Barré syndrome. Phrenic and ocular muscles may also be affected.

Treatment protocols include antibiotics, antitoxin, bed rest, and supportive care of respiratory and cardiac function. Patients with diphtheria must be isolated until three consecutive negative throat cultures have been obtained. Intimate contacts should receive antibiotic prophylaxis and booster immunization if previously immunized or throat culture and antitoxin if not previously immunized. The Schick test for sensitivity to horse serum should be carried out before administration of antitoxin.

The primary anesthetic concerns with this disease center on intubation. Nasal intubation is not recommended, because of bleeding and the potential for sinusitis. Even oral intubation presents concerns about spreading the disease from the pharynx to the larynx. During the third week, when neuritis produces paralysis of the soft palate and difficulty in swallowing, the likelihood of aspiration increases.

## *Clostridium* (Gram-Positive Anaerobic Bacteria)

Clostridia are gram-positive motile rods. They are obligate anaerobes and sensitive to destruction by heat, light, and oxygen. In humans, clinical disease is promoted by the formation of spores that are highly resistant to these destructive forces. When the spores are introduced into supportive tissue, such as the gastrointestinal tract or penetrating wounds, proliferation of the vegetative organism can occur. Conditions that support this transition include reduced oxygen and pH, lack of light, concurrent bacterial infection, and reduced blood flow.

This group of bacteria is responsible for a large variety of diseases in children. The disease may result from local infection with local toxin production, ingestion of preformed toxin, or the elaboration of toxin with systemic effects by vegetative forms.

Clostridial infections are not common, accounting for fewer than 10 percent of all anaerobic infections; however, they have a very high morbidity and mortality, related to the elaboration of highly potent toxins.

### *Clostridium perfringens*

The reservoirs for *C. perfringens* spores include soil, human and animal feces, and raw red meat. These organisms may be found in the bowel and vagina. Ingestion of contaminated meat will produce an acute self-limited illness. The signs of clostridial food poisoning usually begin 8 to 12 hours after exposure and consist of crampy abdominal pain and watery diarrhea with minimal nausea and vomiting or systemic symptoms.[23] In rare cases, a severe necrotizing enterocolitis with bowel perforation and shock may be the result of an invasive clostridial infection. These organisms have been implicated in the development of pneumatosis intestinalis and necrotizing enterocolitis in the infant. Invasive *C. perfringens* infection can also be seen after complicated abortion or delivery and is accompanied by a characteristic massive intravascular hemolysis and shock. *C. perfringens* also produces infection of superficial tissues associated with trauma and wound contamination. Mild cases may be indistinguishable from the cellulitis caused by other organisms.

Gas gangrene, a serious invasive infection of the skin, soft tissues, and muscle, is fatal in up to one-third of cases. Infection is promoted by devitalized tissue, foreign bodies, and other bacteria. Elaboration of a number of local toxins enhances tissue destruction and sustains the infection. Clinically, there is a sudden onset of extreme pain in the area of the wound. Pain exceeds what is expected for the extent of the trauma. The area becomes progressively edematous and discolored. Signs of systemic toxicity and the presence of myonecrosis are diagnostic. Primary therapy is the surgical removal of necrotic tissue without closure of the wound. Antibiotics are also used to eliminate bacterial growth. The use of hyperbaric oxygen is controversial.

### *Clostridium botulinum* (Botulism)

Two distinct age-dependent syndromes are seen as a result of *C. botulinum* food poisoning. In older children and adults, ingestion of preformed toxin results in a descending symmetric paralysis. Botulinum toxin inhibits the release of presynaptic acetylcholine from cholinergic peripheral nerves.[24,25] It does not cross into the central nervous system. Improperly processed home-canned fruits or vegetables are usually implicated. Onset of bulbar palsies, including diplopia, dysarthria, dysphagia, ptosis, dilated pupils, and so forth, without fever or change in mental status, is characteristic and occurs hours to days following ingestion. Severity of illness is inversely related to the interval between ingestion and symptoms. Although most patients experience minimal or no gastrointestinal symptoms, nonspecific nausea, vomiting, abdominal pain, diarrhea, or constipation may occur. If ingestion is recent, gastric lavage is the primary therapy. Antitoxin (horse serum) is available but should be begun only after the onset of neurologic signs. Decreased muscular function (i.e., generalized weakness and loss of deep tendon reflexes) and cholinergic inhibition (i.e., postural hypotension, urinary retention, and constipation) are later symptoms. Respiratory function should be monitored. A similar clinical picture can result from wound contamination by *C. botulinum*. Although wound botulism is rare, the majority of the cases identified have been in children, commonly following compound fractures.

Infant botulism, identified in 1976, occurs in infants less than 12 months of age. Infection follows the ingestion of *C. botulinum* spores, which germinate in the immature intestine to produce vegetative organisms and toxin. Spores may be found in soil, vacuum cleaner dust, corn syrup, and *honey*. Breastfeeding appears to have a protective effect, offering a slower onset and decreased mortality. The interval between ingestion and onset of symptoms may be from 1 day to 1 month; as with older patients, the length of this interval is inversely related to severity of the disease. The clinical progression is more insidious in infants. Facial weakness is difficult to recognize, and constipation, weak cry, and difficulty sucking or feeding are nonspecific signs of illness. Generalized hypotonia with loss of head control suggests neurologic disease but not specifically botulism. Diagnosis requires isolation of the organism or toxin from the gastrointestinal tract or blood. Therapy is supportive. Antibiotics are contraindicated. Massive toxin elaboration in a stagnant bowel can follow organism destruction. Respiratory compromise is a significant risk, and botulism has been postulated as a potential etiology of sudden infant death syndrome.[26]

The only specific anesthetic concern with this disease would be the use of muscle relaxants. There could be a large potassium flux if succinylcholine were used.

### *Clostridium tetani* (Tetanus)

*C. tetani* spores are ubiquitous. The overall occurrence of tetanus has been reduced, but not eliminated, through immunization programs. After the initial immunization protocol (see Table 8-1), booster injections are required every 5 to 10 years to maintain immunity throughout life. Morbidity remains less than 50 percent when tetanus does occur.[27] The vegetative forms do not produce an invasive infection at the site of entry (i.e., skin wound, gastrointestinal tract, tonsillar crypts), but they do elaborate a highly potent neurotoxin. Tetanus toxin binds to the presynaptic membrane of neuromuscular junctions and ascends axons into the central nervous system.[25] Tetanospasmin acts on the peripheral, central, and sympathetic nervous systems. The overall effect is the loss of inhibitory reflexes, with resulting hypertonicity, muscle spasms, and sympathetic hyperactivity. The severity of the disease is related to patient age, rapidity of symptoms following trauma, and type of tetanus (i.e., localized, generalized, or cephalic). Rarely, the muscular hyperactivity may be limited to the area surrounding the injury (local tetanus). Mortality is very low ($\leq 1$ percent). Localized signs may precede generalized involvement. Cephalic tetanus can follow head and neck trauma, including otitis media or nasal foreign body. This is a fulminant syndrome with rapid onset and localization of the signs to this region, including involvement of the cranial nerves. Prognosis is very poor. Occasionally cephalic tetanus may precede the generalized form.

Generalized tetanus is the most common form. In up to 80 percent of cases the initial wound may be insignificant, as small as an insect bite. The onset of illness may be insidious, with vague complaints of headache, restlessness, and irritability. The hallmark sign in 50 percent of cases is the development of trismus, usually bilateral (risus sardonicus).[27] Classic extremely painful spasms or tetanic seizures then become evident. The patient's posture is characterized by opisthotonus, flexion and adduction of the arms with clenched fists, and extension of the legs. The peripheral spasms may be severe enough to cause vertebral compression, hyperthermia, and increased oxygen consumption. The bursts of muscular rigidity can progress to involve pharyngeal and laryngeal muscles. These acute episodes resemble Valsalva efforts, with congestion of the face and head and neck veins; cyanosis and death may result if the event is sustained and an airway is not secured by intubation. The clinical course of generalized tetanus is fulminate and routinely fatal in neonates and heroin addicts. Treatments include débridement of any wound present, neutralization of toxin with immune globulin or antitoxin, antibiotics, intensive care observation, and minimization of excitatory stimuli. Hypnotics, sedatives, and peripheral or central muscle relaxants have all been utilized. Immunization should be started following recovery because development of natural immunity is limited.

The anesthetic implications of this disease are multiple. Surgery during the acute period should be delayed if possible. If surgery cannot be delayed the patient should receive human hyperimmune globulin before surgery to neutralize the circulating endotoxin.[24] The increased activity in the autonomic nervous system may make a smooth inhalation anesthetic difficult to achieve. β-blockers should be readily available. Regional anesthesia offers one way of circumventing much of the difficulty. Another important issue is the use of muscle relaxants. Long-acting or continuous infusion of muscle relaxants is routinely indicated because of the difficulty in ventilating these patients if they are having tetanospasm. These patients may present on benzodiazepine infusions, which should be continued to prevent withdrawal.

### *Clostridium difficile*

*C. difficile* is the pathogen in many cases of antibiotic-associated enterocolitis in children. The onset of abdominal pain and profuse watery, bloody, mucous diarrhea during or following a course of antibiotics signals infection. Clindamycin, penicillin, ampicillin, amoxicillin, cephalosporins, and tetracycline are common offenders. Treatment involves reevaluation of current antibiotic therapy and maintenance of hydration.

## Gram-Negative Bacteria

Gram-negative pathogens are responsible for two types of infections in normal children. Bacilli from the enterobacter group (e.g., *Escherichia coli, Salmonella, Shigella*) predominantly cause gastroenteritis. Progression to systemic infection occurs only in the very young or immunocompromised patient or occasionally as a result of infection with a highly virulent strain. The gram-negative cocci or coccobacilli are associated with invasive and disseminated infection, which often begins as an URTI. These organisms (e.g., *Neisseria meningitidis, Haemophilus influenzae, Bordetella pertussis*) predominantly affect preschool children.

### Enterobacter Gastroenteritis

***Salmonella, Shigella,* and Enterovirulent *Escherichia coli.*** A nonspecific bacterial gastroenteritis can be produced by *Salmonella, Shigella,* and enterovirulent *E. coli.* Transmission occurs only from human to human by means of fecal-oral contamination. Food, water, and flies may serve as intermediaries. Epidemic food-related episodes peak in the late summer and early fall. Gastroenteritis due to these organisms is more common in areas where water contamination and sewage disposal problems are prevalent (e.g., traveler's diarrhea). The clinical presentation is characterized by the acute onset of fever, anorexia, nausea with minimal vomiting, lethargy, malaise, abdominal distention and pain, profuse watery diarrhea, and dehydration within 1 to 3 days of a suspicious ingestion.[28] At the peak of infection, stools may become mixed with blood and mucus. Treatment is mainly supportive, with replacement of fluids and electrolytes. Antibiotics are indicated only for proven *Shigella* infections. The use of antibiotics for *Salmonella* or *E. coli* enteritis may worsen or prolong the course by inhibition of the growth of normal gastrointestinal flora. Symptoms resolve within 1 week.

Complications of bacterial enteritis are most often related to loss of fluids and electrolytes. Some organisms of the *Shigella* species also produce an enterotoxin that facilitates invasion of the gastrointestinal epithelium. This enterotoxin has neurotoxic properties; there is a frequent association of febrile convulsions with *Shigella* enteritis. Reiter syndrome has been noted following *Shigella* enteritis. Toxin-producing species of both *E. coli* and *Shigella* are common precursors of hemolytic uremic syndrome.[28] Severe or invasive infections can occur in infants or immunocompromised children.

***Salmonella typhi* or *paratyphi* (Enteric or Typhoid Fever).** Enteric or typhoid fever is a clinically distinct gastrointestinal infection that has a prolonged incubation period of 1 to 4 weeks; the onset of the disease is insidious rather than acute. Fever, headache, malaise, lethargy, nausea, anorexia, abdominal pain, and splenomegaly develop progressively over 2 to 3 days. The organisms cause minimal local damage to the gastrointestinal epithelium, but are readily absorbed into the bloodstream and harbored intact within the monocytes. The organisms reproduce within and cause inflammation of reticuloendothelial tissues: spleen, liver, lymph nodes. A second septicemia enables disseminated infection. Infection of the gallbladder and lungs, by *S. typhi* or other bacteria, are most common, but osteomyelitis, septic arthritis, meningitis, pyelonephritis, and endocarditis are possible. The risk of gastrointestinal perforation or hemorrhage is significant during the second week of infection. Chloramphenicol is the treatment of choice. A chronic carrier state, uncommon in children, does exist in 5 percent of older patients following this infection. The chronic infection is usually localized to the gallbladder and biliary tract.[29]

### *Haemophilus influenzae*

*H. influenzae* is a common pathogen in preschool children. Unencapsulated (nontypable) strains are responsible for mild infections (e.g., rhinitis, otitis media, sinusitis, conjunctivitis) related to the upper respiratory tract. Nasal carriage rates for noninvasive strains can approach 90 percent in young children. *H. influenzae* type b (HIB) is the encapsulated organism responsible for the great majority (95 percent) of invasive pediatric *H. influenzae* infections. HIB can be cultured from the nasal mucosa of 5 percent of healthy children. HIB is overall the most common cause of bacterial meningitis, and meningitis is the most common HIB infection.[30] Other common invasive infections include pneumonia, epiglottitis, septic arthritis, and cellulitis. The relative frequencies of these invasive infections vary regionally. Overall, 1 in 200 children will acquire an HIB infection before the age of 5 years. Infrequent infections include sepsis, osteomyelitis, pericarditis, epididymitis, peritonitis, and orbital cellulitis. The clinical presentation of HIB invasive infection is not distinguishable from other bacterial pathogens. Children less than 2 years of age demonstrate minimal immunity to HIB following active infection or vaccination and are at greatest risk for invasive disease.[31] Epiglottitis is the only invasive infection that is more common in older children. Children with diminished or absent splenic function, Native Americans, and Alaskan Eskimos are also at increased risk for HIB.[30] Selection of an antibiotic for treatment of invasive HIB infection should presume CNS infection. Knowledge of the regional pattern of HIB antibiotic susceptibility is also important since multiple varieties of antibiotic resistance have been reported.

### *Neisseria meningitidis* (Meningococcus)

Meningococci are gram-negative organisms found in the nasopharynx of 5 percent of asymptomatic carriers. The group at highest risk for meningococcal infection are infants and preschool children because of limited immunity and ease of spread of respiratory secretions. Maternal antibodies are protective for infants in the first few months of life. A correlation has been noted between recent influenza infection and the subsequent development of meningococcemia. Occasionally superficial infections of the nasopharynx, genitourinary tract, or conjunctiva may develop. Encapsulation of the organism predisposes the host to invasive systemic infections.

Invasive infections can follow three different patterns. Nonspecific symptoms of fever, malaise, myalgia, headache, lethargy, and vomiting accompany meningococcal bacteremia without sepsis. This bacteremia can resolve spontaneously with or without antibiotic therapy or progress to a more fulminant meningococcemia. Meningococcemia with meningitis is indistinguishable from other causes of meningitis. The prognosis is better than with isolated meningococcemia without meningitis.

**Meningococcemia.** Meningococcemia

is a life-threatening infection characterized by diffuse vasculitis, disseminated intravascular coagulation (DIC), renal failure, and cardiovascular collapse. A characteristic petechial or purpural rash accompanies most fulminant cases. An endotoxin mechanism has been proposed for the fulminant course of meningococcemia, and septic shock and symptoms often become worse after the start of antibiotic therapy, with resultant release of endotoxin. Infectious complications occurring during the acute course include pneumonia, pericarditis, myocarditis, pleural effusion, arthritis, and internal hemorrhage. The neurologic complications seen with meningitis are multiple and varied. Delayed "hypersensitivity-type" complications may be noted during the convalescent phase of the infection. Arthritis, pericarditis with effusion or tamponade, cutaneous vasculitis, and episcleritis have been reported. Mortality remains at 20 percent despite advances in antibiotic and supportive treatments (see the section on septic shock below). Shock, coma, purpura, neutropenia thrombocytopenia, DIC, and myocarditis apparent at the time of clinical presentation are poor prognosis indicators.

For treatment, penicillin is the antibiotic of choice, although ampicillin may be substituted if the bacteriologic agent is uncertain. Chloramphenicol is selected for penicillin-allergic patients. Prophylaxis of intimate household or nursery school contacts (especially preschool children) with rifampin is indicated. Minocycline may be used in children over 8 years of age. Vaccination is indicated if available for specific serotype during epidemics. Rifampin treatment of patients is also recommended following completion of penicillin to eliminate meningococcus from the nasopharynx and decrease spread.

## *Bordetella pertussis* (Whooping Cough)

Pertussis is an acute infection of respiratory, ciliated epithelium. Asymptomatic carriers do not propagate the disease; respiratory droplets from patients with active infection are necessary. The incidence of this disease has been sharply curtailed through routine immunization of infants. Although there is no transplacentally acquired protection, vaccination protocols initiated during the first 3 to 12 months of life offer adequate, though not complete, protection. Fever and signs of local inflammation at the site of injection are common following vaccination. These symptoms can be minimized by use of acetaminophen. There is also a small risk (< 0.1 percent) of significant complications, which include febrile convulsions and shock.[32] The age group recommended for immunization is at high risk for sudden infant death syndrome or the onset of encephalopathies; the occurrence of these events in relationship to immunization is probably coincidental. Nevertheless, these potential risks have prompted some parents to refuse pertussis vaccination for their children. As the unimmunized population increases, the incidence of clinical disease may also increase. Medical contraindications to pertussis vaccination include the presence of progressive evolving neurologic disease or history of a severe reaction to previous immunization, such as fever of more than 40.5°C, hypotonia and hypotension, anaphylaxis, or prolonged sustained (> 3 hours) inconsolable screaming.

The clinical course of infection is divided into three stages: catarrhal, paroxysmal, and convalescent. The catarrhal phase resembles a mild URTI accompanied by conjunctival injection. This phase lasts 1 to 2 weeks after a similar incubation period. Erythromycin given at this time will significantly attenuate the course of infection. Characteristic paroxysms of coughing occur during the next 2 to 4 weeks. Coughing is usually worse at night and precipitated by eating, drinking, or physical activity. A series of 5 to 30 forceful uninterrupted coughs accompanied by facial cyanosis, tongue protrusion, and streaming of secretions from nose, mouth, and eyes are terminated with the performance of a massive forceful inspiration (whoop). The characteristic whooping sound is frequently not heard in infants. In infants and children, vomiting following a prolonged episode of coughing should suggest pertussis infection. These episodes are uncomfortable and exhausting. Erythromycin given during this phase will limit the period of communicability but not symptomatology. These paroxysms become less frequent and severe but can persist for several months (convalescent phase). Complications of these extended bouts of forceful expiration include epistaxis, melena, petechiae, hernias, rectal prolapse, central nervous system (CNS) subdural hematoma, spinal epidural hematoma, and hypoxia, which may lead to seizures, encephalopathy, or coma. Respiratory complications are also common and include *Pertussis* pneumonia, other secondary bacterial pneumonia, atelectasis, emphysema, or pneumothorax. Pneumonia is the most frequent cause of death.

Important in the anesthetic management of these patients is an antitussive. The paroxysms of coughing may be severe enough to cause significant desaturations. Narcotic infusion of morphine 5 to 25 μg/kg/h is effective in controlling these paroxysms in children under 6 months; older children may take twice this amount.

## Septic Shock

The entry of microorganisms into the bloodstream, or release of their toxins there, initiates a cascade of host responses designed to eliminate the offending agent. Unfortunately, these self-protective responses are nonspecific and may result in the destruction of the host as well as the invading organism. Gram-negative endotoxins are the classic inducers of septic shock and are used as the basis for the experimental study of sepsis. The clinical picture of septic shock induced by other varieties of microbes is indistinguishable. Neonatal pathogens include GBBHS, *E. coli,* and *Listeria monocytogenes.* Common pediatric pathogens after the neonatal period are HIB, *N. meningitides, S. pneumoniae,* and *E. coli.* The incidence of sepsis has been escalating in parallel with progress in medicine and technology. Improved survival in many seriously ill patients with congenital defects, prematurity, instrumentation [vascular, urinary, or cerebrospinal fluid (CSF) catheters], chronic disease, or acute trauma has produced an enlarged population of children at risk for sepsis and a wide variety of bacterial pathogens. In previously healthy children who receive prompt diagnosis and treatment, the mortality associated with septic shock may be as low as 10 percent.[33] Conversely, if therapeutic intervention is delayed or the patient is high risk, death is anticipated in 50 percent to 90 percent of cases.

Recognition of patients at high risk for the development of bacteremia (see Table 8-3) and the early nonspecific clinical parameters that define the sepsis syndrome is the key to prompt diagnosis and treatment in septic shock. Previously normal children with a diagnosis of bacterial meningitis are also at increased risk of bacteremia and septic shock. Sepsis syndrome is defined as sepsis accompanied by alteration in temperature (fever or hypothermia), tachypnea, tachycardia, and signs of decreased perfusion. Subtle signs of decreased perfusion include changes in mental status such as restlessness, irritability, confusion or euphoria, and decreased urine output. These signs often precede the actual development of hypotension.

The development of shock secondary to sepsis is a result of a massive stimulation of numerous cellular and humoral mediators. Activation and aggregation of platelets and leukocytes result in release of their endogenous humoral mediators or degranulation and release of intracellular toxins in addition to the biochemical alterations induced by endotoxin itself. Arachidonic acid pathway metabolites (e.g., thromboxane $A_2$, prostacyclin, leukotrienes), histamine, bradykinin, kallikrein, serotonin, and endorphins, and complement have all been implicated in the pathophysiology of septic shock. Reviews of these mechanisms are available.[34–36]

The net result of septic shock is the development of a progressive metabolic failure. In contrast to other types of shock, the metabolic decompensation in septic shock is primarily attributed to a direct depression of cellular respiration. Altered tissue perfusion is secondary to decreased preload, myocardial depression, AV shunting, or shift of the oxygen-hemoglobin dissociation curve, which potentiates the metabolic defect with inadequate oxygen delivery. Impaired oxygen utilization (i.e., decreased $\dot{V}O_2$ and increased $AV\dot{D}O_2$) in the presence of normal or increased cardiac output is diagnostic of septic shock.

The clinical course of septic shock can be divided into two phases: an early "warm" shock and a late "cold" shock.[36] Early septic shock is thought to be the same as the sepsis syndrome (see above). The characteristic physiologic parameters are compared with those of late shock in Table 8-6. As the infection and host response progress, massive widespread changes in vascular permeability take place. Initially, fluid leakage will progress to include loss of plasma proteins to interstitial tissues. Depletion of intravascular volume initiates the transition to cold septic shock. Organ failure and tissue damage may become irreversible. Although all organs are affected, pulmonary (ARDS), myocardial, and renal dysfunction determine survival or mortality.

Four major therapeutic priorities can be identified[35]:

1. Early diagnosis by recognition of high-risk patients and sepsis syndrome characteristics. Survival is improved by aggressive treatment of the early warning signs.
2. Resuscitation ABCs mandate placement of invasive monitors (arterial, pulmonary, and urinary catheters) and ventilatory support. Fluid resuscitation may be sufficient cardiovascular support in the early phases of septic shock but inotropic medications, calcium, and vasodilators may be necessary in later stages. Subtle changes in respiration precede the development of frank respiratory failure. Progressive lactic acidosis can lead to respiratory exhaustion.
3. Infection identification and control are the cornerstone of treatment in septic shock. Culture of blood and all potential infection sites and surgical drainage of abscesses are necessary to identify the specific infectious agent and its specific antimicrobial sensitivity. Initial antibiotic treatment may be based on the most common pathogens for children of the patient's age, with consideration of factors that increase the susceptibility to infection or the results of rapid identification techniques.
4. Monitoring and correction of frequent chemical and hematic abnormalities. DIC, thrombocytopenia, anemia, lac-

**Table 8-6.** Comparison of Two Phases of Septic Shock

| *Category* | *Value* | *Early "Warm" Shock* | *Late "Cold" Shock* |
|---|---|---|---|
| General/vital signs | Temperature | ↑ or ↓ | ↑ or ↓ |
| | Blood pressure | None or slight ↓ | ↓ ↓ |
| | Respiratory rate | ↑ | ↑ but ↓ depth |
| | Heart rate | ↑ | ↑ |
| | Pulse pressure | ↑ | ↓ |
| | Skin | Warm, dry | Cold, clammy |
| | Mental status | Irritability, minor changes | Major depression → coma |
| Cardiovascular | CVP/PCWP | ↓ | ↓ |
| | PAP | ↑ | ↑ |
| | Cardiac output | None or ↑ | ↓ |
| | SVR | ↓ | ↑ |
| | FVR | None | ↑ |
| | Intravascular volume | ↓ | ↓ |
| | Intravascular protein | None | ↓ |
| | Stroke volume | None | ↓ |
| Respiratory/acid–base | Oxygen | Mild ↓ | ↓ ↓ |
| | Carbon dioxide | ↓ | ↑ |
| | pH | None | ↓ |
| | Lactate | None | ↑ |
| | $\dot{V}O_2$ | ↓ | ↓ ↓ |
| Renal | Urine output | ↓ | ↓ ↓ |
| | BUN | None | ↑ |
| | Cr | None | ↑ |

*Abbreviations:* BUN, blood urea nitrogen; Cr, creatinine; CVP, central venous pressure; FVR, forearm vascular resistance; PAP, pulmonary artery pressure; PCWP, pulmonary capillary wedge pressure; SVR, systemic vascular resistance.

tic acidosis, hypocalcemia, hypophosphatemia, and hypoglycemia or hyperglycemia are common shock manifestations.

Experimental or controversial therapies for septic shock are numerous. Complement antibodies, arachidonic acid inhibitors (indomethacin, ibuprofen), steroids,[37] opiate antagonists, or thyrotropin-releasing hormone can impede the biochemical cascade elicited by endotoxin. Removal of endotoxin from plasma by specific endotoxin antiserum or fibronectin stimulation of phagocytosis is a possible answer. Elimination of substances that cause tissue damage by free-radical scavenging or plasma cleaning via filtration, plasmaphoresis, or exchange transfusion may also be of potential benefit.[36,38,39]

## ANTIBIOTICS

Ideally, the selection of antimicrobial drugs should be specific for the pathogen and its unique drug sensitivities. In clinical practice it is impractical and potentially dangerous to delay therapy pending culture and sensitivity results. Initial antibiotic regimens are selected to provide coverage for the most likely pathogens for a specific patient. Drug toxicity, method of excretion, and cost are additional factors that may modify drug selection. In pediatrics, differences in individual drug cost are reduced in proportion to patient size. Other factors such as preparation time, delivery equipment, dosage interval, and monitoring of side effects may be more important in calculating the total cost of drug delivery.[40]

## β-Lactam Antibiotics

β-lactam antibiotics attack bacterial cell wall synthesis and are inactive against host cells. Therefore, these drugs have a very high therapeutic/toxic ratio. Side effects are rare and are usually immunologically mediated. Penicillins, cephalosporins, monobactams, and carbepenems are included in this classification. With only two exceptions, β-lactams rely on renal excretion (see Appendix).[41] β-lactams are susceptible to inactivation by bacterial β-lactamase enzymes. Clavulanate and sulbactam are two new β-lactams that inhibit extracellular β-lactamase enzymes. These agents are not prescribed alone, but are combined with other β-lactam antibiotics (e.g., ampicillin, ticarcillin) to limit bacterially induced antibiotic resistance. The role of newer cephalosporins in clinical practice is expanding and they may ultimately replace older, more toxic agents in the primary treatment of suspected gram-negative infections.

## Aminoglycosides

Aminoglycosides are effective against a wide variety of gram-negative organisms. Penetration of biologic membranes or into collections of pus is limited, and alternatives are recommended for the treatment of meningitis or abscesses. The major role of aminoglycosides in pediatric practice is in empiric drug regimens that need to provide coverage for possible gram-negative aerobic pathogens, as with septic neonates or oncology patients and children with peritonitis or urologic sepsis. Aminoglycosides are excreted by the kidney. Their main disadvantage is the occurrence of a dose-related nephrotoxicity and ototoxicity that necessitates careful monitoring of serum concentrations. The risk of renal complications is increased if other nephrotoxic drugs are administered concurrently or if there is a prior history of renal disease or aminoglycoside therapy. Renal tubular dysfunction produced by the aminoglycoside is enhanced when enflurane is used as the inhalation agent.[42] However, even halothane will interact with the aminoglycosides, causing significant decreases in total body clearance and apparent volume of distribution and a significant increase in half-life.[43] Aminoglycosides can also produce varying degrees of neuromuscular blockade or potentiation of other neuromuscular-blocking drugs. Aminoglycosides obtain this effect by inhibiting the presynaptic release of acetylcholine and decreasing postsynaptic sensitivity.[44] Recurarization is a danger when these drugs are given in the immediate postanesthetic period.[24] Even when atracurium is used, caution is necessary because of the aminoglycoside potentiation of the block. It does appear to reverse with edrophonium.[45] Aminoglycosides are physically incompatible in solution with most β-lactams and amphotericin B.

## Vancomycin

Vancomycin is experiencing an expanding role in pediatrics because of its efficacy against gram-positive organisms, especially those that are resistant to traditional β-lactam therapy.[46] β-lactam–resistant staphylococcal bacteria are frequent contaminants of indwelling catheters. Vancomycin is indicated in the treatment of these catheter-associated infections and in staphylococcal meningitis, serious gram-positive infections in patients with significant penicillin allergy, and orally for pseudomembranous colitis. Vancomycin displays a pattern for nephrotoxicity and ototoxicity similar to that of the aminoglycosides, and serious allergic reactions are reported as well. Slow intravenous delivery over 60 minutes decreases, but does not eliminate, the occurrence of histamine-mediated side effects, which may be noted in up to 35 percent of children.[41,47–49] Flushing, hypotension, urticaria, pruritus, and bronchospasm are possible manifestations of histamine release that may be reversed with diphenhydramine.[50] Vancomycin also interferes with neuromuscular blocking agents.[51]

## Erythromycin

Erythromycin is used as therapy for a wide range of mild to moderate infections. It is frequently selected for gram-positive cocci in patients allergic to penicillin. Erythromycin is also effective against several unusual organisms, including *Legionella, Mycoplasma, Chlamydia*, and *B. pertussis*. It is the primary agent for uncomplicated pneumonia in school-age children because of its efficacy against the two most common pathogens, *S. pneumoniae* and *Mycoplasma*. Erythromycin also eradicates pertussis from the nasopharynx and is used for prophylaxis of close contacts.

Both IV and PO formulations of erythromycin are available. However, most mild infections are treated with oral therapy on an outpatient basis. Erythromycin PO is complicated by gastrointestinal distress, nausea, or vomiting in up to 1 in every 4 children. Erythromycin is metabolized and excreted by the liver and may interfere with the hepatic metabolism of other drugs. Levels of theophylline, corticosteroids, warfarin, and digoxin can increase during erythromycin therapy. Hepatotoxicity, interstitial nephritis, and aplastic or hemolytic anemia are rare complications of erythromycin. Specific anesthetic interactions with this antibiotic are rarely identified, but the prolongation of the terminal half-life of alfentanil from 84 to 131 minutes following a course of erythromycin administration has been noted.[52]

## Chloramphenicol

Chloramphenicol is effective against many strains of gram-negative bacteria. Its bactericidal effect against *Neisseria* and *H. influenzae* results in its continued use despite its adverse effects on the bone marrow. The changes in the marrow can lead to leukopenia, thrombocytopenia, and even aplasia of the marrow. This fatal pancytopenia, occurring in about 1 in 40,000 patients,[41] is not related to dose but seems to occur in patients who have received the drug multiple times or for prolonged durations. It also causes a reversible erythroid suppression with a decrease in platelets, white blood cells, and reticulocytes. In patients with G-6P deficiency it will exacerbate hemolysis. In neonates high chloramphenicol levels can produce death via the gray baby syndrome. Although its primary route of elimination is hepatic, it is excreted 20 to 30 percent by the kidney, and the dose needs to be adjusted in children with low renal function. It is effectively administered via the oral and gastrointestinal route. It penetrates the CSF well to achieve levels that are 60 percent of plasma levels. It irreversibly inhibits microsomal enzymes of the cytochrome P-450 complex, and thus drugs that rely on this substance for metabolism should be administered with caution.[53] Because of potential drug interactions between chloramphenicol and anesthetic substances, including alteration of metabolism (barbiturates are known to interfere with metabolism of chloramphenicol), levels should be closely followed after any anesthetic. Chloramphenicol can interfere with the metabolism of other drugs, most noticeably phenytoin. If the patient is receiving intravenous chloramphenicol, aminophylline, barbiturates, diphenhydramine, phenytoin, or steroids should not be given in the same intravenous line.[54]

## VIRAL INFECTIONS

The natural history of viral infections is quite different from that of bacterial ones. Most viruses produce minimal physiologic dysfunction in the immunocompetent host, and infection is usually an acute, self-limited, and nonspecific process. Nonspecific signs and symptoms of viral infection include fever, fatigue, malaise, headache, abdominal pain, nausea, anorexia, vomiting, diarrhea, conjunctivitis, coryza, cough, and rash. Fulminant sepsis or organ failure is possible in the newborn or compromised patient. Infants are passively protected from some diseases by maternal antibodies for their first few months. Maternal infections during pregnancy, however, can result in congenital malformations, fetal demise, or fulminant active disease after birth. In this country, the occurrence of many of the common childhood diseases has been minimized through the development and routine usage of effective immunization programs (see Table 8-1). Vaccines are becoming available for other viral pathogens but are currently administered only to specific high-risk populations (see Table 8-2).

Viruses are ubiquitous and spread rapidly through a susceptible population. Although many viruses are spread via oral or respiratory droplets, some require intimate contact with other body products such as blood or feces. Fomites or animal (especially insect) vectors are most important transmitters for viral agents than for bacterial agents. Disease transmission is also facilitated by some specific characteristics of viral infection. For example, active infections can be completely subclinical; patients are frequently contagious for several days before the actual onset of disease symptoms. In some cases, the virus may be excreted for several months after recovery from active disease. Some viruses are never completely eradicated from the host and may be reactivated periodically throughout life.

Viral replication begins in the local tissue after exposure of susceptible tissue. Passage of the virus through regional lymphatic channels results in a primary, minor viremia. The virus is then delivered by the blood to target tissues, which sponsor viral replication. During this phase the patient is contagious but may be asymptomatic or exhibit several mild, nonspecific symptoms. A second, major viremia follows the release of this larger inoculum of viral particles into the bloodstream, and the characteristic signs of a viral disease then become evident.

An interesting concern for the anesthesiologist is the evidence that viral replication and possibly severity of the viral illness may be attenuated by inhalational anesthetic agents.[55–57] However, any potential benefits from the anesthesia must be carefully weighed against the risks of anesthetizing a child who is undergoing the physiologic effects of the virus.

This section reviews the common childhood viral pathogen as well as infections caused by the herpesvirus and enterovirus families. Viral illness that is endemic to other continents but rare in the United States is excluded. Viruses that primarily produce the "common cold" or disease of the lower respiratory tract (e.g., rhinovirus, adenovirus, and influenza), parainfluenza, and respiratory syncytial virus, are not discussed. Information about respiratory disease, hepatitis, and acquired immunodeficiency syndrome (AIDS) is found in other chapters.

## Enterovirus Family

The enterovirus family includes the coxsackie-, echo-, entero-, and polioviruses. These agents undergo their primary replication within the alimentary tract. Transmission occurs by either the oral-oral or fecal-oral route, and virus may be found in the stool for several months after the infection. Clinical infection and major viremia begins 3 to 7 days following exposure. The clinical course of polio will be discussed separately. Enterovirus infection is asymptomatic in as many as 50 percent of patients. These nonspecific febrile illnesses commonly afflict either the respiratory or gastrointestinal tracts and the conjunctiva. Coxsackieviruses are associated with herpangina characterized by a sore mouth and throat with discrete vesicles and ulcers. Similar lesions can be seen on the palms and soles and in the diaper area (hand-foot-and-mouth disease). Rarely, severe cases may be complicated by myocarditis, meningitis, pneumonitis, hepatic or renal necrosis, orchitis, or myositis. An acute paralytic disease similar to mild forms of polio has been reported.

### Poliovirus

Four different clinical expressions are possible as a result of poliovirus infection. Over 90 percent of all polio infections are asymptomatic. A mild, nonspecific febrile illness is seen in an additional 5 to 8 percent of patients (abortive polio); the general symptoms are accompanied by aseptic meningitis in 1 to 2 percent (nonparalytic polio). Fewer than 2 percent of all infections by this virus result in the classical paralytic polio even under epidemic conditions. The availability and use of effective vaccinations has further limited the extreme clinical expression of polio disease.

Paralytic poliomyelitis is usually preceded by one of the milder forms of disease (abortive or nonparalytic) and a subsequent disease-free interval of 1 to 2 weeks. The neurologic deficits of polio do not involve sensation or the sensorium. Initially, there is a loss of superficial reflexes that progresses to affect deep tendon reflexes as well. Ultimately, a flaccid paralysis of involved muscle groups ensues. Paralysis is usually sudden and asymmetrical. Atony of bowel and bladder function or respiratory failure may accompany severe cases. Isolated involvement of bulbar neurons can also occur. The tenth cranial nerve is observed most frequently with resultant difficulties in control of the pharynx, soft palate, and vocal cords. Deltoid weakness is an ominous sign, heralding the onset of central respiratory failure. Myocardial failure may also be seen as a primary process or secondary to respiratory disease.

## Herpesvirus Family

There are six known herpes simplex virus types: HSV-1, HSV-2, HSV-6, Epstein-Barr virus (EBV), cytomegalovirus (CMV), and varicella-zoster virus (VZV). Vesicles are the characteristic skin lesion associated with this group of viruses. The herpesvirus family is distinguished by its potential for reactivation of infection after variable periods of dormancy. Although these viruses are highly contagious, they are quite labile and require intimate contact with body fluids for transmission.

## Herpes Simplex Types 1 and 2

HSV-1 and HSV-2 are pathogens of the mucous membranes and skin. Although HSV-1 mainly attacks the oral mucous membranes and HSV-2 is usually a genital infection, both types may be found at either location. The virus does not infect intact skin but is easily spread to areas where the skin is broken in conditions such as burns, eczema, and thumb-sucking. Close contact with secretions is necessary for transmission. As an occupational hazard, HSV may affect wrestlers (herpes gladiatorum), rugby players, [herpes rugbiorum (scrum pox)], nurses, respiratory therapists, and anesthetists (herpetic whitlow). The incubation period after exposure to HSV ranges from 2 to 20 days, with a mean of 1 week.

The primary infection may be entirely asymptomatic, or an acute febrile gingivostomatitis may develop in young children. Fever, irritability, salivation, foul-smelling breath, and refusal to eat or drink herald the onset of acute gingivostomatitis. Characteristic vesicular lesions then appear in the anterior portion of the mouth on the lips, gums, tongue, and soft palate. The vesicles rupture to form ulcers, which may become covered with crusts on the skin. The entire process lasts for 1 to 2 weeks, and treatment is supportive, with an emphasis on maintaining adequate hydration. Following resolution of primary disease, HSV remains dormant within sensory neurons associated with the area of primary infection and may be reactivated throughout life. The individual recurrent HSV lesions are indistinguishable from primary ones. However, recurrent infections are often less severe and often limited to a small group of vesicles at the mucocutaneous junction.

Other organ systems that can occasionally demonstrate HSV infection are the eyes and the central nervous system. HSV conjunctivitis usually resolves without sequelae. Involvement of the cornea is a more serious threat to vision. Aseptic meningitis can result from primary or recurrent HSV-2 infection. The clinical picture is indistinct from that of other causes of viral meningitis, and prognosis for full recovery is good. HSV-1 is the most common identifiable cause of sporadic encephalitis. HSV encephalitis may begin as a nonspecific febrile illness that may follow a rapidly progressive downhill course to coma and death after the onset of CNS (not meningeal) signs. In the past HSV was often fatal, and survivors demonstrated significant residual neurologic impairment. Early diagnosis and the use of antiviral agents such as acyclovir have improved the prognosis for patients with HSV encephalitis.[58]

Newborn infants may acquire HSV during birth. A few fortunate infants (about 30 percent of those infected) will manifest disease limited to the skin. The remainder will follow a downhill course characterized by shock, pneumonia, encephalitis, and death. Until cutaneous lesions appear, the only signs suggesting HSV as the cause of the sepsis are a positive maternal history.

Most adults have been infected with HSV-1. Currently, no vaccine is available for HSV prevention. In most cases only supportive therapy is necessary. Several potent antiviral agents—acyclovir, vidarabine, and idoxuriodine—have been used to treat serious or disseminated disease.

VZV is discussed in a later section (Other Common Exanthematous Viral Pathogens).

## Epstein-Barr Virus

EBV (infectious mononucleosis) is a common affliction of teenagers and young adults that produces a characteristic pharyngitis, with atypical lymphocytosis, and hepatosplenomegaly. In young children, the symptoms are much milder, and the diagnosis may be overlooked. Viral transmission is not well defined. Viremia results in a selective infection of B lymphocytes. Virus is found in the saliva for several months after an active infection. The incubation period is quite long (1 to 2 months), and a 1- to 2-week nonspecific prodrome precedes a severe, painful, exudative tonsillopharyngitis. The tonsillopharyngitis is often treated with steroids, and the organs may consequently enlarge to become "kissing tonsils." The need for intubation is possible in severe cases. Lymphadenopathy, especially in the posterior cervical region, and petechiae on the palate are also common findings. The acute phase of the illness usually lasts 2 to 4 weeks and may be followed by a convalescent period of several months of disabling fatigue and malaise. Splenomegaly is a cause for concern during the acute phase and has been associated with activity-related splenic rupture. Edema of the eyelids and adverse cutaneous reactions to ampicillin have also been observed.

Complications are relatively common, occurring in 20 percent of patients, but usually resolve without long-term residual sequelae. Airway obstruction or pneumonia can compromise breathing. Hepatitis and myocarditis are additional frequent complications. Neurologic impairment may manifest as seizures, ataxia, meningitis, encephalitis, transverse myelitis, Guillain-Barré disease, Bell's palsy, or the "Alice in Wonderland syndrome" (distortions in perception of size and space). Pancreatitis, orchitis, hemolytic anemia, thrombocytopenia, tonsillar abscess, and Reye syndrome have also been reported. The relationship of chronic EBV infection to lymphoproliferative tumors and a chronic fatigue syndrome is controversial.

### Cytomegalovirus

CMV infection is asymptomatic in 90 percent of normal patients. Occasionally CMV may produce a clinical syndrome similar to the infectious mononucleosis of EBV. Congenital CMV infection is associated with varying degrees of neurologic impairment. CMV is found in many secretions, including saliva, respiratory droplets, blood, urine, feces, semen, and breast milk. CMV has also been identified in leukocytes and donated organs. As many as 60 percent of patients experience seroconversion 3 to 5 weeks following blood transfusion, and the characteristic clinical syndrome has been noted in children following cardiopulmonary bypass with a blood prime.

## Other Common Exanthematous Viral Pathogens

A primary concern for the anesthesiologist regarding pediatric infectious diseases is to keep them from spreading. As the number of children undergoing hospital procedures as outpatients increases, this responsibility becomes correspondingly more important. The crowded outpatient surgical waiting room is an ideal location for the spread of many infectious conditions. It is important to isolate not only patients with the disease but also those children who have been exposed to the virus and are in the final few days of the incubation period. Parents should be queried about exposure to children with chickenpox, measles, mumps, or rubella the day before their child comes to the hospital. Table 8-7 reviews the incubation periods and infectivity of the common viral pathogens.

### Varicella-Zoster Virus

VZV (chickenpox or zoster) is a common pathogen that produces nonspecific signs of viral illness accompanied by a char-

**Table 8-7.** Incubation and Infectivity for Common Infectious Diseases

| *Infection* | *Incubation (days)* | *Infectivity* |
|---|---|---|
| Varicella (VZV, chickenpox) | Range, 11–20<br>Normal 14–18 | 1–2 days before rash through 5 days after the onset of lesions |
| Rubella | Range, 14–21<br>Normal, 16–18 | Most infectious 2 days before rash and 5–7 days after rash; virus in nasopharyngeal secretions 7 days before to 14 days after rash |
| Congenital rubella | | 1+ years in urine and nasopharyngeal secretions |
| Mumps | Range, 12–25<br>Normal 16–18 | 2 days before parotid swelling; 5–9 days after onset |
| Measles | Range, 7–18<br>Normal, 8–12 | 3–5 days before rash; 4 days after rash |

acteristic rash. Ninety percent of the adult population acquired immunity through infection during the early school years. Transmission occurs via respiratory droplets. The incubation period following exposure ranges from 11 to 21 days. A mild prodrome of fever and malaise may be seen without respiratory or gastrointestinal symptoms for 24 hours before the exanthem appears. The skin lesions begin as macules or papules that develop vesicles upon these erythematous bases (e.g., dewdrop on a rose petal) and are identical to the skin lesions of HSV in form but not in distribution and location.[59] Also, VZV lesions are pruritic rather than painful. Skin lesions appear in successive crops beginning on the trunk with subsequent appearance on the face and proximal extremities for 4 to 5 days with older lesions crusting as new lesions appear.

Secondary bacterial infection of the skin is a common complication. Pneumonia is seen in up to 1 in 3 adult patients but is rare in children. Hepatitis and thrombocytopenia are potential complications. In rare cases, visceral dissemination of the VZV may result in cerebritis, encephalitis, meningitis, myocarditis, endocarditis, pericarditis, arthritis, glomerulonephritis, orchitis, myositis, or conjunctivitis. Postviral syndromes (Guillain-Barré and Reye) have been associated with VZV.

Treatment of VZV infection is entirely supportive with an emphasis on antipruritics to provide patient comfort and minimize the outbreak of secondary bacterial infection. Immune globulin or antiviral agents are available. Although vaccination is a routine practice in Japan, the vaccine is currently undergoing clinical trials in the United States.[60] Vaccination is indicated in certain high-risk populations, such as children with leukemia or lymphoma. Acyclovir does improve the clinical course but is not yet routinely recommended.[61]

VZV remains dormant in the dorsal ganglion. Zoster, when reactivated, is also highly contagious. Crops of vesicles appear unilaterally along one to three discrete adjacent dermatome segments. Thoracolumbar dermatomes are usually involved in adults, in contrast to the cervical-sacral distribution seen in children. The clinical course is similar to that of the initial infection except that the lesions are painful and associated with regional lymphadenopathy.

## Rubeola

Rubeola (measles) once was a common acute contagious disease of young school-age children. Mass immunization has decreased the overall occurrence of this disease. However, episodic outbreaks occur in unvaccinated or ineffectively vaccinated teenagers and young adults.[62] The measles virus is transmitted by respiratory droplets, which may deposit in the conjunctiva or nasopharyngeal mucosa. The normal incubation period lasts 10 to 14 days. Contagion must be assumed as early as 7 days after exposure and will continue until 5 days after the measles rash is fully developed.

Low-grade fever, cough, coryza, conjunctivitis with photophobia, and Koplik spots make up the typical prodromal illness, which may last for 3 to 5 days. Koplik spots appear as white-gray punctate lesions on a diffusely erythematous pharyngeal and buccal mucosa. Maximal spread of disease occurs during this prodromal phase. Sudden onset of a high fever and eruption of a diffuse macular rash beginning behind the ears and along the facial hairline announce the actual disease. The rash spreads down and outward to the trunk, arms, and legs within 2 to 3 days and becomes papular and confluent. Defervescence accompanies involvement of the legs and feet. The confluent rash darkens to a nonblanching coppery color, which undergoes a fine desquamation. The rash progresses and disappears in the same order. Otitis media and respiratory complications (e.g., laryngitis, tracheitis, and pneumonia) are common. Mesenteric adenitis may mimic acute intestinal disease. Encephalitis, myocarditis, and Guillain-Barré syndrome occur less frequently. Subacute sclerosing panencephalitis (SSPE) is a rare, slowly progressive, fatal encephalitis associated with persistent CNS measles infection.

Treatment of rubeola infection is primarily supportive. Ribavarin is useful in cases of disseminated disease. No effective treatment is available for SSPE. Vaccination should be undertaken at 15 to 18 months of age. The use of live virus vaccine is contraindicated in pregnancy or cases of severe allergy to eggs or neomycin.

## Rubella

Rubella (German, or 3-day, measles) is clinically quite similar to measles but the acute phases of the disease are shorter and much milder. Up to 25 percent of these infections may be subclinical. After an incubation period of 14 to 21 days, a mild prodrome of low-grade fever, coryza, cough, conjunctivitis, cervical and suboccipital lymphadenopathy, and Forchheimer spots is observed. Forchheimer spots are pinpoint rose discolorations of the soft palate. Within 1 week, the characteristic macular exanthem begins on the face and then spreads to the trunk and legs. The exanthem does not coalesce or become coppery and is entirely resolved by the third day. Complications include arthritis and a self-limited encephalitis. Transplacental transmission of the virus is responsible for a wide variety of severe congenital abnormalities.

## Mumps

Mumps is characterized by painful swelling of the parotid and other salivary glands. Incubation of this virus requires 2 to 3 weeks. Contagion is possible 1 week before and 1 to 2 weeks after the onset of glandular swelling. Prodromal symptoms are nonspecific—fever, headache, malaise, myalgia—and are uncommon in children. Rapid increase in the size and tenderness of one or both parotid glands is associated with fever, edema of the ipsilateral pharynx, and redness and swelling of Stensen's duct. The submandibular gland may be primarily infected in 10 to 15 percent of cases or may accompany parotid disease. Aseptic meningitis and encephalitis are frequent complications (10 percent). Orchitis or oophoritis are seen in postpubertal patients. Male but not female fertility can be compromised. Rare complications include pancreatitis, nephritis, thyroiditis, myocarditis, mastitis, arthritis, and unilateral deafness. A live virus vaccine is available and is usually coadministered with those for measles and rubella at 15 to 18 months. Vaccination is contraindicated in immune-deficient states [such as human immunodeficiency virus (HIV) infection], pregnancy, and severe allergy to eggs.

## OTHER ORGANISMS

### Spirochaetacea *Treponema pallidum* (Syphilis)

Although syphilis is most commonly transferred by sexual contact, it may also be acquired in the womb and by neonatal contact with a chancre. Although most syphilitic disease in children is congenital, about 33 percent is acquired, usually as a result of sexual abuse.[63]

The primary presentation of the acquired disease in children is frequently overlooked, with the solitary chancre going unnoticed. The secondary disease presents 2 to 10 weeks later and resembles many infectious diseases with different causes, displaying fever, sore throat, lymphadenopathy, headache, and a rash. The rash usually involves the hands and soles. There are white patches on mucous membranes, and highly contagious condylomata may occur in moist areas. The patient then enters the latent phase, during which the symptoms appear to go away. From 3 to 10 years after the secondary disease, the patient enters the tertiary stage, in which gummas develop. CNS involvement may occur in the child even in the early stages of the disease. Neurosyphilis usually does not develop until late and may mimic any other neurologic disease (this disease is referred to as one of the great pretenders). Cardiovascular syphilis does not develop for 10 to 40 years after the primary disease and tends to result in arteritis that primarily affects the great vessels.

Congenitally acquired disease usually presents at about 5 weeks of age. Frequently the neonate appears normal until the syphilis presents. The findings are quite variable, but hepatosplenomegaly has the highest incidence of presence. Skeletal involvement is frequent and occurs early; it can be seen on radiographs and typically manifests as painful lesions on the bone.

Rhinitis, another early sign of congenital syphilis, appears as early as the first week of life. The rhinorrhea persists longer than an URTI and is often associated with blood-tinged secretions. Laryngitis is also often associated with the infection. The discharge has a high content of spirochetes and is highly contagious.[64]

The rash follows the rhinitis by 1 week and is most severe on the hands and feet. Fissures may occur around the lips, nares, and anus and are highly characteristic of congenital syphilis. All of these areas are highly contagious. Condylomata may also be seen in this phase.

Late congenital syphilis results form the scarring of early disease and may result in the child's presenting for an anesthetic. The involved systems typically include teeth, bones, eyes, and eighth cranial nerve, with gummas and neurosyphilis.

Despite the symptoms associated with it, congenital syphilis is often difficult to diagnose. The children frequently have other infections, and blood testing may be unreliable, particularly if the infant is born to a mother who had syphilis in the past, was treated, and remained seroactive.

The treatment for syphilis is penicillin whether the disease is acquired or congenital. However, the congenital form needs longer therapy and longer follow-up. The patient must be tested every 3 months for at least the first 15 months. The patient should then be followed at 6-month intervals until reagin testing is negative or stable at a low level. If the child had any signs of CSF syphilis, the CSF must be reevaluated 2 years after treatment.

## Rickettsia

Microorganisms of this family have characteristics common to both bacteria and viruses. They resemble bacteria primarily; like viruses, however, they grow only in living cells. All the acute infectious rickettsial diseases are characterized by fever, headache, and a rash (except for Q fever, with no rash). They are almost always transmitted to humans by arthropods and in the early stages are susceptible to broad-spectrum antibiotics.

Of the four major groups of rickettsial disease the most common is Rocky Mountain spotted fever. Despite its name, it is found nationwide. It is most commonly transmitted by tick bite, but is also reported to have been transmitted by blood transfusion[65] or by aerosol.[66] Rocky Mountain spotted fever is most often seen between April and September, and most cases occur in children under 15.

Fever, headache, and rash are the major symptoms, usually occurring 2 to 8 days after the bite. The tick must be attached and feeding for 4 to 6 hours before being able to transmit the disease.[67] The fever is usually high (40 to 40.6°C with oscillations of 1.8 to 2.8° over a few hours). The lowest temperatures are recorded in the mornings.[68] The rash occurs 2 to 6 days after the fever onset, appearing peripherally at first and spreading to the trunk in a few hours. The rash is regularly found on the palms and soles. The headache is also characteristic; it persists day and night and is intractable to medications. Rocky Mountain spotted fever usually has some effect on intellectual functioning. Cardiac involvement is also common, resulting in congestive heart failure and arrhythmias. Pulmonary involvement occurs in 10 to 40 percent of cases and may manifest in abnormal blood gases. There are myalgias, which are often elicited from pressure to the calf or thigh. Thrombocytopenia develops in most cases, and this may progress to DIC. Negative nitrogen balance may be extreme, and profound hyponatremia is common. The hyponatremia is usually treated by maintenance fluids or slight fluid restriction. The administration of fluids with high sodium content tends to precipitate cardiac decompensation. An important differential diagnosis must be made between this condition and measles or meningiococcemia. The petechial rash on the hands and feet make it unlike measles. Because differentiation between Rocky Mountain spotted fever and meningiococcemia is difficult, a choice of antibiotics should result that will cover both organisms.

### Q Fever

Q fever is another rickettsial infection that is transmitted to humans from animals. It is unique in its primary mode of transmission, which is by inhalation rather than a bite. Humans contract the disease by coming in contact with infected animals or their secretions or tissue. After an incubation of 9 to 20 days, the symptoms start with chills, fever, and intractable headache. The absence of a rash makes Q fever different from other rickettsial infections. Pneumonitis and hepatosplenomegaly are common. Cardiac involvement is rare, but raises the mortality significantly. The symptoms, lasting 1 to 2 weeks, are frequently mild and self-limiting. Like the other infections in this class, it can be treated with chloramphenicol or tetracycline, if the child is old enough to take them.

## *Borrelia*

Lyme disease, another tick-borne disease, is caused by *Borrelia*, a spirochete-like microorganism. The incubation period of the organism is 3 to 32 days. The skin rash is erythema chronicum migrans, which may occur on any part of the body, although the thighs, buttocks, and axilla are the most common.[69] The rash lasts 3 weeks if untreated. The skin lesion is associated with symptoms of malaise, fatigue, headache, stiff neck, and arthralgias. The fever is usually low grade. The most common finding of this disease is arthritis, which usually begins 4 weeks following the rash. The large joints, often those closest to the rash, are affected. The knee is the most commonly involved joint (85 percent).[70] The arthritis usually lasts 1 week, but recurrent attacks are common. Neurologic symptoms usually occur within 4 weeks of the bite, are variable, and include meningitis, chorea, cerebellar ataxia, cranial neuritis, myelitis, and radiculopathies. The symptoms are most often those of aseptic meningitis; CSF findings are consistent with this diagnosis. Cardiac anomalies are seen in 10 percent of patients about 5 weeks after the bite, and have a short duration of 3 to 6 weeks. The symptoms include fluctuating atrioventricular block and left ventricular dysfunction. The cardiac involvement presents as syncope, dizziness, shortness of breath, and chest pain. The cardiac symptoms may present in the absence of other symptoms.[71] Treatment of this disease is with penicillin or, if the patient is allergic to penicillin, erythromycin. Ceftriaxone is effective in refractory cases. Children over 8 years are best treated with tetracycline.

Anesthetic implications of this disease are the careful evaluation of the preoperative electrocardiogram (ECG) and the availability of transvenous pacing equipment should complete heart block present.

## *Candida*

Usually limited to the skin and mucous membranes, *Candida* has taken on increasing importance as a pathogen that can produce life-threatening infections in the patient with a compromised immune system. Other patients at increased risk are those with cancer or organ transplants, premature infants, and those with central lines or who are undergoing major surgery. *Candida* is transmitted by personal contact, contaminated instruments, and airborne particles. Infants are considered to be especially susceptible to candidal infections during the first few months of life and then become relatively resistant. Infection may be acquired as the neonate comes in contact with the vaginal tract. The infection is usually limited to the mouth but may extend into the trachea or down the esophagus. In the normal neonate the disease is self-limiting and clears up in 15 to 59 days with treatment of nystatin.[72] Oral thrush in an older child is more important, as it usually indicates an endocrine or immune disturbance.

Other sites that can present an isolated disease are the bronchial tree, peritoneum, and bladder. Infection in the respiratory passages over long periods of time may result in chronic bronchopulmonary disease (e.g., mycetomas, pneumonia, progressive cavitation, bronchial obstruction, and pulmonary collapse). Candidiasis of the larynx can occur with the pulmonary disease, but is usually seen only with disseminated disease. In young infants this has been reported to cause inspiratory stridor.[73]

Peritoneal candidiasis is usually a result of contamination from peritoneal dialysis. Such infections tend to remain localized, and dissemination is rare. The urinary tract may also become infected, usually after an indwelling catheter placement causing urethritis and cystitis; however, the infection may ascend to pyelonephritis. If it becomes renal candidiasis, it should be considered as disseminated disease.

When the infection becomes systemic this relatively benign organism has an extremely high mortality rate (70 percent if untreated). Treatment of severe disseminated candidiasis with amphotericin B appears most effective, but flucytosine and ketoconazole are also used.[74] *Candida* penetrates the mucous membrane to involve deeper layers of the gastrointestinal tract, oropharynx, and esophagus. The kidney is often involved, and there are increasing reports of central nervous system involvement. The eyes, liver, lungs, heart, blood vessels, joints, and spleen may also become involved. The systemic response to the disease is pyogenic, with microabscess.

Cardiac candidiasis has been temporally related to the introduction of central venous catheters. The valves most commonly involved are the aortic and mitral.

Endophthalmitis caused by candidiasis often appears to be associated with hyperalimentation, and infants of very low birth weight seem to be highly susceptible to it.

Patients with systemic candidiasis treated with amphotericin B present special problems for the anesthesiologist: the drug can cause anaphylaxis and thrombocytopenia, affect renal function (in 80 percent of patients), and produce temperature instability.[75] The fever may become so high that dantrolene may be needed to control the temperature elevation.

## SYNDROMES ASSOCIATED WITH INFECTION

### Mucocutaneous Lymph Node Syndrome

Mucocutaneous lymph node syndrome (also known as Kawasaki disease or MLNS), initially described in Japan, is now recognized worldwide. The etiology is undetermined, although it is presumed to be infectious or mediated by immune complexes generated during an infection. Possible environmental, allergic, or toxic causes have not been entirely eliminated.[76] The mean age of onset is 1.5 years, and males are stricken more often than females. Other risk factors include Japanese ancestry and upper socioeconomic class. Diagnosis is based upon the presence of five of six clinical criteria: prolonged unresponsive high fever, bilateral conjunctival injection, changes of the oral mucosa (i.e., injection, strawberry tongue, or fissuring of lips), peripheral extremity involvement (i.e., edema, erythema, and desquamation), polymorphous rash, and anterior cervical adenopathy. A diffuse vasculitis and perivasculitis is noted pathologically. Acute and long-term morbidity and mortality come from involvement of the heart, coronary arteries, and large arteries. The acute phase begins with the onset of fever and lasts 4 to 10 days. Presenting symptoms persist during the subacute phase (weeks 1 to 3) and are accompanied by leukocytosis, thrombocytosis, increase in acute-phase reactants, and evidence of cardiovascular disease. Defervescence and desquamation of the hands, feet, and diaper region herald the beginning of a convalescent phase.

The spectrum of cardiovascular disease is broad. Abnormal ECGs are noted in the majority of patients. There is a classic involvement of the coronary arteries, with formation of aneurysms or stenosis in 20 percent of cases. These lesions may result in death by rupture or acute myocardial infarction in the subacute phase. Risk factors in the development of significant cardiovascular disease are age under 12 months, male sex, Japanese ancestry, fever lasting more than 16 days, white blood cell count more than 30,000, elevation of erythrocyte sedimentation rate more than 101 or for over 30 days, and abnormal ECG. Coronary artery pathology regresses spontaneously and slowly in the majority of cases. Persistent aneurysms or stenosis may require coronary artery bypass grafting, and valvulitis may impair cardiac function. Sudden death is possible many years after recovery from acute disease.

Additional frequent manifestations of MLNS are arthritis, uveitis, and hydrops of the gallbladder. Necrotic pharyngitis, otitis media, mastoiditis, encephalitis, pleural effusions, myositis, and nephritis are rare complications. Aneurysms of most large arteries have been reported. Axillary aneurysms are the most common peripheral vascular lesion. Rupture of cerebral or renal aneurysms has also been reported.

Aspirin is the current treatment of choice in these patients. Aspirin does not reduce the fever or alter the early clinical course of MLNS, but it does effectively decrease the incidence of coronary and cardiovascular complications. Other drugs with antiplatelet effects have been tried but have not been as successful. During the course of high fever, aspirin absorption is erratic, and doses of 80 to 150 mg/kg/d may be necessary to achieve therapeutic plasma concentrations (15 to 25 mg/dl). The dose is reduced to 30 mg/kg/d after defervescence. At 1 month the dose can be further reduced to 3 mg/kg/d. This regimen can be maintained until the resolution of cardiovascular disease. Immune globulin protocols have produced an improvement in acute symptoms as well as a decrease in coronary disease. Steroids may promote the deleterious cardiac events.

## Reye Syndrome

Reye syndrome is an acute postinfectious encephalopathy accompanied by fatty degeneration of the liver. Disruption of mitochondrial function is found in both the brain and liver. Following recovery from a prodromal febrile illness, there is an acute onset of protracted vomiting and delirium. An URTI is noted in over 90 percent of patients. Varicella is reported as the antecedent in 5 to 7 percent of cases. Diseases described in association with Reye syndrome have included influenza A and B, reovirus, echovirus, coxsackievirus A and B, adenovirus, EBV (although less than HSV), measles, and mumps.

The populations at increased risk for Reye syndrome are young school-age children, whites, and rural dwellers. A strong association with the use of aspirin during the acute febrile illness has been noted. Likewise, there is an increased incidence of Reye syndrome in children who require chronic aspirin treatment for connective tissue disorders.

Alterations in mental status progress over the course of 24 to 96 hours. At this point, the patient either begins to recover or deteriorates toward an irreversible fatal outcome (26 to 42 percent). There are no focal neurologic signs. The progress of Reye syndrome has been divided into five stages. Stages 1 to 3 indicate mild disease and a favorable prognosis. Lethargy and confusion characterize stage 1. Stage 2 manifests as an increase in delirium with agitation. Decorticate and decerebrate posturing are seen in stages 3 and 4, respectively. There is an absence of brainstem reflexes in stage 5. Serologic abnormalities reported include increases in serum glutamic-oxaloacetic transaminase (SGOT), serum glutamote-pyruvate transaminase (SGPT), lactate dehydrogenase (LDH), creatinine phosphokinase (CPK), and ammonia. Gluconeogenesis is impaired, and hypoglycemia is evident in the absence of supplementation. Respiratory alkalosis compensates for a metabolic acidosis. Treatment is supportive.

## Guillain-Barré Syndrome

Guillain-Barré syndrome has become the most common cause of acute paralytic disease since routine polio vaccination. The etiology of this syndrome has not been determined. There is antecedent viral illness in most cases. There is no neurologic involvement during the viral infection. EBV, measles, mumps, echovirus, CMV, coxsackievirus, influenza virus, and mycoplasma have all been implicated.

Guillain-Barré syndrome is an acute demyelinating disease of the peripheral nervous system. Pain and paresthesias of the lower extremities may be described before the onset of a symmetric, ascending, flaccid paralysis with loss of deep tendon reflexes. Cranial nerve deficits are seen in 50 to 75 percent of patients. Sensory impairment is mild, and significant weakness of respiratory muscles necessitates respiratory support in 20 percent of patients. Autonomic nervous system instability may manifest as labile hypertension or hypotension, tachycardia, sweating, flushing, and bowel or bladder dysfunction. The sensorium remains intact. Neurologic dysfunction evolves to a maximum at 3 weeks, when gradual recovery begins. The convalescent phase may last between several months and several years. Seventy-five percent of patients experience slow but complete recovery. Residual neurologic deficits are seen in 20 percent; 5 percent are fatal cases.

It is important not to use succinylcholine for muscle relaxation in these patients. Dysfunction of the autonomic nervous system is also often seen, and medications to treat hypotension, hypertension, tachycardia, or bradycardia must be readily available.

# SUMMARY

The pediatric anesthesiologist must encounter infectious disease issues regularly. Each time infection is an issue, the risks and benefits must be carefully weighed to determine whether the timing is optimal for the surgery in light of the specific infectious process. Other than with URTIs, which are dealt with elsewhere, there are few guidelines as to when anesthesia can be safely provided and when it cannot. Integrating the information from this chapter should allow the anesthesiologist to be prepared for the problems that may be directly related to the infectious process.

Anesthesiologists must also be aware that they are at risk for acquiring some of the infectious agents described here—more likely the viruses than the bacteria—because anesthesiologists cannot predict which procedures will result in contact with body fluids that can transmit disease.[77] The anesthesiologist should take preventive measures (gloves, face mask, and glasses) whenever dealing with patients, particularly those with viral pathogens.

Another real risk for transmission of disease to the anesthesiologist is needlesticks. One study has documented the risk of needlestick injuries and was able to document an increased risk to those in the operating room.[78] The circumvention of this danger in anesthetic practice deserves considerable attention.

## REFERENCES


1. Frenkel LD: Routine immunizations for American children in the 1990s. Pediatr Clin North Am 37:531, 1990
2. Feigin RD, Shearer WJ: Opportunistic infection in children in the compromised host. J Pediatr 87:607, 1975
3. Bellanti A: Basic immunologic principles underlying vaccination procedures. Pediatr Clin North Am 37:513, 1990
4. Bonadio WA, Hogenbarth M, Zachariason M: Correlating reported fever in young infants with subsequent temperature patterns and rate of seroius bacterial infections. Pediatr Infect Dis J 9:158, 1990
5. Hill HR, Zimmerman RA, Reid GVK et al: Food-borne epidemic of streptococcal pharyngitis at the United States Air Force Academy. N Engl J Med 280:917, 1969
6. Rammelkamp CH, Jr: Epidemiology of streptococcal infections. Harvey Lect 51: 113, 1957
7. Hoekelman RA, Blotman S, Friedman SB et al: Primary Pediatric Care. CV Mosby, St. Louis, 1987
8. Levin RM, Grossman M, Jordan C et al: Group A streptococcal infection in children younger than 3 years of age. Pediatr Infect Dis J 7:581, 1988
9. Kaplan EL, Wannamaker LW: Group A streptococcal infections. p. 1312. In Feigin RD, Cherry JD (eds): Textbook of Pediatric Infectious Disease. 2nd Ed. WB Saunders, Philadelphia, 1987
10. Moffet HL: Pediatric Infectious Diseases: A Problem-Oriented Approach. p. 265. JB Lippincott, Philadelphia, 1989
11. Dayani AS, Bisno AL, Chung KJ et al: Prevention of rheumatic fever: a statement for health professionals by the Committee on Rheumatic Fever, Endocarditis, and Kawasaki Disease of the Council on Cardiovascular Disease in the Young, the American Heart Association. Pediatr Infect Dis J 8:263, 1989
12. Griffiths SP, Gersony WM: Acute rheumatic fever in New York City, 1969 to 1988: a comparative study of two decades. J Pediatr 116:882, 1990
13. Anthony BF: Group B streptococcal infections. p. 1322. In Feigin RD, Cherry JD (eds): Textbook of Pediatric Infectious Diseases. 2nd Ed. WB Saunders, Philadelphia, 1987
14. Saez-Llorens X, Ramilo O, Mustafa MM et al: Molecular pathophysiology of bacterial meningitis: current concepts and therapeutic implications. J Pediatr 116: 671, 1990
15. Teele DW: Pneumococcal infections. p. 1243. In Feigin RD, Cherry JD (eds): Textbook of Pediatric Infectious Diseases. 2nd Ed. WB Saunders, Philadelphia, 1987
16. Feigin RD: Staphylococcal infections. p. 580. In Behrman RE, Vaughan III VC (eds): Nelson Textbook of Pediatrics. 13th Ed. WB Saunders, Philadelphia, 1987
17. Oski FA, De Angelis CD, Feigin RD, Warshaw JB (eds): Principles and Practice of Pediatrics. JB Lippincott, Philadelphia, 1990
18. Ferguson MA, Todd JK: Toxic shock syndrome associated with *Staphylococcus aureus* sinusitis in children. J Infect Dis 161:953, 1990
19. Resnick SD: Toxic shock syndrome: recent developments in pathogenesis. J Pediatr 116:321, 1990
20. Rolston RD, Yabek SM, Florman AL et al: Severe cardiac conduction abnormalities associated with atypical toxic shock syndrome. J Pediatr 177:89, 1990
21. Tyson W, Wershey DF, Anderson JD et al: Atypical staphylococcal toxic shock syndrome: two fatal pediatric cases. Pediatr Infect Dis J 8:642, 1989

22. Conway EE, Haber RS, Gumprecht J, Singer LP: Toxic shock syndrome following influenza A in a child. Crit Care Med 19:123, 1991
23. Feingold SM, Arnon SS: Clostridial intoxication and infection. p. 1118. In Feigin RD, Cherry JD (eds): Textbook of Pediatric Infectious Diseases. 2nd Ed. WB Saunders, Philadelphia, 1987
24. Stoelting RK, Dierdorf SF, McCammon RL: Infectious disease. p. 647. In Stoelting RK, Dierdorf SF, McCammon RL (eds): Anesthesia and Co-Existing Disease. 2nd Ed. Churchill Livingstone, New York, 1988
25. Berkowitz FE: Bacterial exotoxins: how they work. Pediatr Infect Dis J 8:42, 1989
26. Feigin RD: Botulism. p. 622. In Behrman RE, Vaughan VC III (eds): Nelson Textbook of Pediatrics. 13th Ed. WB Saunders, Philadelphia, 1987
27. Weinstein L: Tetanus. p. 1126. In Feigin RD, Cherry JD (eds): Textbook of Pediatric Infectious Diseases. 2nd Ed. WB Saunders, Philadelphia, 1987
28. Hornick RB: *Shigella* infections. p. 683. In Feign RD, Cherry JD (eds): Textbook of Pediatric Infectious Diseases. 2nd Ed. WB Saunders, Philadelphia, 1987
29. Hornick RB: *Salmonella* infections. p. 673. In Feigin RD, Cherry JD (eds): Textbook of Pediatric Infectious Diseases. 2nd Ed. WB Saunders, Philadelphia, 1987
30. Mendelman PM, Smith AL: *Haemophilus influenzae*. p. 1142. In Feigin RD, Cherry JD (eds): Textbook of Pediatric Infectious Diseases. 2nd Ed. WB Saunders, Philadelphia, 1987
31. Committee on Infectious Diseases, American Academy of Pediatrics: *Haemophilus influenzae* type B conjugate vaccines: immunization of children at 15 months of age. Pediatrics 86:794, 1990
32. Golden GS: Pertussis vaccine and injury to the brain. J Pediatr 166:854, 1990
33. Jacobs RF, Sowell MK, Moss M, Fiser DH: Septic shock in children: bacterial etiologies and temporal relationships. Pediatr Infect Dis J 9:196, 1990
34. Jardin F, Brun-Ney D, Auvert B et al: Sepsis-related cardiogenic shock. Crit Care Med 18:1055, 1990
35. Wetzel RC: Shock. p. 483. In Rogers MC (ed): Textbook of Pediatric Intensive Care. Williams & Wilkins, Baltimore, 1987
36. Zimmerman JJ, Dietrich KA: Current perspectives on septic shock. Pediatr Clin North Am 34:131, 1987
37. Sprung LS, Caralis PV, Marcial EH et al: The effects of high-dose corticosteroids in patient with septic shock: a prospective, controlled study. N Engl J Med 18:1137, 1984
38. Mink RB, Pollack MM: Effect of blood transfusion on oxygen consumption in pediatric septic shock. Crit Care Med 19: 1087, 1990
39. Gomez A, Wang R, Unruh H et al: Hemofiltration reverses left ventricular dysfunction during sepsis in dogs. Anesthesiology 73:671, 1990
40. Kaplan JM, Goretski SA, Keith S, Calford L: Cost of antibiotic therapy for infants and children. Pediatr Infect Dis J 9:722, 1990
41. Stutman HR, Marks MI: Review of pediatric antimicrobial therapies. In Feigin RD (ed): Semin Pediatr Infect Dis 2:3, 1991
42. Motuz DJ, Watson WA, Barlow JC et al: The increase in urinary alanine aminopeptidase excretion associated with enflurane anesthesia is increased further by aminoglycosides. Anesth Analg 67:770, 1988
43. Smith CM, Steffey EP, Baggot JD et al: Effects of halothane anesthesia on the clearance of gentamicin sulfate in horses. Am J Vet Res 49:19, 1988
44. Sokoll MD, Gergis SSD: Antibiotics and neuromuscular function. Anesthesiology 55:148, 1981
45. Forsyth SF, Ilkiw JE, Hildebrand SV: Effect of gentamicin administration on the neuromuscular blockade induced by atracurium in cats. Am J Vet Res 51:1675, 1990
46. Alpert G, Campos JM, Harris MC et al: Vancomycin dosage in pediatrics reconsidered. Am J Dis Child 138:20, 1984
47. Levy JH, Kettlekamp NB, Goertz P et al: Histamine release by vancomycin: a mechanism for hypotension in man. Anesthesiology 67:122, 1987

48. Lyon GD, Bruce DL: Diphenhydramine reversal of vancomycin-induced hypotension. Anesth Analg 67:1109, 1988
49. Odio C, Mohs E, Sklar FH et al: Adverse reactions to vancomycin used as prophylaxis for CSF shunt procedures. Am J Dis Child 138:17, 1984
50. Best CJ, Ewart M, Sumner E: Perioperative complications following the use of vancomycin in children: a report of two cases. Br J Anaesth 62:576, 1989
51. Huang KC, Heise A, Shrader AK, Tsueda K: Vancomycin enhances the neuromuscular blockade of vecuronium. Anesth Analg 71:194, 1990
52. Bartkowski RR, McDonnell TE: Prolonged alfentanil effect following erythromycin administration. Anesthesiology 73:566, 1990
53. Sande MA, Mandell GL: Antimicrobial agents. p. 1170. In Gilman AG, Goodman LS, Rall TW, Murad F (eds): Goodman and Gilman's Pharmacological Basis of Therapeutics. Macmillan, New York, 1985
54. Flacke WE, Flacke JW: Mechanism: general principles. p. 14. In Smith NT, Miller RD, Corbascio AN (eds): Drug Interactions in Anesthesia. Lea & Febiger, Philadelphia, 1981
55. Tait AR, Du Boulay PM, Knight PR: Alterations in the course of and histopathologic response to influenze virus infections produced by enflurane, halothane, and diethyl ether anesthesia in ferrets. Anesth Analg 67:671, 1988
56. Knight PR, Bedows E, Nahrwold ML et al: Alterations in influenza virus pulmonary pathology induced by diethyl ether, halothane, enflurane, and pentobarbital anesthesia in mice. Anesthesiology 58: 209, 1983
57. Knight PR, Nahrwold ML, Bedows E: Anesthetic action and virus replication: inhibition of measles virus replication in cells exposed to halothane. Antimicrob Agents Chemother 17:890, 1980
58. Kohl S: Herpes simplex virus encephalitis in children. Pediatr Clin North Am 35: 465, 1988
59. Widome MD: Pharyngitis and tonsillitis. p. 1429. In Hoekelman RA, Blotman S, Friedman SB et al (eds): Primary Pediatric Care. CV Mosby, St. Louis, 1987
60. White CJ, Kuter BJ, Hildebrand CS et al: Varicella vaccine (varivax) in healthy children and adolescents: results from clinical trials, 1987 to 1989. Pediatrics 87:604, 1991
61. Balfour HH, Kelly JM, Suarez CS et al: Acyclovir treatment of varicella in otherwise healthy children. J Pediatr 116:633, 1990
62. Farizo KM, Stehr-Green PA, Simpson DM, Markowitz LE: Pediatric emergency room visits: a risk factor for acquiring measles. Pediatrics 87:72, 1991
63. Marks MI: Genitourinary infections. p. 608. In Feigin RD, Cherry JD (eds): Textbook of Pediatric Infectious Diseases. 2nd Ed. WB Saunders, Philadelphia, 1987
64. Ingall D, Dobson SRM, Musher D: Syphilis. p. 365. In Remington JS, Klein JO (eds): Infectious Diseases of the Fetus and Newborn Infant. WB Saunders, Philadelphia, 1990
65. Wells GM, Woodward TE, Fiset P et al: Rocky Mountain spotted fever caused by blood transfusion. JAMA 239:2763, 1978
66. Oster CN, Burke DJ, Kenyon RH et al: Laboratory acquired Rocky Mountain spotted fever. N Engl J Med 297:859, 1977
67. Feigin RD, O'Neil JH: Rickettsial diseases. p. 1878. In Feigin RD, Cherry JD (eds): Textbook of Pediatric Infectious Diseases. 2nd Ed. WB Saunders, Philadelphia, 1987
68. Heldrich FJ: Rocky Mountain spotted fever. p. 1459. In Hoekelman RA, Blotman S, Friedman SB et al (eds): Primary Pediatric Care. CV Mosby, St. Louis, 1987
69. Strechenberg BW: *Borrelia*: Lyme disease. p. 1102. In Feigin RD, Cherry JD (eds): Textbook of Pediatric Infectious Diseases. 2nd Ed. WB Saunders, Philadelphia, 1987
70. Siegel DM, Baum J: Joint pain. p. 1029. In Hoekelman RA, Blotman S, Friedman SB et al (eds): Primary Pediatric Care. CV Mosby, St. Louis, 1987
71. Vlay SC: Complete heart block due to Lyme disease. N Engl J Med 315:1418, 1986

72. Fitzpatrick RE, Newcomer VD: Dermatophytosis and candidiasis. p. 843. In Feigin RD, Cherry JD (eds): Textbook of Pediatric Infectious Diseases. 2nd Ed. WB Saunders, Philadelphia, 1987
73. Jacobs RF, Yashuda K, Smith AL, Benjamin DR: Laryngeal candidiasis presenting as inspiratory stridor. Pediatrics 69: 234, 1982
74. Hughes WT: Candidiasis. p. 1939. In Feigin RD, Cherry JD (eds): Textbook of Pediatric Infectious Diseases. 2nd Ed. WB Saunders, Philadelphia, 1987
75. Sande MA, Mandell GL: Antimicrobial agents. p. 1219. In Gilman AG, Goodman LS, Rall TW, Murad F (eds): The Pharmacological Basis of Therapeutics. Macmillan, New York, 1985
76. Rauch AM, Glode MP, Wiggins JW et al: Outbreak of Kawasaki syndrome in Denver, Colorado: associaton with rug and carpet cleaning. Pediatrics 87:663, 1991
77. Kristensen MS, Sloth E, Jensen TK: Relationship between anesthetic procedure and contact of anesthesia personnel with patient body fluids. Anesthesiology 73: 619, 1990
78. McGeer A, Simor AE, Low DE: Epidemiology of needlestick injuries in house officers. J Infect Dis 162:961, 1990

# 9

# Renal Diseases

**Renal Function in Infants and Children**

- Renal Function in the Fetus
- Transition and Maturation
- Neonatal Renal Function
- Assessment of Renal Function

**Renal Disease in Neonates**

- Congenital Renal Disease
- Nonrenal Causes of Acquired Renal Disease
- Mortality and Morbidity in Infants with Acute Renal Failure

**Renal Diseases in Older Infants and Children**

- Hemolytic-Uremic Syndrome
- Vesicoureteral Reflux
- Glomerulonephritis
- Nephrotic Syndrome
- Flank Masses
- Diabetes and Renal Disease

**Acute and Chronic Renal Failure**

- Acute Renal Failure
- Chronic Renal Failure
- Medical Management of Renal Failure
- Hemodialysis and Peritoneal Dialysis
- Preoperative Assessment of the Child with End-Stage Renal Disease

(*Continues*)

**The Child with a Kidney Transplant**

Renal Transplantation
Growth and Development of Young Children Receiving Renal Transplants
Seizures and Renal Transplantation

**Miscellaneous Issues**

Thyroid Function in Children with End-Stage Renal Disease
Association of Renal Disease with Severe Viral Infections
Renal Disease Associated with Nonsteroidal Antiinflammatory Drugs
Long-Term Parenteral Nutrition and Renal Function

# 9

# Renal Diseases

*Frederic A. Berry*

Renal disease in infants and children includes diseases unique to the neonate as well as many of the diseases of the adult. This chapter reviews renal function in infants and children, transition and maturation of renal function, and assessment of the patient with renal disease, including the various laboratory studies. The remainder of the chapter describes some diseases specific to the neonate, as well as those renal diseases that are found in infants and children.

## RENAL FUNCTION IN INFANTS AND CHILDREN

The object of this section is to give an overview of renal function in infants and children. For detailed information about specific urologic problems and their management, the reader should consult a pediatric urology text.[1] The kidney is a primary organ involved in the control of the volume and composition of the fluid compartments of the body. The content of these fluid compartments depends upon a highly complicated balance of intake of fluids, cardiovascular function, renal function, and normal or abnormal losses of fluids from the body. Abnormal losses may be due to disease states such as burns, trauma, gastrointestinal disease, bleeding, and disorders of renal function. The kidney receives approximately 25 percent of cardiac output, which supplies the metabolic requirements of the kidney as well as a large flow for selective ultrafiltration of the plasma. The process of selective ultrafiltration depends upon glomerular filtration and active tubular reabsorption excretion. The kidney has an enormous reserve in its ability to compensate for fluid losses even with some decreased renal function.

The renal tubules are involved in the process of resorption of enormous quantities of solute and fluid, approximately 98 percent of those that are filtered. At the same time, the tubules also control that which is excreted. This can either be done indirectly (i.e., by not resorbing filtered substances), or it can be a direct process, whereby substances are actively excreted by the tubule. Hormones can directly and indirectly affect the dynamics of glomerular filtration and tubular function, including the catecholamines, those of the renin-angiotensin-aldosterone system, atrial natriuretic factor, and antidiuretic hormone. Drugs also may either directly or indirectly effect renal function, as may circulatory insufficiency, hypoxia, and central nervous system trauma.

## Renal Function in the Fetus

The placenta is a hemodialysis unit for the fetus. Approximately 50 percent of the cardiac output of the fetus perfuses the placenta. The fetus swallows amniotic fluid and produces urine, which is then excreted into the amniotic fluid. Thus amnionic fluid is formed both by fetal urine and the maternal placenta. Disorders of amniotic fluid production may be associated with some congenital defects. Renal agenesis or malformation decrease the formation of amniotic fluid and may result in oligohydramnios. Oligohydramnios may also be associated with impairment of pulmonary development. This condition has been well documented in Potter's syndrome (the triad of prune-belly, pulmonary abnormalities, and major renal anomalies). Polyhydramnios may be the result of a defect in swallowing by the fetus, which may be due to an upper gastrointestinal (GI) tract obstruction such as tracheoesophageal fistula or duodenal atresia. The only fetal requirement for renal blood flow, which is about 5 percent of fetal cardiac output, is for the growth and development of the kidney. All of the nephrons of the kidney are developed by 34 weeks' gestation.

## Transition and Maturation

All infants must pass through the transition from the fetal to the newborn to the neonatal state. The newborn period is defined as the first 24 hours of life; a neonate is within the first 30 days of life. Transition of the circulatory system involves the closure of the fetal vascular shunts (i.e., the ductus venosus, ductus arteriosus, and foramen ovale), thereby establishing the pathway of the adult circulation. Initially, the circulatory changes occur because of initiation of ventilation and the associated changes in intra-atrial pressure that close the foramen ovale and the sensitivity of the ductus arteriosus to oxygen. With time, these shunts become anatomically closed. However, it is well known that the foramen ovale remains functionally open in approximately 10 percent of adults.[2]

Renal function at the time of birth and in the first week of life depends upon the conceptual age of the neonate as well as the extent of transition.[3] If a neonate is born before 34 weeks, there will be incomplete renal development and a decreased number of nephrons; after 34 weeks, all of the nephrons are developed. After birth, there is an increase in renal blood flow up to 20 to 25 percent of cardiac output, which provides for the additional requirements for increased ultrafiltration of the plasma. The initial electrolyte values of the newborn reflect placental function since the placenta is the kidney of the fetus, and are similar to those of the mother. Thus, the creatinine of the premature or full-term infant is often in the range of 0.8 to 1.2 mg/dl. Increased renal blood flow, because of both an increase in systemic pressure and a decrease in renal vascular resistance, results in a rapid improvement in renal function as reflected in the ability to dilute and concentrate the urine. This results in a reduction in the serum creatinine levels. By the end of the first month of life, the serum creatinine will be in the neighborhood of 0.2 to 0.3 mg/dl (see Table 9-1 for normal values).

## Neonatal Renal Function

### Urine Concentration

In the first several days of life in a full-term infant, there is a diminished ability to concentrate urine. Urine osmolarity ranges somewhere in the neighborhood of 700 to 800 mOsm/L. In the premature

**Table 9-1.** Mean Plasma Creatinine (Cr) Concentration

| *Age* | *Cr (mg/dl)* | *Standard Deviation* |
|---|---|---|
| Birth | .8–1.4[a] | |
| 1 month | .2 | .05 |
| 6 months | .3 | .05 |
| 1 year | .4 | .07 |
| 3 years | .43 | .1 |
| 5 years | .48 | .12 |
| 7 years | .5 | .11 |
| 9 years | .53 | .11 |
| 11 years | .57 | .13 |
| 13 years | .61 | .13–.19 |

[a] Maternal levels.

infant, the ability to concentrate is impaired even further, with the maximum concentrating ability somewhere around 500 mOsm/L. With normal dietary intake, there is a rapidly increasing ability to concentrate the urine, as evidenced by a concentrating ability of 1,200 mOsm/L at approximately 6 months. The mature value of 1,400 mOsm/L is achieved at approximately 1 year of age. The ability to dilute the urine is quite good, even in the premature infant. The major need for diluting the urine is in cases of excessive fluid administration. In general, this not a problem. However, in small premature infants, it has been shown that an excessive rate of fluid administration is associated with an expanded extracellular fluid and an increased incidence of a patent ductus arteriosus.[4] This finding has been challenged by others, so the issue is unresolved.[5] The definition of *excessive* may be at the heart of the controversy. The challenges in the neonatal period to the kidney are mainly those due to the need for surgery. When a fluid deficit develops due to GI tract obstruction or hemorrhage, the kidney needs to be able to conserve fluid by concentrating the urine and resorbing sodium from the distal tubule. The concentrating mechanism of the kidney is established by the accumulation of urea in the interstitium of the kidney in order to develop an osmotic gradient so that water may be reabsorbed against the gradient. The metabolism of protein produces the urea.

### Sodium Conservation

Most newborns at birth have an excess volume of extracellular fluid, and the first several days of life is characterized by diuresis of this extra fluid. In the face of other additional reductions in extracellular fluid volume (i.e., intestinal obstruction, blood loss, etc.), the normal homeostatic mechanisms of the kidney are required to conserve fluid, which is done primarily through the almost complete resorption of sodium and water in the distal tubule to restore the extracellular fluid volume. The neonate has normal quantities of aldosterone but would appear to have a relatively immature distal tubule, because even in the face of a sodium deficit, the neonate will continue to excrete sodium in the urine. This is referred to as the obligatory loss of sodium in the urine and is the reason that neonates require sodium in all fluids that are administered.[6] This rate of sodium excretion can be measured by what is termed the fractional excretion of sodium (FE-Na). This is calculated by measuring the amount of sodium filtered in the glomerulus and that is excreted in the urine. That fraction of sodium excreted in the urine is referred to as the FE-Na. In the premature infant, this may represent 2 to 6 percent of filtered sodium, while in a full-term neonate the FE-Na is 2 to 3 percent. After 3 months of age, the FE-Na is less than 1 percent of the filtered load, which is the normal mature value. From a practical viewpoint, the kidney is 50 percent mature at 4 to 6 weeks of age and therefore has no limitations from the standpoint of renal function.

## Assessment of Renal Function

The anesthesiologist is faced with three different clinical situations in which renal function is a priority item in an evaluation of the patient: (1) the child with a stable history of renal disease for elective surgery; (2) the child with acute alterations in renal function, which are secondary to dehydration and/or hypovolemia or to renal damage; and (3) the child with a history of renal disease who also has a superimposed acute problem. When attempted corrections of acute alterations in renal function that are thought to be secondary to dehydration or hypovolemia do not respond in the expected way, then the clinician should be very suspicious that there is underlying renal disease.

The assessment of the child with renal disease includes the triad of history, physical, and laboratory studies. Clinical evidence of renal disease appears late in the development of renal pathology, indicating that 75 percent of the nephrons are nonfunctional.[7] The history and physical examination of an infant or child with renal disease is usually unremarkable. Many children present with lethargy and pallor, and history of poor feeding. In older children the symptomatology may precipitate an earlier concern by the parents if the child complains of specific problems such as headache, not feeling well, and so forth. In an infant, some of the subtle signs may be attributed to other conditions such as a "cold" or "mild touch of the flu," or "diarrhea." Thus renal disease in infants and children is often not recognized early. A good example is the hemolytic uremic syndrome, in which the presenting problem is usually diarrhea. Hypertension may be an indicator of renal disease. The history of the amount and character of the urine can be helpful in the evaluation of the fluid status of the child as well as in diagnosing renal disease. Decreased urine output is usually an indicator of the volume status. The color of the urine is also helpful in the evaluation of the fluid status, since a darker yellow color indicates concentrated urine. A history of red or "Coke"-colored urine would suggest either glomerulonephritis or myoglobinuria, while turbid urine might suggest the presence of nephrosis.

It is impossible to evaluate the child with renal disease without a urinalysis and blood chemistry studies.

### Urine Output

Urine output is similar in infants of all ages. In the first 24 hours of life normal infants will have their first voiding regardless of gestational age. Afterwards, normal infants will have 1 to 2 ml/kg/h of urine output. Oliguria has long been recognized as a sign of renal impairment, and is usually defined as urine output less than 0.6 ml/kg/h. Anuria is defined as a urine output less than 1 ml/kg/d.[8] This is a general figure that can be used for neonates as well as older children.

### Urinalysis

The urinalysis usually consists of an evaluation of specific gravity as well as protein, glucose, and sediment content. Fluid restriction in a normal child will cause the specific gravity of the urine to increase. This ability to concentrate the urine depends upon tubular function. A specific gravity of 1.018 or greater in the absence of protein and/or sugar indicates that tubular function is essentially normal. Repeated urine specific gravities of 1.010 indicate a state of isosthenuria. This is the specific gravity of plasma; with severe renal damage, there is an inability of the kidney to dilute or concentrate the urine.

## Sickle Cell Anemia

Inability to produce maximally concentrated urine is the most consistent feature of sickle cell nephropathy and occurs in both homozygous (SS) and heterozygous (AS) states. When the erythrocytes containing hemoglobin are exposed to a hyperosmotic environment such as that found in the inner medulla, sickling occurs, which leads to scarring and patchy interstitial fibrosis of the inner medulla and papillae. The result is a loss of the ability to concentrate the urine so even with a normal glomerular filtration rate (GFR) and tubular function, there is a reduced ability to concentrate the urine. Similar states in which there may be a reduced ability to concentrate the urine occur in patients with a low protein intake and those receiving diuretics, which cause additional water to be excreted, thereby diluting the urine.

## Routine Urinalysis in Hospitalized Pediatric Patients

There has been considerable debate in the literature about routine testing. The Joint Commission for the Accreditation of Hospitals has denounced the "routine test" and stated that only tests that are indicated should be performed. However, many hospital bylaws require a urinalysis in all patients admitted. A recent study on pediatric patients evaluated the results of such a policy.[9] Children with symptoms felt to be in the least way related to the urinary tract were excluded. Thus the urinalysis performed on the remaining children was simply a "screening" urinalysis. The patients included both same-day–admission surgical patients as well as inpatient admissions. Twenty percent of the "screening" urinalyses were abnormal, the commonest abnormality being either pyuria or hematuria. It was of interest that in only 38 percent of the patients was there any followup urinalysis or any other diagnostic study based upon the abnormal "screening" urinalysis. In the patients in whom a followup urinalysis was obtained, 58 percent showed persistent abnormalities. It was concluded that "screening" urinalysis was not useful, in that abnormal results were either unappreciated or not pursued. None of the patients with an abnormal urinalysis had any immediate problems because of the lack of followup. The issue of an adequate followup would have been much more applicable to the long-term renal problems that these patients may develop. This issue, however, was not pursued.

## Hematuria

Hematuria is the presence of red blood cells in the urine. Microscopic hematuria is that which requires a microscope and/or a biochemical test, whereas macroscopic hematuria may be seen with the naked eye. Occasional microscopic hematuria is not unusual in neonates or in very active older children. However, persistent hematuria is distinctly abnormal at any age. The causes of persistent hematuria include glomerulonephritis, cystitis, trauma, tumors, bleeding disorders, vascular problems, and congenital anomalies. A limited number of red blood cells in the urine is normal, but the exact definition of what constitutes "significant" hematuria is unclear. Microscopic hematuria occurs transiently at times of extreme exertion, trauma, illness, or fever. On the other hand, recurrent hematuria is quite another matter. In a study by Miller et al.[10] in 100 children with recurrent hematuria for more than 1 year, the outcomes were different: 5 of the 100 children ended up with end-stage renal failure, 5 had hypertension, and 27 had significant proteinuria. In an apparently well child with persistent microscopic hematuria and a negative medical history, the most likely cause is glomerulonephritis. Meadow[11] is of the opinion that glomerulonephritis is present in approximately 1 percent of children and suggests that even though it may be relatively benign in childhood, it may not be so on long-term follow-up of adults.

## Proteinuria

Small amounts of protein are often excreted in the first several days of life and generally by the second week of life reflect normal mature concentrations. Protein is normally found in the urine. It is the quantity of protein and the conditions under which it is found that differentiate the normal amount of protein in the urine from that found in disease. Proteins are both filtered by the glomerulus as well as secreted by the urinary tract and accessory sex glands. The proteins that are filtered by the glomerulus are almost completely resorbed by the renal tubules.

**Glomerular Filtration of Protein.** Two factors play a role in the ability of proteins to cross the glomerular barrier into the ultrafiltrate: the molecular charge and the size of the protein. The surfaces of both the glomerular endothelial and epithelial cells are lined with proteins that have a negative charge.[12] Since albumin has a negative charge at a pH of 7.4, transglomerular filtration is minimized. The small proteins, like albumin, are filtered in low concentrations, while the larger proteins such as globulins cannot pass through the normal glomerular membranes. Some of the smaller proteins like growth hormone or insulin, which are peptide hormones, can easily penetrate the glomerular barrier. The filtered proteins are resorbed through the proximal convoluted tubules almost completely, but a small amount will pass through into the urine. The presence of albumin in the urine is a highly sensitive indicator of abnormalities in glomerular permeability. In the normal subject it represents approximately 25 percent of the urinary protein. As is discussed later in the section on diabetes and renal function, proteinuria plays an important role as a predictor of nephropathy in diabetic children. There are other proteins that are indicators of tubular function. For example, the protein lysozyme is a bacteriolytic enzyme of low molecular weight that is freely filtered by the glomerulus and almost completely resorbed in the proximal tubule. It has been used as a measure of tubular dysfunction. Therefore, characterizing the specific protein in the urine is a useful technique for characterizing renal damage. Increases in albumin point to glomerular disease, whereas increases in lysozyme would indicate tubular dysfunction.[13] Approximately 60 percent of the protein in normal urine is derived from plasma protein, while the remaining 40 percent is of tissue origin (i.e., secreted by the urinary tract and accessory sex glands).

**Frequency.** It is evident from the discussion above that there is a great deal of variability in the amount of protein in the urine, depending on factors such as exercise, whether the patient is febrile, and the time of day. Urine that is quite dilute may give a false-negative test in a person with renal disease, but when the concentration of the urine is normal, the result might be positive. Conversely, in the face of a greatly reduced urine output with a resulting concentration of the urine, the protein test may be false positive. There is no absolute limit for the normal value for protein, but the range is somewhere between 60 and 150 mg/m$^2$/d. In the first few months of life, the amount of protein present in the urine may be as high as 240 mg/m$^2$/d. One guideline for normal values for proteinuria in children suggests that if the urine is collected with the patient at rest and afebrile, urinary protein content should not exceed 60 mg/m$^2$/d.[12] It has been shown that children tested for protein during the day have a much higher value than those tested at night, when at rest and supine. Approximately 15 percent of patients have "postural proteinuria"; increased proteinuria occurs when they are upright, but when they are in a supine position the amount of protein is normal. It should be evident from this discussion that the intermittent isolated occurrence of proteinuria is not an indicator of renal disease. On the other hand, persistent proteinuria is usually considered to be of glomerular origin and if found along with other microscopic urinary findings is strongly suggestive of underlying renal disease.

**Screening Techniques.** The simplest technique for measuring protein is by the dipstick. Measurement of the urinary albumin to creatinine ratio (Ualb/Ucr), which is expressed as the ratio of micrograms of albumin to milligrams of creatinine, has been used to assess glomerular permeability and tubular function. These techniques are extremely important for the nephrologist who is in the process of evaluating renal function in patients. In general, the anesthesiologist is best served by simpler methods for determining abnormal protein in the urine, which may well be a reflection of both glomerular filtration as well as tubular dysfunction; this is accomplished by the dipstick.

Use of the dipstick has enabled the clinician to measure the amount of protein in the urine with a great deal of accuracy from a protein concentration as low as 10 to 15 mg/dl to more than 1,000. The test is much better for albumin than it is for some of the other proteins such as globulins. Some interobserver error occurs because of differences in the interpretation of color, but for the purposes of screening, the test is quite satisfactory. False negatives can occur with dilute urine, and false positives can occur with concentrated urine, hematuria, and pyuria, and from contamination with cleansing agents.

## Glomerular Filtration and Tubular Function

For purposes of discussion and evaluation, kidney function will be divided into glomerular filtration and tubular function, but it is obvious that the two functions are interrelated. Screening the urine for proteins, although specific for the presence of renal disease, does not quantitate the degree of either glomerular or tubular dysfunction quite as accurately as do blood chemistries and other specialized laboratory techniques. The usual blood chemistries that are used to assess glomerular filtration are creatinine and blood urea nitrogen (BUN). The normal BUN level in infants and children is between 10 and 20 mg/dl. However, it should be realized that the BUN may not be an accurate reflection of glomerular filtration for several reasons. In patients on high-protein diets as well as in patients who have gastrointestinal bleeding, when hemoglobin is digested and absorbed, there is an elevated BUN. In addition, BUN levels will increase in hypermetabolic states, as well as in states in which there is slow movement of fluid through the renal tubules with increased reabsorption of urea. However, the plasma creatinine usually remains normal in this situation. Regardless of its limitations, however, a BUN greater than 50 mg/dl is strongly suggestive of renal disease. In the usual situation, blood chemistries are adequate for evaluation of renal function, but at times it becomes necessary to delineate more clearly the degree of impairment of renal function; then the creatinine clearance is performed. The problem with this test in infants and children is that the usual method for creatinine clearance requires accurate urine collection. Schwartz and Gauthier[14] devised a technique for calculating the GFR in boys using the plasma creatinine value and a formula that was directly related to the height of the patient in centimeters. However, with usage it was found that this formula overestimated the creatinine clearance in full-term and preterm infants and that it underestimated the creatinine clearance in adolescent boys. It was found that the sample population could be more accurately analyzed by regression techniques. This seems a bit cumbersome for the anesthesiologist, and for purposes of evaluation of glomerular filtration the serum creatinine values would appear to be quite adequate (see Table 9-1). The reason for the higher excretion of creatinine per kilogram of body weight in adolescent boys compared with adolescent girls is that they have an increase in muscle mass.

Creatinine and BUN reflect glomerular filtration and remain as standard techniques for estimating GFR. The blood creatinine values are related to the production of creatinine, which is relatively constant. Therefore acute interruptions in renal function may not be reflected immediately in an elevated creatinine value—rather it may take a period of 8 to 24 hours for the creatinine to begin to rise, depending upon the degree of impairment of glomerular filtration. Normal values based on age are shown in Table 9-1. The serum creatinine of the newborn is a direct reflection of the mother's creatinine level but by the age of 1 month drops to normal levels of approximately 0.2 mg/dl. It slowly increases to mature values by age approximately 16 to 20 years. It should be remembered that it takes a 50 percent or greater decrease in GFR to cause an increase in serum creatinine.

**Glomerular Filtration Rate.** The GFR is usually expressed in terms of ml/min/1.73 $m^2$. Using this value it takes until approximately the first year of life for an infant's glomerular function to achieve what has been termed the mature levels. However, when considered in terms of milliliters per minute per kilogram of body weight, then the levels of maturity are arrived at more quickly.

**Tubular Function.** Urine specific gravity is a good indicator of tubular function. FE-Na has also been used as an indicator of tubular function. Urine specific gravity is directly related to concentrating ability, which is directly related to the creation of a hypertonic medullary interstitium by the presence of urea. This takes several weeks to develop in the normal infant, but by a month or so the infant is able to concentrate urine relatively efficiently. In the mature state, the ability to concentrate the urine specific gravity above 1.018 after an overnight fast reflects relatively normal tubular function.

## Radioisotopes

Of more interest in recent years has been the use of various imaging techniques in order to study renal function. The use of the isotope technetium-99m to estimate renal perfusion has been an important advance in the assessment of renal perfusion and GFR in young infants and toddlers. The individual rates of renal perfusion can be established separately for each kidney and hence can be a reflection of the GFR of each kidney.

## Evaluation of Dehydration and/or Hypovolemia

The medical and/or surgical problems that are causing dehydration and/or hypovolemia may occur over varying time periods. The problem may be one that develops over a period of several days, and the course of dehydration will proceed through a period of decreased output followed by the development of the clinical picture of dehydration and hypovolemia (see Table 9-2 for the clinical findings ac-

**Table 9-2.** Degree of Dehydration (Reduction of Extracellular Fluid)

| *Clinical Findings* | *Mild* | *Moderate* | *Severe* |
|---|---|---|---|
| Body weight | 5% ↓ | 10% ↓ | 15% ↓ |
| Skin turgor | ↓ | ↓ ↓ | ↓ ↓ ↓ |
| Mucous membranes | Dry | Very dry | Parched |
| Urine | Reduced | Oliguria | Marked oliguria and azotemia |
| Blood pressure | Normal | ± Normal | Reduced |
| Pulse | Normal | ↑ | ↑ ↑ |

companying varying degrees of slowly developing hypovolemia). The problem may be one that develops acutely over a matter of hours. In this case, the acute loss of circulating blood volume and/or other body fluids may result in rather dramatic changes in the circulation, which may manifest in orthostatic hypotension, tachycardia, or hypotension. The history and physical findings will then depend upon the acuteness of the fluid loss and the body's compensatory mechanisms.

The history-taking and physical examination of a child with dehydration and/or hypovolemia are directed to the presence of vomiting and/or diarrhea, bleeding, lethargy, pallor, and orthostatic hypotension. There may be a decrease in urine output following decreased oral intake, as well as discolored urine (i.e., hematuria, myoglobinuria). The physical examination will depend upon the degree of dehydration, as suggested in Table 9-2.

**Laboratory Findings in Dehydration.** In the face of untreated dehydration, the usual findings are those of an increasing urine specific gravity, and a decreasing urine sodium. There is hemoconcentration, which will result in normal electrolyte values, a slightly elevated urea and creatinine, and an increased hematocrit. Fluid therapy to correct the dehydration may or may not correct the laboratory and/or physical abnormalities unless it is appropriate for the fluid being lost. As an example, an infant with duodenal atresia, who has had several days of vomiting and losing isotonic fluid (i.e., gastric juice mixed with bile) and who receives replacement with a hypotonic solution such as quarter-strength saline, may well develop acute hyponatremia with lethargy, convulsions, and potential CNS damage. The creatinine usually rises very slowly with dehydration since the creatinine levels usually reflect the amount of creatinine produced in addition to the baseline blood creatinine values. Very little creatinine is excreted daily, and because of this lack of excretion, dehydration will have a relatively small effect on the blood level. On the other hand, the BUN will rise more rapidly with dehydration, since there is a greater daily excretion of urea relative to creatinine. Therefore, in this situation, the BUN is a better reflection of the state of hydration than is the creatinine. The BUN level will respond more rapidly to rehydration than will the creatinine level.

## RENAL DISEASE IN NEONATES

Renal disease in neonates can be arbitrarily divided into two major categories, congenital and acquired.[15–18]

## Congenital Renal Disease

Examples of congenital disease are renal malformations, such as renal agenesis, polycystic kidneys, Wilms tumor, and the various obstructive disorders of the urinary tract. It has been reported that 10 percent of all infants are born with some anomaly of the genitourinary tract (kidney, ureters, urethra, bladder, and the genital system).[19] This figure represents about 30 percent of all congenital malformations. Since the placenta of the mother has acted as a hemodialysis unit for the fetus, it takes several days for conditions involving abnormal renal function to become evident.

## Nonrenal Causes of Acquired Renal Disease

There are three major categories of acquired renal disease: (1) birth asphyxia; (2) neonatal medical illnesses that cause hypoxia and/or hypotension; and (3) drugs. The primary etiology of the renal disease in the former two conditions is varying degrees of hypoxia of the kidney. The hypoxia may be due to ventilatory insufficiency or to reduced blood flow to the kidney either because of thrombosis or hypotension that may be the result of a number of causes. The disease that ensues may be transitory renal failure, which can be handled conservatively, or permanent renal failure requiring peritoneal or hemodialysis and ultimately renal transplantation. Renal failure in the neonate may present as a decrease in urinary output, the development of edema, weight gain, or abnormal urinalysis or blood chemistries. A rising serum creatinine is highly suggestive of renal disease.

Examples of neonatal disorders that can cause acquired renal disease due to hypoxia and/or hypotension are respiratory failure, sepsis, and heart failure. Indomethacin is an example of a drug that can magnify or cause renal disease. Indomethacin, which is used to close a patent ductus arteriosus, can also lead to a reduction in renal blood flow, which can cause various perturbations of renal function. This type of renal disease is almost always temporary and reversible.

## Mortality and Morbidity in Infants with Acute Renal Failure

Acute renal failure is a severe deterioration in renal function that leads to a disturbance in the homeostasis in fluid, electrolyte, and acid base status of the infant. It is characterized biochemically by an increase in creatinine and BUN concentrations. It should be remembered, however, that a high BUN can also be seen in several states such as high protein intake, tissue necrosis, sequestered bleeding (i.e., GI tract), and hypercatabolic states. The mortality rate of acute renal failure in neonates is on the order of 70 percent.[17] Parenchymal renal disease in the infant will result in abnormalities in the urinalysis, proteinuria, hematuria, and an elevated urinary sodium due to an increase in the fractional excretion of sodium, as well as biochemical abnormalities in the blood. Urinary sodium increases occur because a damaged tubule cannot resorb sodium effectively.

Treatment of acute renal failure in neonates has progressed rapidly in the last several years; nevertheless, the incidence of residual renal disease is high (approaching 50 percent). Therefore any patient with a history of renal failure as an infant must have the renal status evaluated, with at least a serum creatinine, in order to determine if there is any residual renal disease. If the child has been followed for a period of 6 months or more and the serum creatinine and renal function have stabilized, no additional tests are required for elective surgery. However, in case of emergency surgery, it may be useful to document the state of preoperative renal function since there may be a perioperative decrement in renal function. The problems of hyperkalemia and those relating to the various forms of dialysis will be discussed later.

## RENAL DISEASE IN OLDER INFANTS AND CHILDREN

### Hemolytic-Uremic Syndrome

Hemolytic-uremic syndrome is beginning to be recognized as the most common cause of acute renal failure in childhood.[20,21] This syndrome is characterized by a prodrome of gastroenteritis and hemorrhagic colitis. In one study, diarrhea was present in 95 percent, bloody diarrhea in 74 percent, vomiting in 67 percent, fever in 32 percent, and seizures in 10 percent of patients.[22] The gastrointestinal prodrome is followed several days later by the triad of the hemolytic-uremic syndrome, consisting of a microangiopathic hemolytic anemia, thrombocytopenia, and acute nephropathy. The disease mainly occurs between the ages of 6 months and 5 years but affects children through the teenage years. It also appears to be slightly more frequent in girls. Multiorgan involvement can occur. Some patients demonstrate central nervous system (CNS) dysfunction characterized by seizures, coma, and occasionally cerebral infarction with secondary hemiparesis. The mortality rate approximates 3 percent. The causes of mortality include pulmonary hemorrhage, acute respiratory insufficiency, sudden cardiac arrest, and cerebral edema with increased intracranial pressure. In one study, 16 percent had seizures after admission to the hospital. Approximately 40 to 45 percent of the children will require dialysis.

A recent study in Canada documented a strong association of hemolytic-uremic syndrome with *Escherichia coli* 0157:H7 infection.[22] There was a higher incidence in the summer, and regional differences were discovered. The major sources of the *E. coli* were thought to be either rare or undercooked beef and through person-to-person spread. Severe renal failure or death correlated with certain risk factors: shorter, more severe prodromal period, CNS symptoms at admission, and either oliguria exceeding 15 days or anuria lasting longer than 8 days. Oliguria or anuria always led to chronic disease. Of interest was the fact that even in the absence of oliguria or anuria some children still developed chronic renal disease.

The anesthesiologist may become involved with a hemolytic-uremic syndrome patient either during the acute presentation of the syndrome or at a later date. Some of these children may require access for urgent peritoneal or hemodialysis because of renal failure, or they may have an acute surgical emergency. At a later date, the child may present for surgery with a known past history of the syndrome. It should be recognized that a complete recovery can only be determined through laboratory studies. There is quite a significant incidence of chronic problems persisting after an apparently normal recovery. In one study in which 18 percent originally presented with hypertension as part of the syndrome, 5 percent had residual hypertension, which is often associated with proteinuria and a low creatinine clearance. In a group of 61 patients who were studied an average of 6.6 years after disease occurrence, 39 percent had one or more abnormalities such as proteinuria, a decreased creatinine clearance, and/or hypertension.[21] The residual pathophysiology in the kidney appears to be glomerulosclerosis, which results in a progressive loss of nephrons. There is a compensatory enlargement of the surviving glomeruli, which may result in hyperfiltration with proteinuria. It is not clear whether the hyperperfusion and proteinuria may cause more sclerosis of the nephrons. Some of these children have a loss of kidney function progressing to end-stage renal disease needing dialysis and/or transplantation. These patients need a serum creatinine to determine if there is any residual renal disease.

## Vesicoureteral Reflux

One of the most frequent urologic conditions in infancy and childhood is vesicoureteral reflux. A relationship has long been suspected between this condition and the development of hypertension and end-stage renal disease. However, there are no good studies that clearly delineate this association. In one recent review of the literature, the severe methodologic limitations of the available studies were clearly defined.[23] The anesthesiologist should be aware that the incidence of hypertension in vesicoureteral reflux may range up to 38 percent, whereas the incidence in the general pediatric population is less than 2 percent. This means that in the perioperative evaluation of these children, careful attention must be paid to the blood pressure measurements and if any degree of perioperative hypertension occurs, this certainly needs to be followed up by the pediatrician. The issue is not so much what to do about the blood pressure during the perioperative period but the long-term consequences of hypertension.

## Glomerulonephritis

Glomerulonephritis is a disease in which inflammation and proliferation of cells within the glomerulus are the major pathologic findings. It may occur as a primary disease or secondary to a systemic disorder such as systemic lupus erythematosus, diabetes mellitus, or sickle cell anemia. The etiology of the glomerular injury may be by immune or nonimmune mechanisms. The immune complex-related glomerular injury is the most common form of glomerulonephritis in children, and its most frequent cause is streptococcal infection with a group A hemolytic *Streptococcus*, followed by IgA nephropathy, idiopathic membranous glomerulopathy, and membranoproliferative glomerulonephritis. The major evidence of damage to the glomerular capillary filter mechanism is proteinuria, but the patients may also develop hematuria. The result varies from very mild changes to a frank nephrotic syndrome, with hypoalbuminemia, hypertension, and impaired renal function. Poststreptococcal acute glomerulonephritis may be confused with chronic glomerulonephritis with an acute infectious component.

The aspect of acute glomerulonephritis that is of concern to the anesthesiologist should emergency surgery be necessary is the potential for hypertension and hypervolemia due to a reduction in renal function with fluid retention.

For the vast majority of patients with acute glomerulonephritis, symptoms and blood pressure will normalize within 1 month, while it may take up to 6 to 12 months for the abnormal urinary findings to resolve completely. In the case of poststreptococcal acute glomerulonephritis, it is difficult to be specific about long-term prognosis because it may be hard to differentiate a child with this conditions from a child with underlying chronic renal disease plus an acute infection. In general, the prognosis for the condition is good; greater than 90 percent of patients should recover without any significant alteration in renal function. Unfortunately, however, 0.5 to 2 percent may progress rapidly to end-stage renal disease within weeks or months.[24] The remainder develop chronic stable renal disease.

## Nephrotic Syndrome

Persistent or progressive glomerular injuries in children may lead to nephrotic syndrome, which is a heterogeneous group of glomerular diseases characterized by massive proteinuria, hypoalbuminemia, edema, and hyperlipidemia. Approximately 65 percent of children with the nephrotic syndrome present between the ages of 1 to 5 years, with the vast majority contracting the illness before the age of 10 years. The majority of cases are due to what has been called "minimal change nephrotic syndrome," referring to a pathologic characteristic of the disease (no abnormality of the glomerular tuft by light microscopy). The remainder of the causes are listed in Table 9-3. The occasional patient will present with acute renal failure. Management of this situation will be discussed later. Occasionally, the severe hypoproteinemia leads to severe edema or anasarca with symptoms of respiratory insufficiency and hypotension. The most frequent cause of death in patients with the primary nephrotic syndrome is infection.

**Table 9-3.** Classification of Nephrotic Syndrome

| *Lesion* | *Approximate Incidence (%)* |
|---|---|
| Minimal change nephrotic syndrome | 75 |
| Membranoproliferative glomerulonephritis | 6 |
| Other proliferative glomerulonephritis | 5 |
| Congenital nephrotic syndrome | 1.5 |
| Other causes | 13.5 |

The current principal therapy in primary and chronic nephrotic syndrome is the use of steroids. Patients are treated with 1 to 2 mg/kg of prednisone on alternate days until the urine clears of protein and then for several weeks thereafter. There are many other treatment modalities at the present time. Occasional patients with minimal change nephrotic syndrome may prove to be resistant to corticosteroids and therefore the cytotoxic alkylating agents cyclophosphamide and chlorambucil are added to control the disease. These drugs are not considered as effective for the other types of nephrosis. The most frequent side effects of steroids are hypertension, slowed growth, infection, GI hemorrhage, osteoporosis, and adrenal suppression. The major effects of the cytotoxic drugs are secondary to bone marrow depression and include infections and GI irritation.

### Congenital Nephrotic Syndrome

Congenital nephrotic syndrome refers to a heterogenous group of diseases, either primary or secondary, that cause symptoms in the first months of life. Affected infants may develop edema, and the urinalysis will demonstrate proteinuria. The etiology may include primary renal disease such as minimal change nephrotic syndrome, but it may also include such secondary diseases as Wilms tumor and nephroblastoma.

### Outcome of Primary Nephrotic Syndrome

The prognosis for patients with primary nephrotic syndrome varies with both the etiology and the initial response to treatment. The best outcome follows minimal change nephrotic syndrome; complete remission may occur in up to 60 percent of patients. The short- and long-term prognosis in patients whose nephrotic syndrome is due to other etiologic factors is less favorable. The death rate in primary nephrotic syndrome has been reported to be as high as 20 percent, and there is a fairly high incidence of persistent proteinuria, continuing relapses, and renal failure.

## Flank Masses

During the neonatal period, flank masses are most commonly due to a unilateral multicystic kidney or congenital hydronephrosis secondary to an obstructed ureter.[25,26] The usual treatment for unilateral multicystic kidney is removal to prevent problems of infection. However, with a hydronephrotic kidney, even if there is considerable hydronephrosis, a conservative form of therapy is usually indicated. Hydronephrosis with infection usually presents with fever.

The two most common solid intraabdominal malignant tumors in childhood are neuroblastoma and nephroblastoma (Wilms tumor), with the latter being the more common. Patients with flank masses may also present with other findings such as hypertension, anemia, renal failure, and so forth. Hypertension may occur with neuroblastoma as well as nephroblastoma. There is an enormous variability in the size of a Wilms tumor, from a small unilateral tumor to bilateral tumors extending into the aorta and inferior vena cava with metastasis in the brain, lung, and liver. The evaluation of these patients requires computed tomography (CT) and/or magnetic resonance imaging (MRI) in order to determine the extent of the involvement. This will determine the extent of operation required as well as the anesthetic technique. There has been a concern that children who have a unilateral nephrectomy as part of the treatment for Wilms tumor may develop a decrease in renal function secondary to the long-term consequences of glomerular hyperfiltration. However, a recent 15-year followup study in a group of 12 survivors of Wilms tumor demonstrated no evidence of a glomerular hyperfiltration injury.[26]

## Diabetes and Renal Disease

Insulin-dependent (type 1) diabetes mellitus is the most frequent endocrine disease of children. Because of its frequency and the severity of the disease process, it has the highest morbidity and mortality of any of the pediatric endocrine diseases. A major complication of insulin-dependent diabetes is diabetic glomerulopathy, also known as diabetic nephropathy.[27,28] Diabetic nephropathy usually begins within 10 years of the onset of the disease, and eventually 30 to 50 percent of diabetics will be afflicted with nephropathy. All diabetics will eventually have abnormalities of glomerular function, but the progressive form only develops in 30 to 50 percent. This diabetic nephropathy is responsible for 25 to 30 percent of all new cases of end-stage renal disease in adults. It is usually characterized by three stages. The first stage is a occult process that cannot be diagnosed by conventional laboratory methods and is characterized by an elevation of the GFR and an increase in renal plasma flow. This glomerular hyperfiltration is accompanied by an increase in urinary albumin excretion, from 15 to 50 μg, which is less than that detectable by conventional techniques. This first stage usually lasts approximately 10 years. Two subsequent clinically demonstrable stages of progressively severe glomerular injury then follow, which usually terminate in renal failure. Stage II is intermediate and is characterized by the development of a proteinuria that can become considerable. During this stage, there is a declining GFR and the development of hypertension and edema. Stage III is advanced and represents the terminal 2 or 3 years of what is typically a 20- to 25-year process.

There has long been a theory that there is a relationship between hyperglycemia and the development of the complications of diabetes. Recent evidence strongly suggests that the nephropathy as well as diabetic retinopathy are related to poor glucose control.[27] One of the first signs of diabetic nephropathy is the presence of proteinuria. This proteinuria has prognostic significance, since 50 to 80 percent of diabetic patients with persistent proteinuria will develop end-stage renal disease within 10 years. One of the problems with testing for proteinuria is that many of the tests for proteinuria only determine protein when it appears in quantities of 0.3 to 0.5 g/24 h. However, by the time this degree of persistent proteinuria is present, little can be done either to reverse the nephropathy or prevent is relentless progression. Recent studies in children have evaluated the relationship of small amounts of albumin in the urine to blood glucose control.[27,28] The laboratory values evaluated were glycosylated hemoglobin ($HBA_1C$) and albumin excretion rate (AER), measured by a radioimmunoassay for albumin. The AER is expressed as a Ualb/Ucr ratio (milligrams of albumin to grams of creatinine). Normal amounts of albumin in the urine are up to 20 to 40 mg/24 h. Higher levels have been shown to be associated with a progression of diabetic nephropathy. Most of the recent studies that compared the mean glycosylated hemoglobin and albuminuria have found that lower glycosylated hemoglobin levels correlated with a lower albumin and decreased incidence in the frequency of nephropathy. One of the mechanisms that may link hyperglycemia to diabetic complications is the glycosylation of the various proteins of the body. Proteins can be nonenzymatically glycosylated, the degree of this glycosylation being directly related to the degree of hyperglycemia. This process is a direct reflection of the average glucose concentration to which the protein (e.g., in the red blood cell) is exposed throughout its life span. Glycosylation occurs on a continuous basis within the red blood cell and results in hemoglobin A being converted to hemoglobin $A_1C$. Early studies do not prove that there is a cause-and-effect relationship between hyperglycemia and nephropathy but do suggest that better control of blood glucose levels as reflected in maintaining hemoglobin $A_1C$ values at no more than 9 percent (1.5 times the upper limit of normal) may delay the onset of and/or decrease the likelihood of development of nephropathy.

## ACUTE AND CHRONIC RENAL FAILURE

There is little difference between acute and chronic renal failure in the effects on fluid volume, electrolyte concentrations, and hypertension. However, chronic renal failure is characterized by the presence of uremia, defined as the accumulation of nitrogenous waste products in the blood, plus a symptom complex that results from the failure of various organ systems. Children with chronic renal failure may have various combinations of organ failure or dysfunction including anemia, osteodystrophy, peripheral neuropathy, cardiac dysfunction, and uremic pneumonitis. Most will also have varying degrees of hypertension. In addition, pediatric patients, many because of their chronic problems, have some difficult psychosocial problems.

## Acute Renal Failure

Acute renal failure is a sudden decline in renal function due to rapid deterioration in the GFR and/or tubular function. The result is a disturbance in fluid and electrolyte homeostasis, possibly with hypertension, and at times disturbances of central nervous function with seizures. Acute renal failure results in the retention of nitrogenous wastes; usually there is an increase in both creatinine and BUN. It should be recognized, however, that the BUN may also be elevated in hypercatabolic states, high protein intake, tissue necrosis, and GI bleeding. Therefore the main blood chemical value used to assess renal function is the creatinine level. It should be recognized that acute renal failure can occur in a background of chronic renal failure so that the previous baseline creatinine value may also be elevated. Serum creatinine values change dramatically in the neonatal period and vary during the rest of the infant and child's life, so there is no one value of creatinine normal for all ages (see Table 9-1).

### Oliguric and Nonoliguric Acute Renal Failure

A broad definition of oliguria is less than 1 ml/kg of urine output per day. Normal urine output or even polyuria may occur in acute renal failure. As a matter of fact, approximately 50 percent of adult and pediatric cases will be nonoliguric; although the urine output is normal, there is a decrease in kidney function as evidence by a steadily increasing creatinine and BUN. Aminoglycoside toxicity, for example, may cause renal tubular dysfunction, which will result in polyuria. Acute tubular necrosis is also characterized by a diuretic phase.

### Classification of Acute Renal Failure

Renal failure can be classified as follows: (1) prerenal, (2) intrinsic, and (3) postrenal.[29] Prerenal acute renal failure is due to reduced perfusion of the kidneys, through cardiac failure, hypovolemia, or hypoxia leading to decreased cardiac output. The end result of decreased renal blood flow is reduced oxygen delivery resulting in kidney damage. Patients with prerenal acute renal failure usually present with oliguria; this disorder may be rapidly reversed with correction of the circulatory and/or hypoxic conditions. Intrinsic renal failure results when the kidney has sustained sufficient primary glomerular or tubular damage to alter renal function. The causes of the damage may be either infectious or immunologic or may be the result of prolonged ischemia, which results in acute tubular necrosis, one of the leading causes of intrinsic renal failure. Severe asphyxia, septic and hemorrhagic shock, and disseminated intravascular coagulation are major causes of glomerular damage, which is characterized by proteinuria. Postrenal failure is generally due to obstruction of the urinary tract and in the infant may be due to such causes as posterior urethral valves.

## Chronic Renal Failure

The first stage of chronic renal failure is that of decreased reserve, representing a loss of 50 to 60 percent of renal function (Table 9-4). It is evident that the serum creatinine levels used to determine this stage are age dependent and therefore, unlike decreased reserve in adults, no absolute number can be given. The patient has no renal symptoms, and the diagnosis may be made incidentally. Renal insufficiency is the next stage, with loss of function between 80 and 90 percent and a GFR of 25 to 50 percent. There is a loss

**Table 9-4.** Stages of Chronic Renal Failure

| *Stage* | *Creatinine Levels* | *Glomerular Filtration Rate* |
|---|---|---|
| 1. Decreased reserve | < 2 | > 50 |
| 2. Renal insufficiency | 2–8 | 25–50 |
| 3. Renal failure | 8–20 | 10–25 |
| 4. Uremia | > 20 | < 10 |

of the urinary concentrating ability and the appearance of azotemia and anemia. The final stage is renal failure, with less than 10 percent of normal renal function; patients have symptoms of progressive azotemia, anemia, acidosis, and fluid imbalance. Those patients with uremia may have progressive CNS dysfunction.

Thus chronic renal failure is a spectrum of disease that results in a chronic elevation of creatinine. Remember that it takes at least a 50 percent decrease in renal function to result in a doubling of the serum creatinine. At one end of this disease spectrum is the child whose only finding is an elevated serum creatinine, with no systemic manifestations of illness. At the other end is the child with end-stage renal disease and multisystem involvement, possibly terminating in death. It is evident that chronic renal disease (which may be mild and static) and chronic renal failure (which may be progressive and fatal) are not the same thing, although they are potentially interrelated.

## Medical Management of Renal Failure

It is important for the anesthesiologist to understand not only the pathophysiology of the development of renal failure but also its medical management.

### Medical Complications

The major complications of renal failure are alterations in the extracellular fluid volume, characterized by problems with either hypo- or hypervolemia. Alterations in serum electrolyte levels are characterized by hyperkalemia, hyponatremia, and hypocalcemia; and derangements of acid–base balance occur, usually in the form of metabolic acidosis. There may be disturbance of the central nervous system, either because of the acute uremic syndrome or secondary to the hypertension that may accompany acute renal failure. The anesthesiologist may become involved in the care of a patient with acute renal failure because of a need for access for peritoneal or vascular dialysis or because of an acute surgical problem. Usually, if the patient presents with an acute medical problem, and if dialysis has recently been completed, the electrolytes will be within the normal range but the patient will be relatively hypovolemic. On the other hand, if the patient has an acute surgical problem and dialysis cannot be accomplished before the surgical procedure must be undertaken, it is safer to assume that the patient is hypervolemic. Following the patient's recent and current weight will help to establish which problem may face the anesthesiologist.

**Hyperkalemia.** Hyperkalemia is the most frequent electrolyte abnormality in acute and chronic renal failure, resulting from a reduction in the elimination of potassium. Hyperkalemia causes peaked T waves on the electroencephalogram (ECG). The treatment for hyperkalemia depends upon the severity of the disturbance and the resulting symptomatology. Severe hyperkalemia, with cardiovascular dysfunction characterized by peaked T waves, may progress at times to complete circulatory collapse. The acute treatment would be a β-agonist such as epinephrine, which will rapidly shift potassium into the cells. Other drugs that will cause the immediate shift of potassium into cells or antagonize the effects of potassium include sodium bicarbonate and calcium. Glucose and insulin take at least 30 minutes to become effective, but may be appropriate to treat a less acute hyperkalemic state. Glucose should not be given in the face of hypoxia because of the known augmentation of central nervous system damage when glucose is administered in the hypoxic state.[30,31]

**Hyponatremia.** As part of the dietary and fluid management of the patient with renal failure, the admonition to reduce or avoid sodium is often given. The fear that sodium administration will result in fluid overload has caused some physicians to avoid or reduce the administration of sodium in surgical patients and to use a hypotonic solution such as $D_5W$ or $D_5/0.25$ percent NS, with the result that the patient develops a further dilutional hyponatremia. This type of acutely developing hyponatremia needs to be differentiated from chronic hyponatremia, which, in general, is not a serious problem. It is acute hyponatremia, occurring over 12 to 24 hours, that leads to the symptom complex of acute dilutional hyponatremia; central nervous system dysfunction characterized by vomiting, lethargy, and seizures; and the resulting potential for brain damage. Asymptomatic patients with hyponatremia do not need acute treatment; therapy for this condition should be gradual. On the other hand, acute *symptomatic* hyponatremia must be treated immediately with the use of hypertonic saline solution. The most readily available hypertonic saline solution is sodium bicarbonate, which is a 6 percent sodium solution. In the face of seizure activity due to acute hyponatremia, 1 to 2 ml/kg of sodium bicarbonate should be administered rapidly over a period of 1 to 2 minutes.

## Renal Control of Blood Pressure

The kidneys excrete and are affected by a whole host of hormones and enzymes that are vasoactive. As an example, renin is secreted by the kidney and activates the renin angiotensin aldosterone system. This system is responsible for the elaboration of various mineral corticoids and aldosterone, which then affect the sodium and water reabsorption by the kidney as well as the production of angiotensin II, an extremely potent vasoconstrictor. The kidneys also produce prostaglandins, some of which are vasodilators. The kidneys are in turn affected by various natriuretic factors that are important in the regulation of salt and water excretion by the kidney. The atrial natriuretic factor causes natriuresis by increasing glomerular filtration as well as inhibiting the tubular reabsorption of sodium. Many of the drugs that are used to treat the hypertension of renal disease are specifically aimed at these various hormones and enzymes in an attempt to control not only the vascular component of hypertension but also the regulation of sodium, potassium, and water by the kidney.

## Renal Disease and Hypertension

Hypertension is usually divided into two categories depending upon etiology.[32] In essential or primary hypertension, no specific etiology can be found. In secondary hypertension, the etiology can be identified. In children under 10 years of age, hypertension is usually due to renal disease; 70 percent of cases are due to renal parenchymal disease (e.g., pyelonephritis), and 10 percent are due to renal vascular disease. Other etiologies include endocrine disease and coarctation of the aorta or other cardiovascular disease. In teenage patients, there is a higher incidence of essential and obesity-associated hypertension.

In renovascular hypertension, the primary problem is either constriction of the renal artery or thrombosis of the renal vein. The hypertension is thought to be secondary to renin release. Renal parenchymal disease, the most frequent cause for hypertension in children, is also thought to be a renin-induced hypertension. The most frequent causes of parenchymal disease are the hemolytic uremic syndrome, chronic pyelonephritis, and chronic glomerulonephritis. Nephroblastoma, a tumor of renal origin, is thought to cause hypertension either by the direct production of renin or by the distortion of the renal vessels, leading secondarily to the release of renin. Hypertension due to catecholamine excess is found in pheochromocytoma, neuroblastoma, or ganglioneuroma. These tumors are usually associated with a symptom complex characterized by episodic headaches, sweating, nausea and vomiting, and visual disturbances.

The hypertension of acute renal failure is generally due to the retention of salt and water and can usually be controlled by dietary salt restriction and diuretics, but some patients may require either hemo- or peritoneal dialysis. Infrequently, the hypertension is secondary to renin release from the damaged kidney (referred to as renin-dependent hypertension). Diet, medications, and surgery are used to control the hypertension.

## Medical Management of the Child with Renal Hypertension

The hypertension that occurs in association with renal disease can be arbitrarily divided into two major groups: (1) hypertension secondary to chronic renal insufficiency and/or renal vascular disease, and (2) hypertension in association with excess sodium and fluid retention developed by patients with end-stage renal disease. It is important to control such hypertension because it is thought that this condition may itself accelerate the progression of chronic renal insufficiency, probably by glomerulosclerosis caused by hyperperfusion of the remaining glomeruli. Figure 9-1 is a flow chart showing blood pressure control measures in chronic renal failure. For patients suffering from chronic renal insufficiency, the first step is dietary sodium restriction. The second step is diuretic therapy, and, if this is not effective, the use of angiotensin-converting enzyme inhibitors (ACEI). These drugs are cleared by the kidney, and elevated blood levels may occur. The other complication is that of hyperkalemia. It should be remembered that if the various steps in the treatment of the hypertension are unsuccessful and the hypertension remains refractory to all forms of medical therapy, then nephrectomy may be necessary to correct the problem.

In patients who are undergoing dialysis, one of the major steps in the control of hypertension is the removal of excess sodium and water. Some patients, however, do not respond and they require antihypertensive therapy. The first choice for this group are adrenergic blockers and vasodilators. The dilators may be either calcium channel blocking agents, hydralazine, or prazosin. When the hypertension still does not respond to dialysis and medications, it usually indicates excess renin release from the kidney; the next step is use of the ACEIs. As suggested for blood pressure control, after all other avenues have been explored, the last measure is nephrectomy.

Many children develop hypertension following renal transplantation; treat-

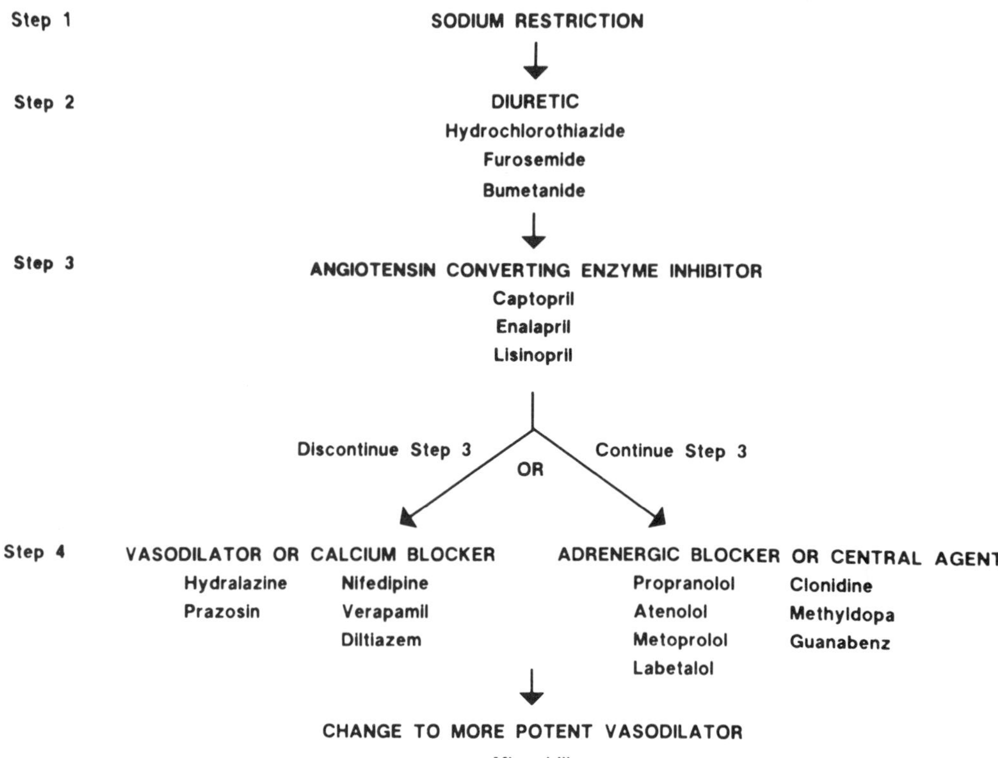


**Fig. 9-1.** Measures for controlling blood pressure in chronic renal failure. (From Hanna et al,[32] with permission).

ment will depend upon identification of the cause, which may be steroids, stenosis of the renal artery, acute rejection, hydronephrosis with obstruction, and so forth. Drugs used for the treatment of hypertension are listed in the Appendix with the various dosages and associated complications.

## Hemodialysis and Peritoneal Dialysis

It is estimated that approximately 500 children a year receive a renal transplant in North America. Although dialysis has been used to manage acute as well as chronic end-stage renal disease, renal transplantation is the definitive procedure for these patients. Two forms of dialysis are used to treat children with end-stage renal disease and prepare them for surgery, hemodialysis, and peritoneal dialysis. Both techniques can be carried out either in the hospital or as outpatients in the home, but it should be understood that neither form of dialysis will correct all aspects of chronic renal failure.

### Hemodialysis

Patients on chronic hemodialysis may have normal growth, but in general there is significant stunting of growth as well as a delay in puberty, often coupled with osteomalacia. Aluminum toxicity has been reported in patients with chronic renal failure,[33] in the form of bone disease as well as an encephalopathy. Aluminum toxicity has been reported in infants and children with impaired renal function whether or not they have been dialyzed. This may be related to oral phosphate binding therapy, which consists of large doses of aluminum compounds. In addition, many of these children are on vitamin D, which is known to increase intestinal absorption of aluminum. Patients who are on either peritoneal or hemodialysis may be at increased risk because of the aluminum content of the dialysis fluid.

Children with end-stage renal disease on hemodialysis are often anemic for several reasons. There is a continued small loss of blood with each dialysis, coupled with other metabolic derangements, including a decreased production of erythropoietin. Severe degrees of anemia with hemoglobins in the 6 to 9 range (Hct, 18 to 27 percent) may result.

Most of the hypertension in end-stage renal disease is due to salt and water overload so that the hypertension usually responds to dialysis. However, some of the patients have renin-dependent hypertension and therefore require bilateral nephrectomies in order to control the hypertension. Dialysis itself is not completely benign due to the need for vascular access as well as the dialysis process itself. Catastrophic events, such as cardiac arrest and pulmonary edema, may occur during dialysis.

## Peritoneal Dialysis

There have been remarkable advances in peritoneal dialysis over the last several years, including techniques of continuous ambulatory peritoneal dialysis and continuous cycling peritoneal dialysis. The advantage of continuous cycling peritoneal dialysis is that the major exchanges can occur overnight, with one long-time, daytime dwell left in the abdomen. This allows the child to attend school. One of the major problems with peritoneal dialysis is recurrent infection resulting in peritonitis, which can greatly decrease the effectiveness of the dialysis and is the major factor limiting the long-term success.

### Limitations of Peritoneal Dialysis

*Hypogammaglobulinemia.* Adults and older children undergoing peritoneal dialysis have normal levels of immunoglobulins. However, infants with uremia undergoing peritoneal dialysis have low levels of gammaglobulin. Peritoneal dialysis results in the loss of proteins through the peritoneal membrane, and these losses are relatively greater in infants less than 2 years of age than in older children and adults. A recent study suggested that in addition to the increased amounts of immunoglobulins lost through peritoneal dialysis, uremia suppresses immunoglobulin synthesis.[34] Infants in the study had a relatively high incidence of complications due to infection, and it was suggested that prophylactic immunoglobulin replacement therapy should be considered.

*Hypertension.* As with hemodialysis, most of the cases of hypertension can be controlled, but since peritoneal dialysis is not as effective as hemodialysis, more dietary restrictions are required. Patients with renin-dependent hypertension still require medication and occasionally bilateral nephrectomies in order to control the blood pressure.

*Anemia.* There is no loss of blood with peritoneal dialysis, and the problems of severe anemia are not as great as in hemodialysis, but there may be anemia due to the erythropoietin-suppressing effects of uremia.

*Growth and Bone Disease.* Growth is improved by peritoneal dialysis, but it is not normalized. Bone disease remains a major problem, as it is with hemodialysis.

Patients with end-stage renal disease are usually managed with some form of dialysis, as long as it is effective and the child can maintain reasonable degrees of growth and health. However, at some point renal transplantation needs to be considered. The current opinion is that the earlier the transplant is done, then the better the growth and overall health of the child.[35]

## Preoperative Assessment of the Child with End-Stage Renal Disease

Children scheduled for renal transplantation and other forms of surgery often have a complicated medical history due to the multiorgan system failure associated with end-stage renal disease. The child may have a while host of cardiovascular, pulmonary, and central as well as peripheral nervous system derangements, in addition to anemia.

### Anemia

Many patients with end-stage renal disease have varying degrees of anemia. The level of hemoglobin, depending upon dialysis and so forth, is usually from seven to ten. The cause of anemia in end-stage renal disease is thought to be multifactorial. The primary cause is considered to be a relative deficiency of erythropoietin. Erythropoietin is produced in the kidney and then circulates to the bone marrow where it interacts with membrane receptors on the erythroid progenitors, and thus regulates red blood cell formation. Other factors of importance include shortened red blood cell life span; such factors are considered secondary.

Many patients with hemoglobins below 9 to 10 who have symptoms of anemia are candidates for treatment with recombinant erythropoietin.[36] This drug has recently become available and has been quite successful in treating patients with the anemia of end-stage renal disease, generally by intravenous administration three times a week. As a result, the hemoglobin will usually be 10 to 12 g/dl. Other effects (most commonly the development of an iron-deficiency anemia) are not caused by the erythropoietin but by correction of the anemia. Such patients require preventative supplemental iron. The most worrisome side effect of erythropoietin is either the development or exacerbation of the hypertension. The mechanism is not clear; it is thought to be the result of improvement in the oxygen-carrying capacity of the blood, which results in a decrease in the elevated cardiac output and precipitates an increase in peripheral vascular resistance. Any child being treated with erythropoietin needs careful blood pressure monitoring in order to assess the effects of therapy. One other potential disadvantage is that some patients improve their appetite with correction of the anemia but do not improve renal function; hence dietary potassium intake has to be carefully evaluated. Erythropoietin is an expensive drug.

### Cardiovascular System

The circulation is usually hyperdynamic secondary to anemia, increased extracellular fluid volume resulting in increased cardiac output, and often arteriovenous shunting. These changes are frequently accompanied by a cardiomyopathy, congestive heart failure, accelerated atherosclerosis, and arrhythmias. In addition, of course, these patients may be hypertensive.

### Pulmonary System

There may be primary and secondary interference with the pulmonary system. The primary reason for difficulties within the pulmonary system is that hypertension and cardiomyopathy may result in varying degrees of congestive heart failure. In addition, patients who are chronically uremic may develop a uremic pneumonitis. The major cause for mortality in end-stage renal disease is infection, and these patients are susceptible to pulmonary infection.

### Central and Peripheral Nervous System

There may be disease in the central and peripheral nervous system secondary to the uremia or secondary to the condition that precipitated the end-stage renal disease (e.g., diabetes). In addition, there may be alterations within the autonomic nervous system. Signs and symptoms of CNS involvement may be due to psychological problems compounding central nervous system dysfunction and can result in personality and intellectual changes. In its most life-threatening form, CNS disease may result in seizure activity and coma.

### Other Blood Disorders

Some patients may have thrombocytopenia and platelet dysfunction secondary to the uremia. A small number of patients may have acquired serious infections due to their frequent need for transfusions. They may represent a health-care risk for the medical team since they may be infected with hepatitis B or acquired immunodeficiency syndrome (AIDS) virus. The electrolyte disorders have already been discussed previously; the major concern is that for hyperkalemia.

### Preoperative Dialysis

Patients with end-stage renal disease scheduled for surgery should have dialysis in the period prior to the surgery. It is usually the goal of dialysis to leave patients on the "dry side," with normal serum potassium levels, corrected acid–base balance, and a hemoglobin between 6 and 8. Any significant coagulopathy should be corrected at this time. The reason that leaving these patients on the "dry side" is a major problem for the anesthesiologist is that when this is coupled with the fear of oversalting and overhydrating renal failure patients, hypotension may follow the administration of anesthetic agents. This should be minimized by normalizing the extracellular fluid volume with an infusion of balanced salt solution.

### Steroid Therapy

Patients with renal disease and transplants usually have been or currently are on steroid regimens. At the present time, there is much controversy about the correct steroid supplementation. There are few objective studies on this issue but those that have appeared have demonstrated little relationship between the management of steroid therapy and development of perioperative hypotensive problems. The major concern should be to use the appropriate replacement fluid (i.e., balanced salt solution to maintain an appropriate intravascular volume). All replacement regimens are arbitrary. My current practice is to continue the patient on the usual daily dose of steroid, given orally early in the morning. It should be noted that the steroid overdosing that often occurs may result in hypertension.[37]

## THE CHILD WITH A KIDNEY TRANSPLANT

The major issue in evaluating the patient with a renal transplant is the level of function provided by the transplanted kidney. At one end of the spectrum is the child with a poorly functioning transplant who requires intermittent dialysis and at the other end of the spectrum, the child with a renal transplant with normal renal function. Many of these children are or have been on steroids, and the same caveats exist as were just discussed. One special caveat for patients with a renal transplant is that renal function depends upon adequate circulation. Many physicians maintain patients with marginal renal function on the "dry side" so they do not "overload" the renal system with sodium and water that may need to be dialyzed later. This may result in a relatively or actually hypovolemic patient who is more susceptible to hypotension, decreased cardiac output, and resulting decreased renal blood flow. Efforts need to be made to normalize the extracellular fluid volume status in these patients and to be quite generous in the administration of balanced salt solution in order to maintain a normal circulating blood volume and perfusion of the renal system.

## Renal Transplantation

There have been great improvements in renal transplantation in children since the late 1980s, particularly in the infant. In the not too distant past, renal transplantation below age 5 had a poor outcome and for this reason was discouraged. However, the current improvement in care has resulted in more and more transplants being done in the first year of life, with good results.[38]

## Growth and Development of Young Children Receiving Renal Transplants

It has been shown that children who develop renal failure and uremia before 1 year of age have a greater degree of developmental delay and CNS dysfunction when compared with children who develop uremia at a later age.[35] Although the more conservative management of dialysis allows these infants to continue to grow, they do so at the suboptimal rate, which results in delay of cognitive development and brain growth. For this reason, renal transplantation is encouraged in young infants in order to avoid the adverse effects of end-stage renal disease on the maturing brain. It is felt that the combined effects of uremia, malnutrition, and possibly aluminum toxicity are the responsible etiologic factors and that renal transplantation can eliminate these problems. A study of 37 children undergoing transplantation at or before 30 months of age demonstrated a postoperative improvement in psychomotor and mental development scores and an increase in occipital frontal circumference.[35] It would therefore appear that even though renal transplantation is technically more difficult in the younger infant, the trade-off of a better development of the uremic child may outweigh this increased risk.

## Seizures and Renal Transplantation

One of the perioperative concerns in patients with end-stage renal disease who are undergoing transplantation is the problem of seizure activity. In one review, 31 percent of children who received renal transplants had seizure activity either before or after transplantation.[39] It was of interest that of the children having seizure activity, 60 percent had only one seizure. In this particular study, hypertension was felt to be the most frequent etiologic factor. In 12 percent of the children who had seizure activity, the seizure was a manifestation of a serious underlying brain injury, and in this group there were serious neurologic sequelae. Therefore it would appear that in this group of patients close attention needs to be paid in the preoperative period to the control of blood pressure and that aggressive measures should be taken to treat any hypertensive episodes. When seizure activity was triggered by hypertension, there was little in the way of prodromal symptoms, such as headache, confusion, disorientation, visual disturbances, or lethargy.

## MISCELLANEOUS ISSUES

### Thyroid Function in Children with End-Stage Renal Disease

Since children with end-stage renal disease often have significant growth retardation, delayed bone age, and some of the clinical features as well as the biochemical changes compatible with hypothyroidism, there has been interest in determining whether or not these patients suffer from a primary disorder of thyroid function.[40,41] There are nonspecific clinical symptoms of hypothyroidism that are also found in chronic and end-stage renal disease. These include growth retardation, poor appetite, constipation, dry skin, and cold intolerance. Biochemical changes found in thyroid disorders have not been uniformly or consistently found in patients with end-stage renal disease, since end-stage renal disease and chronic renal failure have very complex effects that may be reflected in measurements of thyroid function. These patients in general are on a whole host of drugs such as immunosuppresants, antihypertensive medication, and so forth. In addition, the effects of uremia, malnutrition, and dietary protein restriction, as well as dialysis, may all affect thyroid measurements. At the present time, in spite of some biochemical studies suggesting the presence of hypothyroidism or evidence of hypothalamic-pituitary thyroid abnormalities, patients with end-stage renal disease have a normal metabolic state, which does not justify treatment with thyroid hormone.

### Association of Renal Disease with Severe Viral Infections

Renal disease has been reported to be associated with serious viral infections such as chronic hepatitis B as well as AIDS.[42,43] The first report of an association of membranous glomerulonephritis and chronic hepatitis B appeared in 1974. Membranous glomerulonephritis may either resolve spontaneously or progress to chronic nephrosis, which may in turn progress to end-stage renal disease. The association of renal disease with AIDS has long been recognized in the adult patient, in whom the incidence of end-stage renal disease varies up to 6 percent. A recent report of 164 children with AIDS documented the occurrence of the nephrotic syndrome in 15. The disease usually appears 1 to 2 years after the clinical appearance of AIDS. Twelve of the patients with nephrotic syndrome were treated with prednisone, but none responded. Three were treated with cyclosporine, and these three patients did go into remission. Three of the children with end-stage renal disease were treated with maintenance peritoneal dialysis with the hope of improvement of the quality of life.

### Renal Disease Associated with Nonsteroidal Antiinflammatory Drugs

The incidence of renal abnormalities related to the use of nonsteroidal antiinflammatory drugs is 1 to 2 percent in adult patients. The types of renal disease that these patients develop include the nephrotic syndrome, hypertension, and interstitial nephritis. In a recent study of children who had long-term treatment of juvenile rheumatoid arthritis, the incidence of renal disease was extremely low.[44] In a series of 226 children, only one child developed a urinary tract abnormality that could be directly related to the nonsteroidal antiinflammatory drugs. Another child had renal disease, but the association was uncertain. This is a much lower incidence than that reported in adults.

## Long-Term Parenteral Nutrition and Renal Function

It has been well recognized that long-term parenteral nutrition is associated with various clinical and biochemical abnormalities. Perhaps the most worrisome is that of hepatobiliary dysfunction. Other problems include metabolic bone disease. Recently a decrease in the GFR was described in children who had been on long-term total parenteral nutrition.[45] The decrease in GFR ranged from 20 to 50 percent, but was not enough to cause changes in either the serum creatinine or the BUN.

## REFERENCES


1. Gillenwater JY, Grayhack JT, Howards SS et al: Adult and Pediatric Urology. 2nd Ed. Mosby Year Book, St. Louis, 1987
2. Hagen PT, Scholz DG, Edwards WD: Incidence and size of patent foramen ovale during the first 10 decades of life: an autopsy study of 965 normal hearts. Mayo Clin Proc 59:17, 1984
3. Berry FA: The renal system. p. 93. In Gregory G (ed): Pediatric Anesthesia. 2nd Ed. Churchill Livingstone, New York, 1989
4. Bell EF, Warburton D, Stonestreet BS: Effect of fluid administration on the development of symptomatic patent ductus arteriosus and congestive heart failure in premature infants. N Engl J Med 302:598, 1980
5. Green TP, Thompson TR, Johnson D, Lock JE: Letter to the editor: fluid administration and the development of patent ductus arteriosus. N Engl J Med 303: 337, 1980
6. Berry FA: Practical aspects of fluid and electrolyte therapy. p. 89. In: Anesthetic Management of Difficult and Routine Pediatrics Patients. 2nd Ed. Churchill Livingstone, New York, 1990
7. Stoelting RK, Dierdorf SF: Renal disease. p. 289. In: Anesthesia and Co-Existing Disease. 3rd Ed. Churchill Livingstone, New York, 1993
8. Arbus GS, Farine M: Acute renal failure in children. p. 197. In Postlethwaite RJ (ed): Clinical Paediatric Nephrology. Wright, Bristol, 1986
9. Mitchell N, Stapleton FB: Routine admission urinalysis examination in pediatric patients: a poor value. Pediatrics 86: 345, 1990
10. Miller PFW, Speirs NI, Aparicio SR et al: Long term prognosis of recurrent haematuria. Arch Dis Child 60:420, 1985
11. Meadow SR: Haematuria. p. 26. In Postlethwaite RJ (ed): Clinical Paediatric Nephrology. Wright, Bristol, 1986
12. Houser MT: Characterization of proteinuria using random urine samples. Int J Pediatr Nephrol 7:197, 1986
13. Robson AM, Vehaskari VM: Proteinuria. p. 42. In Postlethwaite RJ (ed): Clinical Paediatric Nephrology. Wright, Bristol, 1986
14. Schwartz GJ, Gauthier B: A simple estimate of glomerular filtration rate in adolescent boys. J Pediatr 106:522, 1985
15. Dauber IM, Krauss AN, Symchych PS et al: Renal failure following perinatal anoxia. J Pediatr 88:851, 1976
16. Anand SK, Northway JD, Crussi FG: Acute renal failure in newborn infants. J Pediatr 92:985, 1978

17. Cepero-Akselrad AE, Ramirez-Siejas F, Castaneda AM et al: Acute renal failure in the newborn. Int Pediatr 5:328, 1990
18. Grylack L, Medani C, Hultzen C et al: Nonoliguric acute renal failure in the newborn: a prospective evaluation of diagnostic indexes. Am J Dis Child 136:518, 1982
19. Vaughan ED, Middleton GW: Pertinent genitourinary embryology: review for practicing urologist. Urology 6:139, 1975
20. Milford DV, White RHR, Taylor CM: Prognostic significance of proteinuria one year after onset of diarrhea-associated hemolytic-uremic syndrome. J Pediatr 1818: 191, 1991
21. Siegler RL, Milligan MK, Burningham TH et al: Long-term outcome and prognostic indicators in the hemolytic-uremic syndrome. J Pediatr 118:195, 1991
22. Rowe PC, Orrbine E, Wells GA et al: Epidemiology of hemolytic-uremic syndrome in Canadian children from 1986 to 1988. J Pediatr 119:218, 1991
23. Shanon A, Feldman W: Methodologic limitations in the literature on vesicoureteral reflux: a critical review. J Pediatr 117:171, 1990
24. Gill DG, Turner DR, Chantler C et al: The progression of acute proliferative post-streptococcal GN to severe epithelial crescent formation. Clin Nephrol 8:449, 1977
25. Raffensperger JG, Morgan ER: Renal masses. p. 347. In Raffensperger JG (ed): Swenson's Pediatric Surgery. 5th Ed. Appleton & Lange, East Norwalk, CT
26. Bhisitkul DM, Morgan ER, Vozar MA et al: Renal functional reserve in long-term survivors of unilateral Wilms tumor. J Pediatr 118:698, 1990
27. Roe TF, Costin G, Kaufman FR et al: Blood glucose control and albuminuria in type 1 diabetes mellitus. J Pediatr 119: 178, 1991
28. Travis LB: Editor's column—prevention of renal disease in insulin-dependent diabetes mellitus: a "responsibility" for the pediatrician? J Pediatr 119:273, 1991
29. Byrick RJ, Rose DK: Review article: pathophysiology and prevention of acute renal failure: the role of the anaesthetist. Can J Anaesth 37:457, 1990
30. Nakakimura K, Fleischer JE, Drummond JC: Glucose administration before cardiac arrest worsens neurologic outcome in cats. Anesthesiology 72:1005, 1990
31. Hoffman WE, Braucher E, Palligrino DA et al: Brain lactate and neurologic outcome following incomplete ischemia in fasted, nonfasted, and glucose-loaded rats. Anesthesiology 72:1045, 1990
32. Hanna JD, Chan JCM, Gill JR: Medical progress: hypertension and the kidney. J Pediatr 118:327, 1991
33. Wills MR, Savory J: Aluminum and chronic renal failure: sources, absorption, transport and toxicity. Crit Rev Clin Lab Sci 27:59, 107, 1989
34. Katz A, Kashtan CD, Greenberg LJ et al: Hypogammaglobulinemia in uremic infants receiving peritoneal dialysis. J Pediatr 117:258, 1990
35. David ID, Chang PN, Nevins TE: Successful renal transplantation accelerates development in young uremic children. Pediatr 86:594, 1990
36. Ad Hoc Committee for the National Kidney Foundation: Statement on the clinical use of recombinant erythropoietin in anemia of end-stage renal disease. Am J Kidney Dis XIV:163, 1989
37. Koch F: Anesthesia for the steroid-dependent child. p. 373. In Berry FA (ed): Anesthetic Management of Difficult and Routine Pediatric Patients. 2nd Ed. Churchill Livingstone, New York, 1990
38. Beebe DS, Belani KG, Mergens P et al: Anesthetic management of infants receiving an adult kidney transplant. Anesth Analg 73:725, 1991
39. McEnery PT, Nathan J, Bates SR et al: Convulsions in children undergoing renal transplantation. J Pediatr 115:532, 1989
40. LaFranchi S: Editor's column—thyroid function in children with chronic renal failure. J Pediatr 118:896, 1991
41. Pasqualini T, Zantleifer D, Balzaretti M et al: Evidence of hypothalamic-pituitary thyroid abnormalities in children with end-stage renal disease. J Pediatr 118: 873, 1991
42. Ingull E, Tejani A, Fikrig S et al: Nephrotic syndrome associated with ac-

quired immunodeficiency syndrome in children. J Pediatr 119:710, 1991

43. Jonas MM, Ragin L, Silva MO: Membranous glomerulonephritis and chronic persistent hepatitis B in a child: treatment with recombinant interferon alfa. J Pediatr 119:818, 1991
44. Szer IS, Goldstein-Schainberg C, Kurtin PS: Paucity of renal complications associated with nonsteroidal antiinflammatory drugs in children with chronic arthritis. J Pediatr 119:815, 1991
45. Moukarzel AA, Ament ME, Buchman A et al: Renal function of children receiving long-term parenteral nutrition. J Pediatr 119:864, 1991

# 10

# Special Considerations for the Pediatric Oncology Patient

# 10

# Special Considerations for the Pediatric Oncology Patient

*Joseph D. Tobias*

Despite a relatively low incidence overall, malignancies rank second to trauma as a cause of death in children. Long-term survival is now possible due to increased use of aggressive therapy with toxic agents. These advances in therapy have resulted in a new population of patients requiring frequent anesthetic care. The pediatric oncology patient may need care for relatively minor procedures such as central line placement, or for major operations aimed at total surgical excision or debulking of solid tumors. Cancer can occur at any age, and the anesthesiologist must provide for patients of varying age, weight, maturity, and clinical status. This chapter focuses on the impact of childhood malignancies and their therapy on the various organ systems.

## THE CARDIOVASCULAR SYSTEM

The cardiovascular system of the pediatric oncology patient may be affected by the disease process itself or by radiation or chemotherapy. Symptoms may manifest simply as an electrocardiographic disturbance or by significant alteration in function. Direct cardiac effects may occur with solid tumors of the anterior mediastinum, but disease-related problems occur more commonly with leukemias and lymphomas as a result of malignant pericardial effusions. Therapy is aimed at palliative treatment of the effusion by pericardiocentesis and institution of effective chemotherapy to halt disease progression. Conduction abnormalities may be related to myocardial infiltration by malignant cells.

A more common concern to the anesthesiologist is the cardiotoxicity of many of the chemotherapeutic agents. Although most frequently occurring with the anthracyclines (doxorubicin and daunorubicin), cardiac effects may also been seen with several other chemotherapeutic agents (Table 10-1). Chemotherapy-related effects may present early, during the infusion of the drug, or several months to years after cessation of therapy.

Doxorubicin (Adriamycin) and daunorubicin are the most commonly used anthracyclines and are components of the chemotherapeutic regimens for acute

**Table 10-1.** Chemotherapeutic Agents Associated with Cardiac Toxicity

| |
|---|
| Anthracyclines—doxorubicin, daunorubicin |
| Cyclophosphamide |
| 5-Fluorouracil |
| Amsacrine |
| Cisplatin |
| Mithramycin |
| Mitomycin C |
| Vincristine |
| Actinomycin D |

myelogenous leukemia, Hodgkin's lymphoma, and various solid tumors of childhood. Acute cardiovascular effects described during anthracycline infusion include disturbances in cardiac rhythm and conduction manifested by supraventricular tachycardia, premature ventricular contractions, and atrial tachyarrhythmias.[1,2] Although the majority of rhythm disturbances are transient and subside with a decrease in the infusion rate, sudden death has occurred during doxorubicin infusion.[3]

A second manifestation of acute anthracycline toxicity is a pericarditis-myocarditis syndrome[4] that affects patients without a previous history. Although pericarditis may be the sole manifestation, many patients will also have myocarditis. The myocardial damage may be severe, resulting in overt cardiac failure and death. Histologic examination reveals acute necrosis of myocardial cells. Both arrhythmias and the pericarditis-myocarditis syndrome occur acutely, during the infusion, and are not dose related. The third acute toxic effect of the anthracyclines is congestive cardiac failure. This finding is more common in patients with underlying cardiac dysfunction and occurs as a result of drug-induced, transient left ventricular depression that is not dose related.

Chronic congestive cardiac failure and subclinical left ventricular dysfunction may also occur following anthracycline administration. This phenomenon is dose related, occurring in as many as 25 percent of patients who receive cummulative doses exceeding 550 mg/m$^2$. Although chronic congestive cardiac failure is dose related, several additional factors may place the patient at an increased risk, and cardiac decomposition may then occur at a lower total dose (Table 10-2). Preoperative echocardiography is indicated in patients with these additional risk factors when smaller doses of anthracyclines have been administered.

The clinical signs and symptoms of anthracycline-induced cardiomyopathy may occur during therapy, but generally appear 1 to 6 months following cessation of therapy.[5] Recent reports have documented the onset of congestive cardiomyopathy 6 to 10 years following therapy.[6] This late-onset cardiomyopathy is thought to occur as a result of failure of myocardial growth to match somatic growth. In such patients, repeated echocardiography demonstrates no increase in left ventricular wall thickness despite increases in body surface area and weight. Therefore patients treated earlier in life

**Table 10-2.** Factors that Increase the Risk of Anthracycline Cardiotoxicity

1. Doses in excess of 550 mg/m$^2$
2. Preexisting myocardial dysfunction
3. Uncontrolled hypertension
4. Extremes of age (< 1 or > 70 years)
5. Mediastinal irradiation
6. Concurrent use of other chemotherapeutic agents
   - Cyclophosphamide
   - Cisplatin
   - 5-Fluorouracil
   - Vincristine
   - Actinomycin D
   - Mithramycin
   - Mitomycin C
   - Amsacrine
7. Other drugs
   - Propranolol
   - Calcium channel blockers

may be at risk for the development of congestive cardiomyopathy as they grow, due to the failure of myocardial growth to keep pace with somatic growth.

Regardless of the age of onset, clinical findings include those common to congestive failure of other etiologies and include tachycardia, cough, edema, orthopnea, and exertional dyspnea. There is dilated cardiomyopathy with biventricular enlargement, and the chest radiography reveals cardiomegaly and pulmonary edema. Histologic examination of the myocardium reveals a dilated sarcoplasmic reticulum with intracellular vacuolization and dropout of myofibrillar elements. Several possible mechanisms have been postulated for anthracycline-induced cardiotoxicity, including carnitine depletion, disruption of oxidative phosphorylation, calcium overload, free radical formation, and indirect effects through the release of vasoactive substances such as histamine or endogenous catecholamines.

Prevention of cardiotoxicity by periodic monitoring of cardiac function and by limitation of the total dose in patients with evidence of myocardial dysfunction is the objective, as there is no specific treatment. Once symptoms occur therapy is the same as for congestive failure of any etiology and includes cardiac glycosides, diuretics, and the judicious use of afterload reduction. In more severe cases, invasive monitoring and intravenous inotropic agents may be required. Despite aggressive therapy, mortality is high once symptoms occur and has been estimated to range from 30 to 60 percent.[7] Although left ventricular dysfunction generally progresses in adults, some recovery of function may occur in children, and therefore aggressive supportive care may be indicated.[8]

Several modalities are available for monitoring anthracycline cardiotoxicity, including electrocardiography, echocardiography, measurement of systolic time intervals, nuclear angiography, and cardiac catheterization with endomyocardial biopsy.

Electrocardiographic changes are relatively nonspecific and are late findings of anthracycline-induced cardiotoxicity. Findings such as decreased voltage are nonspecific and may occur with other disease processes such as pericardial effusion or myocarditis. Despite these restrictions, Bender et al[9] have suggested that the Q-T interval may be a relatively sensitive indicator of myocardial damage from the anthracyclines. They found that Q-T prolongation preceded the echocardiographic findings of myocardial dysfunction and suggested that routine electrocardiograms may be used to screen for anthracycline toxicity.

The principal test used for monitoring is echocardiography. Although relatively nonspecific (i.e., significant myocardial damage may occur prior to echocardiographic changes), the test is noninvasive and can be used serially to follow cardiac function. Once abnormalities occur on echocardiography, more complex tests such as nuclear angiography or endomyocardial biopsy may be indicated if further anthracycline administration is clinically indicated.

Without a doubt, the most sensitive measure of myocardial damage is endomyocardial biopsy. Bristow et al[10] demonstrated that histologic changes are linearly related to dose. The histologic changes are specific for anthracycline toxicity. However, in children this procedure is invasive, may require general anesthesia, and is associated with significant morbidity. Therefore its use is limited. Routine monitoring includes repeated echocardiography and consideration of more invasive tests (radionuclide angiography or endomyocardial biopsy) when the shortening fraction falls to less than 25 to 27 percent, especially if further use of anthracyclines is considered.

Aside from limitation of dose, prolonged continuous infusion rather than bolus dosing has been suggested as a means of limiting anthracycline toxicity.[11] Based on endomyocardial biopsies, Legha et al[11] found a significant reduction in histologic damage to myocardial cells in patients receiving continuous infusions when compared with bolus dosing of doxorubicin. These effects were noted without any change in clinical antitumor effects of the agent. Other methods of reducing anthracycline cardiotoxicity include the concomitant administration of agents (i.e., vitamin E) known to have free radical scavenging properties, but such reports are preliminary. New anthracycline compounds that lack cardiotoxicity are in phase I and II trials.

The anesthetic implications of anthracycline therapy are relatively straightforward. The anesthesiologist must know the cumulative dose administered and whether other "cardiotoxic" agents have been used, including radiation therapy. Preoperative echocardiography may serve to identify those patients with cardiac dysfunction who may require invasive hemodynamic monitoring. Invasive monitoring with a pulmonary artery catheter may be indicated in certain scenarios (Table 10-3). Aside from such monitoring, it has also been suggested that halothane be avoided,[12] based on the histologic findings of decreased numbers of β-adrenergic receptors on myocardial cells and the postulation that a hyperadrenergic state compensates for cardiac dysfunction in these patients. The blunting of this hyperadrenergic state by halothane is one mechanism proposed for intraoperative cardiac failure.[12]

**Table 10-3.** Indications for Invasive Monitoring in Patients Receiving Anthracyclines

| |
|---|
| Overt congestive cardiomyopathy |
| History of congestive cardiomyopathy |
| Significant alteration in function on preoperative echocardiography |
| Major surgical procedures in patients that have received large doses (250 μg/m² or 150 μg/m² if combined with mediastinal radiation) |

Although the anthracyclines have received the most attention as cardiotoxic agents, severe cardiovascular manifestations can also occur with other agents, including cyclophosphamide, cisplatin, amsacrine, and 5-fluorouracil (see Table 10-1). They are associated with acute cardiac disturbances and will also potentiate the cardiotoxicity of the anthracyclines. Cyclophosphamide-induced cardiac toxicity is manifested by acute congestive failure that is not dose related.[13] Electrocardiographic findings include loss of R-wave progression and ST-T wave changes. Histologic examination reveals hemorrhagic necrosis of cardiac cells.

In addition to the acute cardiovascular effects of the concomitant administration of cyclophosphamide and halothane, laboratory evidence suggests that effects of combining these drugs may be lethal.[14] Although no alterations in cyclophosphamide pharmacokinetics could be identified with the administration of halothane, the mortality in the animals receiving halothane and cyclophosphamide was significantly higher than the group receiving halothane alone. Histologic evaluation failed to reveal any morphologic reason for death. Despite the lack of hard evidence as to the mechanism responsible for the interaction of these two agents, it seems appropriate to avoid the administration of general anesthesia to patients receiving cyclophosphamide.

Three other potential cardiotoxic agents deserve special mention: 5-fluorouracil (5-FU), cisplatin, and amsacrine.

Although much of the evidence concerning the cardiotoxicity of these agents is anecdotal, the clinical significance cannot be ignored. 5-FU inhibits DNA synthesis through its incorporation into the tumor cell genome. Although most commonly used in solid tumors in the adult population, it is also used in some relatively uncommon malignancies of childhood such as carcinoma of the colon. The toxicity of 5-FU is not dose related and is manifested by acute myocardial ischemia with chest pain and electrocardiographic changes.[15] This toxicity occurs in 1 to 2 percent of patients and has a mortality rate of 10 to 15 percent. Possible mechanisms for the ischemia include coronary vasospasm, inhibition of myocardial cell DNA synthesis, and depletion of high-phosphate compounds. 5-FU is metabolized to fluorocitrate, which inhibits aconitase, an enzyme of the Krebs cycle, leading to citrate accumulation and depletion of high-energy phosphate compounds. In addition to the acute ischemic changes associated with 5-FU administration, acute cardiac failure has also been described.[16] Clinical manifestations include hypotension and cardiac failure occurring during 5-FU administration. These changes occurred without electrocardiographic evidence of ischemia or alterations in cardiac enzymes.

Anecdotal evidence also supports the potential cardiac toxicity of cisplatin.[17,18] Cardiac effects have included congestive failure, with electrocardiographic evidence of myocardial ischemia, myocarditis, and alterations in cardiac conduction (left bundle branch block). The exact cardiotoxic mechanism of cisplatin is difficult to define, as anecdotal reports have included patients who were receiving several different chemotherapeutic agents.

The most recently introduced agent associated with cardiotoxic effects is amsacrine (AMSA). AMSA is an acridine derivative that inhibits DNA synthesis, with activity in various hematologic and solid malignancies. The toxicity of this new agent is acute (both arrhythmias and congestive failure).[19] Arrhythmias have occurred during the infusion and have been both atrial and ventricular in origin. Ventricular premature beats and, more importantly, ventricular tachycardia and fibrillation have been reported. Acute congestive failure may also occur, especially in patients who have received previous doses of anthracyclines. In particular, patients who have received more than 400 mg/m$^2$ of anthracycline, those receiving more than 200 mg of AMSA, and those receiving a total dose of the two agents more than 900 mg/m$^2$ are at risk for cardiotoxicity.

Although the toxic effects of most chemotherapeutic agents relate to the direct effects of the drugs on cellular metabolism, other mechanisms may lead to cardiovascular compromise in the pediatric oncology patient. The epipodophyllotoxins (VM-26 and VP-16) are commonly used in a variety of pediatric malignancies including salvage therapy for treating hematologic relapse of acute lymphocytic leukemia. Although the major toxicity of these agents lies in their suppressive effects on the bone marrow, adverse reactions may also occur due to the solute vehicle involved. Both of these agents are insoluble in water and therefore are administered in an oil-based vehicle. Acute anaphylactic reactions with cardiorespiratory compromise may occur during administration. Because of the drugs' insolubility in water, they are administered as a dilute solution (1 mg/ml), the solubility of which is increased by the addition of ethyl alcohol. Although the dose of ethyl alcohol is generally low, the use of escalating doses of the epipodophyllotoxins, based on pharmacokinetic profiles, has resulted in acute ethanol intoxication, with cardiovascular compromise.[20]

Radiation therapy can also have significant adverse effects on the cardiac system, including alterations in both function and rhythm such as congestive failure, conduction block, pericarditis, and sick sinus syndrome.[21,22] Such effects are generally transient, but permanent alterations in conduction and potentiation of the toxic effects of various chemotherapeutic agents may occur with mediastinal irradiation.

## THE RESPIRATORY SYSTEM

Pulmonary dysfunction in the pediatric oncology patient may be related to the underlying disease and its complications, chemotherapeutic agents, and alterations accompanying surgical procedures. Leukemia and lymphoma may lead to the production of large pleural effusions, alveolar-capillary block due to leukemic infiltration, and leukostatic vascular obstruction as a result of severe elevations in white cell count. Chemotherapy and the primary disease process both place the patient at risk for pulmonary hemorrhage from bleeding diathesis, and there is the ever-present risk of infection due to opportunistic organisms.

A more common cause of mortality in the pediatric oncology patient is respiratory failure. Although this is commonly due to infection, chemotherapeutic agents may also have deleterious effects on the pulmonary system. Bleomycin causes pulmonary toxicity, which may be divided into acute and chronic forms. The chronic form of bleomycin toxicity is a progressive, restrictive disorder that presents with rales, dyspnea, and cough. Pulmonary function testing reveals restrictive disease with a decrease in diffusion capacity. Several predisposing factors for bleomycin toxicity have been described, including preexisting pulmonary disease, age over 70 years, total dose greater than 450 U/m$^2$, administration of other pulmonary toxic chemotherapeutic agents, and concurrent use of radiation therapy. Of these factors, total dose is the most consistent factor in the prediction of pulmonary toxicity; there is little risk (less than 3 percent) with doses less than 450 U/m$^2$ and an incidence of 10 to 15 percent in patients who have received 450 to 550 U/m$^2$.[23]

Of prime importance to the anesthesiologist is the acute toxicity of bleomycin, which presents as an exaggerated form of oxygen toxicity. Shortly after its introduction as a chemotherapeutic agent, Goldiner and Schweizer[24] described the development of adult respiratory distress syndrome following surgery in patients who had received bleomycin. Unlike the chronic toxicity, the acute toxicity is not dose related. The five patients described by Goldiner et al.[25] had received doses ranging from 135 to 595 U, with the last dose 6 to 12 months before surgery. The five patients were receiving chemotherapy for testicular cancer and developed adult respiratory distress syndrome (ARDS) following retroperitoneal node dissection. Based on this experience, Goldiner and associates altered their anesthetic care for the next 12 patients. They were matched for age, bleomycin dose, and preoperative pulmonary function status, and the inspired fraction of oxygen was maintained between 0.21 and 0.25 (in the previous five patients the inspired fraction of oxygen ranged from 0.35 to 0.42). All 12 survived. Based on these findings, Goldiner et al.[25] postulated that bleomycin predisposes patients to exaggerated oxygen toxicity, even with low inspired concentrations. It is also noteworthy that the survivors received less intraoperative fluid (3.87 ml/kg/h versus 5.86 ml/kg/h), and more of the fluid administered was colloid.

**Table 10-4.** Chemotherapeutic Agents Associated with Pulmonary Toxicity

| |
|---|
| Alkylating agents: busulfan, cyclophosphamide, chlorambucil |
| Azathioprine |
| Methotrexate |
| 6-Mercaptopurine |
| Cytosine arabinoside |
| Bleomycin |
| Mitomycin C |
| Nitrosureas: methyl CCNU, BCNU |
| Procarbazine |

The mechanism of the acute pulmonary toxicity related to bleomycin may involved free radical formation. Bleomycin complexes with iron and oxygen, leading to free radical formation. The quantity of free radical production and the cytotoxicity of bleomycin increases in the presence of increased oxygen concentration.[26] Additional factors that may increase the risk of acute respiratory failure following excess oxygen administration in bleomycin-treated patients include advanced age, smoking, and previous radiation therapy. Acute postoperative respiratory failure, similar to that seen with bleomycin, has been described following mitomycin C.[27]

Several other chemotherapeutic agents have been implicated as causative agents in respiratory dysfunction (Table 10-4). Regardless of age, the presentation of the chronic toxicity of chemotherapeutic agents is similar, with the development of a progressive, restrictive disorder with a nonspecific pneumonitis that progresses to pulmonary fibrosis.

One of the more common agents that may lead to pulmonary fibrosis is busulfan, an alkylating agent used in the treatment of myelogenous leukemias and in the preparatory regimens for bone marrow transplantation. Toxicity is dose related, and the disease generally progresses to respiratory failure and death despite discontinuation of the agent. Chronic restrictive lung disease has also been described with BCNU, methotrexate, and mitomycin C. Subtle differences exist between the toxicity of these agents. The toxic effects of methotrexate generally respond to corticosteroid treatment and discontinuation of therapy.

Although the pulmonary toxicity of chemotherapeutic agents is characteristically a chronic restrictive disorder, acute disturbances may also occur. In addition to its chronic toxic effects, high-dose methotrexate therapy also may cause chest pain due to an acute chemical pleuritis.[28] Noncardiogenic pulmonary edema has been described during cytosine arabinoside (ara-C) administration and following the combination of vinblastine and mitomycin.[29,30] Although the vinblastine-mitomycin C toxicity is anecdotal in two patients, Haupt et al.[30] have described their experience with ara-C-related pulmonary edema in 51 patients. Postulated mechanisms included a hypo-oncotic state related to gastrointestinal losses of albumin, direct toxic injury to the alveolar-capillary membrane, or a potentiating effect of other causes of noncardiogenic pulmonary edema (i.e., sepsis).

Recent advances in the treatment of various malignancies frequently include a multimodality approach (combination of chemotherapy and radiation therapy). Although such a combination often improves survival, radiation therapy can have deleterious effects on respiratory function. When radiation passes through cells, chemical bonds are disrupted and damage occurs to the DNA. If this damage is not repaired, cellular death occurs. Frequently dividing cells, including malignant cells, are particularly sensitive to radiation. However, normal constituents of the body that also divide frequently, including type II pneumocytes, are also damaged by the harmful effects of radiation.

Radiation pneumonitis occurs in an acute and a chronic phase. Clinical symptoms, which occur in about 10 percent of treated patients, are related to the dose of radiation, area of the lung field irradiated, and concomitant chemotherapy (e.g., dactinomycin[31]). The acute phase occurs 6 to 12 weeks following therapy, with the rapid onset of cough, fever, and dyspnea. Although usually self-limited, it may progress to respiratory failure. In such cases, high-dose corticosteroid therapy may halt the progression of the disease process. The chronic phase consists of a progressive, restrictive disorder occurring 6 to 12 months following therapy.

Another modality that may significantly impact on respiratory function is repeated thoracotomy for excision of the primary or metastatic disease. Repeated thoracotomy with resection of pulmonary tissue can lead to a significant impairment of pulmonary function, thereby increasing the risk of postoperative respiratory complications. Data in adults suggest that patients with significant pulmonary dysfunction are at increased risk of postoperative complications.[32–35] However, these studies primarily concern patients with obstructive disease and there is little information concerning restrictive disease, especially in children.

One review evaluating the postoperative course following thoracotomy in 32 children with diminished preoperative pulmonary function[36] found that although there was a significant postoperative decrease in pulmonary function, the decrease was not greater in patients with more severe preoperative pulmonary dysfunction. Morbidity was limited even in patients with moderate [forced expiratory volume in 1 second ($FEV_1$) or forced vital capacity (FVC) less than 60 percent predicted for age] or severe ($FEV_1$ or FVC less than 40 percent predicted for age) preoperative pulmonary dysfunction.

What is clear is that although conservative prohibitive limits have been suggested by some authors,[37] later outcome studies have demonstrated that limited morbidity and mortality occurs even in patients with severely compromised preoperative pulmonary function.[38,39] It is necessary to identify patients at risk so that aggressive preoperative and postoperative respiratory care can be instituted. Thus surgical intervention, when it offers the possibility of a cure, should be considered even in patients with severely impaired preoperative pulmonary function.

## THE NERVOUS SYSTEM

Several disease- and treatment-related conditions may affect the central and/or peripheral nervous system in the pediatric oncology patient. Increased intracranial pressure, with headaches, seizures, and alterations in mental status, are common presenting symptoms of intracranial tumors. Such tumors are second to acute lymphocytic leukemia as the most common malignancy of childhood. The histologic type and location vary depending on the age of the patient. Posterior fossa tumors are most common in the younger child, and supratentorial lesions predominate in those 10 years of age and older. Central nervous system effects may also occur due to lymphoma or leukemic cell infiltration. Once therapy is instituted, infectious and hemorrhagic complications involving the central nervous system may also occur.

In addition to direct effects on the nervous system due to space-occupying lesions, several paraneoplastic syndromes have been described. For the most part, these have involved the peripheral nervous system and display a combination of motor and sensory effects. Myasthenia gravis has been associated with thymoma and various types of lung cancer. In such cases, the myasthenic symptoms may begin before, at the same time, or after the presentation of the primary malignancy. Clinical symptoms and electromyographic findings are the same as for myasthenia gravis in patients without a concomitant malignancy. Most patients present with muscle weakness and ptosis. Other paraneoplastic syndromes, more commonly described in adult patients, are the Eaton-Lambert syndrome and a generalized peripheral neuropathy. The Eaton-Lambert syndrome occurs most commonly with small cell carcinoma of the lung. Clinical manifestations include motor weakness without the ptosis or respiratory insufficiency that is commonly seen in myasthenia gravis. Characteristic electromyographic findings include normal nerve conduction velocity with an increase in the force of muscular contraction upon repetitive stimulation. The peripheral neuropathy seen with malignancy may be related to the disease itself, to chemotherapy, or to a combination of the two and may affect motor, sensory, or autonomic function.

Toxic effects to both the central and peripheral nervous systems have been described with several chemotherapeutic agents (Table 10-5). Alterations in mental status (somnolence or agitation) and/or seizures have occurred with 5-FU, asparaginase, procarbazine, and, most recently, ifosfamide.[40] These effects generally occur during or shortly after administration of the drug; although they may require supportive care and anticonvulsant therapy, they are usually reversible with time and reduction in dose of the chemotherapeutic agent. The risks of neurotoxicity may be increased by concomitant administration of other medications such as narcotics or antiemetics and by prior chemotherapeutic therapy.[40]

**Table 10-5.** Chemotherapeutic Agents Associated with Neurotoxicity

| |
|---|
| Vincristine |
| Vinblastine |
| Cisplatin |
| Procarbazine |
| Methotrexate |
| 5-Fluorouracil |
| L-asparaginase |
| Ifosfamide |
| Busulfan |

In addition to the effects occurring with the intravenous administration of chemotherapeutic agents, the intrathecal administration of chemotherapy may also cause seizures, mental status changes, and progressive neurologic degeneration. With childhood malignancies, the central nervous system is one of the primary locations that may harbor malignant cells despite eradication of the malignancy from the bone marrow. Therefore, despite an apparent cure, central nervous system relapse may occur. In an effort to obtain a cure, intrathecal administration of chemotherapy including methotrexate and ara-C has become an integral component of many therapeutic regimens, and this may be combined with radiation therapy to the neuroaxis. Although such an approach increases the chance of eventual remission and cure, neurotoxicity may occur. The acute effects of seizures and alterations in mental state are generally transient, but permanent dysfunction such as learning disability and a progressive leukoencephalopathy may occur. Leukoencephalopathy is more common in patients who have received both intrathecal methotrexate and craniospinal irradiation.

In addition to central nervous system effects, chemotherapeutic agents may have profound effects on the peripheral nervous system. Such effects may cause various combinations of motor, sensory, or autonomic dysfunction. Peripheral neuropathy may occur with cisplatin, procarbazine, and the vinca alkaloids (vincristine/vinblastine). Clinical manifestations include decreased sensation, paresthesias, and decreased deep tendon reflexes. These effects are generally transient and subside with reduction or discontinuation of the medication.

While many drugs have been implicated in peripheral neuropathy, the most common agent is vincristine.[41] The mechanism involves a direct toxic effect on the neuron with axonal degeneration. The earliest clinical manifestations include paresthesias of the distal extremities and loss of deep tendon reflexes in the lower extremities. In addition, jaw pain is a frequent complaint. As with the other agents, these signs and symptoms are generally reversible upon withdrawal of the medication. Although less common, autonomic and motor effects may also occur. Motor neuropathy is generally manifested by weakness in distal muscle groups, with wrist or foot drop. Autonomic dysfunction most commonly leads to alterations in gastrointestinal transit time with constipation or ileus. An uncommon manifestation of vincristine's effects on the autonomic nervous system is the occurrence of isolated vocal cord paralysis and stridor.[42]

## THE RENAL/ GENITOURINARY SYSTEM

Chemotherapeutic agents may compromise several different functions of the renal/genitourinary system. Renal activity may be further depressed by the administration of other nephrotoxic agents including aminoglycoside antibiotics and diuretics such as furosemide. Damage to the nephrons may be confined to the glomerulus, leading to alterations in renal function with elevated blood urea nitrogen and creatinine. Otherwise, it may be confined to the renal tubules, with the development of Fanconi syndrome and increased urinary losses of calcium, magnesium, sodium, and phosphorous.

**Table 10-6.** Chemotherapeutic Agents Associated with Nephrotoxicity

| |
|---|
| Cisplatin |
| Ifosfamide |
| Cyclophosphamide |
| Methotrexate |
| 6-Mercaptopurine |
| Mithramycin |
| Streptozocin |

Several of the commonly used chemotherapeutic agents are potentially nephrotoxic (Table 10-6). In general, the toxicity is dose related and resolves with cessation of therapy. However, the use of other nephrotoxic agents such as aminoglycoside antibiotics may lead to renal insufficiency at lower than anticipated doses. Monitoring should include repeated checks of creatinine clearance prior to each course of chemotherapy, since alterations in blood urea nitrogen and creatinine may not occur until the glomerular filtration rate (GFR) is reduced to 25 to 30 percent of normal. In view of the potential efficacy of these agents, especially cisplatin, methods to decrease their nephrotoxicity have been investigated including hydration and mannitol diuresis. The use of prolonged low-dose infusion of cisplatin has also been assessed.[43] Currently, the use of hydration and mannitol diuresis is most common in clinical practice.

In addition to their effects on the GFR, several of the chemotherapeutic agents (including ifosfamide, cyclophosphamide, and cisplatin) may alter tubular function. Tubular dysfunction is manifested by urinary losses of sodium, calcium, magnesium, bicarbonate, and phosphate. Such losses may lead to hypocalcemic tetany, metabolic acidosis, and rickets.[44] In addition, tubular damage may result in loss of urinary concentrating abilities, with obligate isosthenuria.

Further adverse effects associated with both cyclophosphamide and ifosfamide include hemorrhagic cystitis. The damage to the bladder mucosa is produced not by these compounds directly, but rather by their metabolites. Treatment includes hydration and, most recently, the administration of mesna, an agent that binds the toxic metabolites and thus prevents damage to the bladder mucosa. If hemorrhagic cystitis develops despite these maneuvers, cessation of therapy is indicated. Other more aggressive therapy may be indicated if hemorrhagic cystitis continues despite drug withdrawal.[45]

## THE HEPATIC SYSTEM

Alterations in hepatic function may be due to primary disease (hepatic tumor), metastatic disease, or infiltration from a hematologic malignancy. However, more commonly hepatic dysfunction is related to infectious causes or chemotherapeutic drug effects. Several of the commonly used chemotherapeutic agents are hepatotoxic (Table 10-7). Their toxicity may be either hepatocellular, cholestatic, or a combination of the two. Alterations in hepatic function are generally manifested by elevations in liver enzymes, serum bilirubin, or evidence of cholestasis.

In addition to cholestasis or hepatocellular injury, chemotherapeutic agents may affect the synthetic functions of the liver. This is most commonly manifested as alterations in the coagulation status, but alterations in serum pseudocholinesterase levels may also occur. This enzyme is responsible for the hydrolysis of the depolarizing muscle relaxant succinylcholine. Deficiencies of the enzyme may be genetically acquired; however, several disease states include cancer and the administration of chemotherapeutic agents (cyclophosphamide, thiotepa, and nitrogen mustard) may alter serum levels.

**Table 10-7.** Chemotherapeutic Agents Associated with Hepatotoxicity

| |
|---|
| Methotrexate |
| 6-Mercaptopurine |
| Adriamycin |
| Cyclophosphamide |
| Asparaginase |
| Nitrosureas |

Perhaps an even greater risk to the pediatric oncology patient, who already has a chronic immunosuppressed state, is infectious hepatitis. Multiple blood products are administered, resulting in exposure to several blood-borne diseases including cytomegalovirus, hepatitis B, and non-A, non-B hepatitis. Additionally, children receiving chemotherapeutic agents have an increased risk of becoming chronic $HB_sAg$ carriers and remain $HB_eAg$ positive for a longer period of time, which makes them more infectious.[46]

Two additional causes of liver dysfunction in the pediatric oncology patient are veno-occlusive disease (VOD) and graft versus host disease (GVHD) of the liver. VOD can occur following several different chemotherapeutic agents, but is seen most commonly in bone marrow transplant patients. Although it clinically resembles Budd-Chiari syndrome, histologic examination reveals occlusion and fibrosis of small hepatic venules. Clinical characteristics include hyperbiliribinemia, hepatomegaly, ascites, and weight gain with only slight elevations in hepatic enzymes.[47] Onset is generally within the first 21 days following transplantation. Treatment is supportive, but patients with severe involvement have limited survival. VOD represents the third leading cause of death following allogeneic transplant (after infection and GVHD) and the second leading cause following autologous transplantation (following infection). The exact etiology has not been determined, although in most instances it is thought to be related to the preparatory regiment for bone marrow transplantation (combination of radiation and chemotherapy).

GVHD is recognized as one of the major contributing factors to mortality in patients receiving bone marrow transplants. The disease results from the presence of immunocompetent T cells in the donor marrow that recognize host antigens as foreign. The risk of developing GVHD depends on the degree of match (number of HLA antigens) between the host and recipient. Although ideally all HLA antigens should be matched, many candidates for transplant do not have haplotype-identical donors and therefore varying degrees of antigen mismatch or matched unrelated donors are used. In such cases the risks of GVHD are high.

The onset of end-organ dysfunction is used to classify the disease as acute or chronic. The skin, liver, lungs, and gastrointestinal tract may be involved. Acute GVHD tends to affect the liver, skin, and GI tract, while chronic disease presents more as progressive pulmonary fibrosis (bronchiolitis obliterans) and a scleroderma-like picture of the GI tract and skin. Treatment modalities are aimed at limiting the activity of the donor T cells, including either immunosuppressive agents or T-cell depletion of the donor marrow prior to reinfusion. Pharmacologic agents used to prevent and/or treat GVHD include corticosteroids, methotrexate, and cyclosporine.

## THE GASTROINTESTINAL SYSTEM

The GI tract contains some of the most rapidly dividing cells in the body, and many of the chemotherapeutic agents have significant effects on this system. Aggressive chemotherapeutic regimens such as those used to treat neuroblastoma, acute leukemia, and the preparation for bone marrow transplantation can lead to severe ulceration at various points along the GI tract. Stomatitis, dysphagia, and diarrhea with blood and protein loss through the GI tract may occur. Mucositis and ulcerations of the mouth may further complicate enteral nutrition. The nutritional status of many patients is already compromised due to cachexia from the primary disease process, and nausea and vomiting from chemotherapy.

In addition to this effect on nutrition, GI ulcerations and inflammation compromise the normal host barrier against infection. The majority of these infectious episodes are caused by gram-negative enteric organisms, but there is an association of oral mucositis and α-streptococcal sepsis in patients receiving high-dose cytosine arabinoside for treatment of acute myelogenous leukemia.[48]

Direct tumor effects may also occur in the GI system. Large intra-abdominal masses may compress the intestine and alter GI transit time, leading to increased gastric volume and acidity. Several paraneoplastic effects may be caused by vasoactive substances produced by tumors, including gastrin production by pancreatic tumors, which leads to diffuse peptic ulceration (Zollinger-Ellison syndrome), and profuse diarrhea in patients with neuroblastoma.

## THE HEMATOPOIETIC SYSTEM

The bone marrow contains some of the most actively dividing cells of the body, and, without a doubt, the greatest impact of chemotherapeutic agents is on the hematopoietic system. Prior to blood transfusion, hemorrhage was the leading cause of death in oncology patients; today infection is the number one cause.

Although hemorrhage from thrombocytopenia and/or liver dysfunction is more common, a thrombotic tendency can also occur in the oncology patient. It has been described in association with several malignancies including pancreatic carcinoma, prostatic carcinoma, and adenocarcinoma. Although these malignancies are uncommon in children, a thrombotic tendency can also occur with promyelocytic leukemia, and many chemotherapeutic protocols call for heparin during induction therapy. A hypercoaguable state with increases in factor VIII antigen levels (Willebrand factor) may also be seen with the administration of asparaginase.

Although the consequences and treatment of bone marrow suppression are relatively straightforward, some discussion of the use of colony-stimulating factors [granulocyte (G)-CSF and granulocyte-macrophage (GM)-CSF] in the treatment of neutropenia is warranted since these agents can have significant adverse effects.[49] The hematopoietic growth factors regulate the development and differentiation of bone marrow stem cells into erythrocytes, granulocytes, and megakaryocytes. These factors are a heterogenous family of glycoproteins that are now available for clinical use through the technology of DNA cloning. Six are currently in common clinical use or in clinical trials, including G-CSF, GM-CSF, macrophage (M)-CSF, and interleukins 1, 2, and 3 (IL-1, IL-2, and IL-3).

To date the largest experience is with the myeloid-stimulating factors, which include G-CSF and GM-CSF. These agents have been administered to patients with neutropenia of various etiologies including aplastic anemia, idiopathic neutropenia, congenital agranulocytosis, chemotherapy-induced neutropenia, and marrow aplasia following bone marrow transplantation. Aside from reducing the period of neutropenia and thereby limiting the risk of infection, these agents allow for more aggressive chemotherapeutic regimens, which may improve long-term survival.

Mild toxic effects are bone pain and flu-like symptoms, including fever, rash, anorexia, and myalgias. More severe effects include alterations in fluid balance and disruption of capillary-endothelial integrity, with pleural and pericardial effusions. In addition to the pleural and pericardial effusions, a capillary leak syndrome with noncardiogenic pulmonary edema has been described with IL-2.[50] Proposed mechanisms for this syndrome include tumor necrosis factor released from macrophages or possibly the production of vasoactive substances that alter neutrophil-endothelial interactions. Regardless of the etiology, progressive respiratory failure may occur.

The frequency with which these adverse reactions occur depends on several factors including the dose and the source of the particular recombinant product (mammalian, yeast, or bacterial). With the use of the mammalian product, capillary leak is more common when doses exceed 16 μ/kg/d.

In addition to the more common chronic effects of these agents, an acute first-dose phenomenon has been described.[51] Manifestations include hypoxemia without radiographic abnormalities, hypotension, tachycardia, and syncope. A small subset of patients also develops decreased peak expiratory flow rates suggestive of bronchoconstriction. These adverse effects may be the result of an unidentified humoral factor, since no change is found in levels of complement, histamine, or tumor necrosis factor.

One final complication reported with the administration of CSF is thrombosis around the central venous catheter. Although the clinical significance and etiology is yet to be determined, one death due to pulmonary embolism has been reported in a patient receiving GM-CSF.[52]

## THE ENDOCRINE SYSTEM

Hypertension is not an uncommon finding in the pediatric oncology patient and may usually be related to drug administration (steroids, cyclosporine), renovascular compression from an intra-abdominal tumor, or humoral factors produced by the tumor (catecholamines, aldosterone). Hypertension following steroid or cyclosporine administration resolves once the agents are discontinued and can usually be effectively controlled with a combination of diuretics and vasodilators.

More severe hypertension is seen with renovascular compression or catecholamine production. In such cases, surgical excision of the tumor is usually indicated. Although severe hypertension has been classically described with pheochromocytoma, catecholamine excess may also occur with neuroblastoma. Despite the fact that hypertension has been described in up to 30 percent of patients with neuroblastoma,[53] its severity is generally not that of patients with pheochromocytoma.

Radiation and chemotherapy can also impact on other aspects of the endocrine system. Prolonged administration of corticosteroids can lead to alterations in glucose homeostasis, hypokalemia, growth retardation, and suppression of the pituitary-adrenal axis. Craniospinal irradiation may lead to hypothyroidism and hypopituitarism. Such effects generally do not occur acutely, but may have their onset years after the initial diagnosis.

## FLUID AND ELECTROLYTE HOMEOSTASIS

The effects of malignant diseases and their therapy on many metabolic processes warrant a separate discussion. Because of the cachectic effects of cancer, mucositis, and recurrent vomiting with chemotherapy, many patients require prolonged parenteral nutrition. Careful adjustment of sodium, potassium, and other cellular anions and cations is necessary to maintain homeostasis. Normal losses may be magnified by abnormal urinary losses due to renal tubular damage from previous chemotherapy (see renal considerations above) or the administration of antibiotics. In particular, amphotericin B may lead to exaggerated urinary losses of magnesium and potassium, while the aminoglycosides may lead to phosphate and magnesium depletion. Sodium homeostasis may be affected by renal tubular dysfunction or the secretion of antidiuretic hormones following the administration of several chemotherapeutic agents including vincristine, cyclophosphamide, or ifosfamide.

Disturbances of glucose homeostasis may occur related to therapy or on occasion to the tumor itself. Although uncommon in children, soft tissue sarcomas have been associated with hypoglycemia because of the production of insulin-like compounds or glucose uptake by the tumor. More commonly, hyperglycemia may occur during steroid administration or with the combination of prednisone and asparaginase during induction therapy for acute lymphocytic leukemia. Due to its direct toxic effects on pancreatic islet cells, asparaginase decreases insulin release. Insulin therapy may be needed, but the effect is generally transient and subsides following cessation of therapy. Hyperglycemia with asparaginase therapy is particularly common in patients with trisomy 21.

Although the majority of electrolyte disturbances are relatively easy to manage, acute life-threatening conditions may occur with tumor lysis syndrome, as in hematologic malignancies (Burkitt's lymphoma, acute leukemias) with a large tumor mass. Such patients frequently have white blood cells counts in excess of 200,000/mm$^3$ or large lymphomatous masses. Chemotherapy results in rapid cellular death and the release of intracellular contents, leading to hyperkalemia, hyperphosphatemia, hypercalcemia, and hyperuricemia. Therapy is targeted at the various end products of tumor destruction. Initial treatment may include reduction of tumor burden by leukaphoresis prior to the administration of chemotherapy. Hydration and the administration of aluminum-containing antacids will help prevent hyperphosphatemia. Urinary alkalinization increases the solubility of uric acid, thereby decreasing the risks of precipitation in renal tubules, while allopurinol administration blocks uric acid formation through the inhibition of xanthine oxidase. Treatment of hyperkalemia includes the administration of ion exchange resins (Kayexalate), maintenance of diuresis, and administration of sodium bicarbonate, glucose, and insulin. Hemodialysis may be required if hyperkalemia, hyperuricemia, and hyperphosphatemia cannot be controlled medically.

Hypercalcemia may also be seen either with tumor lysis syndrome or as an isolated finding in patients with malignancies. Hypercalcemia may be related to bony metastatic disease or to ectopic parathormone or vitamin D production by the tumor. Regardless of the etiology, the goals of therapy include enhancing renal excretion, inhibiting accelerated bone resorption, and treating the underlying disease. The first step in therapy is to correct dehydration and initiate a saline diuresis with normal saline administration and furosemide. This results in an increased exchange of calcium for sodium in the renal tubules. Thiazide diuretics are contraindicated as they inhibit calcium excretion. Further therapy may be required when saline diuresis does not lower serum calcium levels. Other pharmacologic agents used in the treatment of hypercalcemia include mithramycin, calcitonin, the biphosphonates, gallium nitrate, prostaglandins, phosphate, and glucocorticosteroids.

Both the biphosphonates and gallium nitrate inhibit bone resorption by binding to and inhibiting the dissolution of hydroxyapatite crystals. Both agents, especially gallium nitrate, are potentially nephrotoxic; therefore monitoring of renal function is suggested. Although phosphates will effectively lower serum calcium levels, their use is contraindicated because of the risk of deposition of calcium phosphate crystals in blood vessels, lungs, and kidneys.

Mithramycin acts through the inhibition of RNA synthesis in osteoclasts. Although it may be toxic to the liver and kidneys, adverse effects are uncommon with short-term use. Advantages include a rapid onset (8 to 12 hours) and efficacy in hypercalcemia of diverse etiologies. Calcitonin is a naturally occurring peptide that increases renal excretion of calcium and inhibits bone resorption. Its onset of action is rapid (1 to 2 hours), and it is relatively free of significant adverse effects. Common clinical practice includes the early use of calcitonin to lower serum calcium quickly followed by other agents that have a slower onset (gallium nitrate).

## REFERENCES

1. Lefrak EA, Pitha J, Rosenheim S, Gottleib JA: A clinicopathologic analysis of Adriamycin cardiotoxicity. Cancer 32:302, 1973
2. Mason JW: Anthracycline cardiotoxicity: recognition, management, and avoidance. Comp Ther 5:64, 1979
3. Wortman JE, Lucus VS, Shuster E et al: Sudden death during doxorubicin administration. Cancer 44:1588, 1979
4. Bristow MR, Billingham ME, Mason JW, Daniels JR: Clinical spectrum of anthracycline antibiotic cardiotoxicity. Cancer Treat Rep 62:873, 1978

5. Goorin AM, Borow KM, Goldman A et al: Congestive heart failure due to Adriamycin cardiotoxicity: it's natural in children. Cancer 47:2810, 1981
6. Goorin AM, Chauvenet AR, Perez AR et al: Initial congestive heart failure, six to ten years after doxorubicin chemotherapy for childhood cancer. J Pediatr 116:144, 1990
7. Lenaz LN, Page JA: Cardiotoxicity of Adriamycin and related anthracyclines. Cancer Treat Rev 3:111, 1976
8. Dresdale A, Bonow RO, Wesley R et al: Prospective evaluation of doxorubicin induced cardiomyopathy resulting in postsurgical adjuvant treatment of patients with soft tissue sarcomas. Cancer 52:51, 1983
9. Bender KS, Shematek JP, Leventhal BG, Kan JS: QT prolongation associated with anthracycline cardiotoxicity. J Pediatr 105:442, 1984
10. Bristow MR, Masow JW, Billingham ME, Daniels JR: Doxorubicin cardiomyopathy: evaluation by phonocardiography, endomyocardial biopsy, and cardiac catheterization. Ann Intern Med 88:168, 1978
11. Legha SS, Benjamin RS, Mackay B et al: Reduction of doxorubicin cardiotoxicity by prolonged continuous intravenous infusion. Ann Intern Med 96:133, 1982
12. Borgeat A, Chiolero R, Baylon P et al: Perioperative cardiovascular collapse in a patient previously treated with doxorubicin. Anesth Analg 67:1189, 1988
13. Mills BA, Roberts RW: Cyclophosphamide-induced cardiomyopathy. Cancer 43: 2223, 1979
14. Bruce DL. Anesthetic-induced increase in murine mortality from cyclophosphamide. Cancer 31:361, 1973
15. Labianca R, Beretta G, Clerici M et al: Cardiac toxicity of 5-fluorouracil: a study on 1083 patients. Tumori 68:505, 1982
16. Misset B, Escudier B, Leclercq B et al: Acute myocardiotoxicity during 5-fluorouracil therapy. Intensive Care Med 16: 210, 1990
17. Jakubowski AA, Kemeny N: Hypotension as a manifestation of cardiotoxicity in three patients receiving cisplatin and 5-fluorouracil. Cancer 62:266, 1988
18. VonHoff DD, Schilsky R, Reichert CM et al: Toxic effects of cis-dichlorodiammineplatinum in man. Cancer Treat Rep 63: 1527, 1979
19. Steinherz LJ, Steinherz PG, Mangiacasale D et al: Cardiac abnormalities after AMSA administration. Cancer Treat Rep 66:483, 1982
20. Tobias J, Zuckerman S: Ethanol intoxication following teniposide administration. Clin Intensive Care 2:235, 1991
21. Applefield M, Wiernik P: Cardiac disease after radiation therapy for Hodgkin's disease. Am J Cardiol 51:1679, 1983
22. Pohjola-Sintonen S, Totterman KJ, Kupari M: Sick sinus syndrome as a complication of mediastinal irradiation therapy. Cancer 65:2494, 1990
23. Blum RH, Carter SK, Agre K: A clinical review of bleomycin: a new antineoplastic agent. Cancer 31:903, 1973
24. Goldiner PL, Schweizer O: The hazards of anesthesia and surgery in bleomycin-treated patients. Semin Oncol 6:121, 1979
25. Goldiner PL, Carlon GC, Cvitkovic E et al: Factors influencing postoperative morbidity and mortality in patients treated with bleomycin. Br Med J 1:1664, 1978
26. Burger RM, Peisach J, Horwitz SB: Mechanism of bleomycin action: in vitro studies. Life Sci 28:715, 1981
27. Franklin R, Buroker TR, Vaishampayan GV, Vaitkeviciuns VK: Combined therapies in esophageal squamous cell carcinoma. Proc Am Assoc Cancer Res 20:223, 1979
28. Urban C, Nirenberg A, Caparros B et al: Chemical pleuritis as the cause of acute chest pain following high dose methotrexate treatment. Cancer 51:34, 1983
29. Rao SX, Ramaswamy G, Levin M, McCravey JW: Fatal acute respiratory failure after vinblastine-mitomycin therapy in lung carcinoma. Arch Intern Med 145: 1905, 1985
30. Haupt HM, Hutchins GM, Moore GW: Ara-C lung: non-cardiogenic pulmonary edema complicating cytosine arabinoside therapy of leukemia. Am J Med 70:256, 1991
31. Cohen IJ, Loven D, Schoenfeld T et al: Dactinomycin potentiation of radiation

pneumonitis: a forgotten interaction. Pediatr Hematol Oncol 8:187, 1991
32. Stein M, Koota GM, Simon M, Frank HA: Pulmonary evaluation of surgical patients. JAMA 181:765, 1962
33. Latima RG, Dickman M, Day WC et al: Ventilatory patterns and pulmonary complications after upper abdominal surgery determined by preoperative and postoperative computerized spirometry and blood gas analysis. Am J Surg 122:622, 1971
34. Gracey DR, Divertie MB, Didier EP: Preoperative pulmonary preparation of patients with chronic obstructive pulmonary disease. Chest 76:123, 1979
35. Stein M, Cassara EL: Preoperative pulmonary evaluation and therapy for surgery patients. JAMA 211:787, 1970
36. Tobias JD, Bozeman PM, Mackert WM, Rao BN: Postoperative outcome following thoracotomy in the pediatric oncology patient with diminished pulmonary function. J Surg Oncol (in press)
37. Williams CD, Brenowitz JB: Prohibitive lung function and major surgical procedures. Am J Surg 132:763, 1976
38. Milledge JS, Nunn JF: Criteria of fitness for anesthesia in patients with chronic obstructive lung disease. Br Med J 3:670, 1975
39. Reichel J: Assessment of operative risk of pneumonectomy. Chest 62:570, 1972
40. Pratt CB, Goren MP, Meyer WH et al: Ifosfamide neurotoxicity is related to previous cisplatin treatment for pediatric solid tumors. J Clin Oncol 8:1399, 1990
41. Rosenthal S, Kaufman S: Vincristine neurotoxicity. Ann Intern Med 80:733, 1974
42. Tobias JD, Bozeman PM: Vincristine-induced laryngeal nerve paralysis. Intensive Care Med 17:304, 1991
43. Womer RB, Pritchard J, Barratt TM: Renal toxicity of cisplatin in children. J Pediatr 106:659, 1985
44. Burk CD, Restaino I, Kaplan BS, Meadows AT: Ifosfamide-induced renal tubular dysfunction and rickets in children with Wilms tumor. J Pediatr 117:331, 1990
45. Klein FA, Smith MJV: Urinary complications of cyclophosphamide: etiology, prevention, and management. South Med J 76:1413, 1983
46. Hovi L, Saarinen MV, Jalanko H et al: Characteristics and outcome of acute infection with hepatitis B virus in children with cancer. Pediatr Infect Dis J 10:809, 1991
47. Jones RJ, Lee KSK, Beschorner WE et al: Venoocclusive disease of the liver following bone marrow transplantation. Transplantation 44:778, 1987
48. Sotiropoulos SV, Jackson MA, Woods GM: Alpha-streptococcal septicemia in leukemic children treated with continuous or large dosage intermittent cytosine arabinoside. Pediatr Infect Dis J 8:755, 1989
49. Tobias JD, Furman WL: Anesthetic considerations in patients receiving colony-stimulating factors (G-CSF and GM-CSF). Anesthesiology 75:536, 1991
50. Rosenberg SA, Lotze MT, Muul LM: Observations on the systemic administration of autologous lymphokine-activated killer cells and recombinant interleukin-2 to patients with metastatic cancer. N Engl J Med 313:1485, 1985
51. Lieschke GJ, Cebon J, Morstyn G: Characteristics of the clinical effects after the first dose of bacterially synthesized recombinant human granulocyte-macrophage-stimulating factor. Blood 72:834, 1989
52. Steward WP, Scarffe JH, Austin R et al: Recombinant human granulocyte-macrophage-colony stimulating factor given as daily short infusions: a phase I dose toxicity study. Br J Cancer 59:142, 1989
53. Grosfeld JL: Neuroblastoma: a 1990 overview. Pediatr Surg Int 6:9, 1991

# 11

# Cardiopulmonary Resuscitation

# 11

# Cardiopulmonary Resuscitation

*Andrew M. Woods*

In infants and children, cardiac arrest is rarely a primary event; it is usually secondary to prior failure of the respiratory or, less commonly, the circulatory system. Thus, when faced with a child in cardiac arrest, it is critical that the underlying etiology be promptly identified and properly treated. This chapter presents three cases involving pediatric patients requiring cardiac resuscitation, each of which an anesthesiologist might expect to confront in a hospital setting. All are situations in which successful resuscitation and a potentially good clinical outcome can be expected if appropriate measures are promptly initiated. As this usually depends upon assessment and management of the underlying etiologies for cardiac arrest, that is the focus of this chapter. It is also important to be able to recognize prearrest syndromes (i.e., shock, electrolyte disorders) and to institute management designed to prevent cardiac arrest.

The case method used in this chapter is similar to the format utilized in the Pediatric Advanced Life Support (PALS) courses sanctioned by the American Heart Association (AHA).[1] It should be noted that the guidelines set forth by the various subcommittees of the AHA are just that, and may not always reflect recent advances in the field. Guidelines are not standards, and even standards do not necessarily represent the highest level of care, but the best care that can be expected at a given point in time. For example, very shortly after the introduction of the pulse oximeter into clinical practice, it became clear that it provided an improved level of care. However, it took several years (during which time oximeters were manufactured, distributed to hospitals, used extensively, and reported favorably upon in peer-reviewed publications) for the use of pulse oximetry to evolve to the level of "standard of care" for patients undergoing general anesthesia. Thus, some of the concepts introduced in this chapter do not represent guidelines of the AHA, but the best judgment of the author and editors, all active pediatric practitioners.

The pace of the scenarios that follow may not parallel actual situations because of the need for didactic discussion in the material presented. Obviously, in real life, a child in full cardiopulmonary arrest presents little time for discourse. Our hope is that the thoughtfulness applied to these simulations will allow for more goal-directed action in the event of a true arrest.

## CASE 1: RESUSCITATION IN THE DELIVERY ROOM

You are called emergently to the operating room in the delivery suite. The anesthesiology resident has already intubated the trachea of a parturient whom you are informed has a diagnosis of placental abruption accompanied by severe fetal bradycardia (heart rate < 30 bpm for 5 minutes). The mother is a healthy 20-year-old with no other medical problems, and the pregnancy is at term. The mother is being adequately volume resuscitated and is hemodynamically stable. The pediatrician has been called at home but has not yet arrived.

### Who Should Direct the Resuscitation?

The most experienced available person in the room should direct the resuscitation. In this case, since your primary patient, the mother, has one-on-one care by a resident and is stable, you may be considered available. In some cases, nurse specialists or respiratory therapists may be more experienced than you in neonatal resuscitation, and, if present, such individuals should take the leadership role. The most important thing is to decide who will assume what roles, so that each person knows what is expected of her or him (manage the airway, feel for pulses, draw up medications, etc.) and to assign these tasks in the brief period before the infant is delivered.

The obstetrician delivers via cesarean section a flaccid and ashen-appearing female infant. The baby is placed beneath an overhead radiant heater and immediately dried with a warm blanket. The nurse informs you that she cannot palpate a pulse in the umbilical cord and the infant makes no response as a bulb syringe is used to clear the airway. *Elapsed time: 10 seconds.*

### Do You Wait for a One-Minute Apgar Score Before Further Intervention?

This infant has sustained prolonged intrauterine asphyxia based upon the clinical evidence of severe intrauterine bradycardia and absent pulses after delivery. There is no need to wait for a one-minute Apgar score before beginning appropriate resuscitative efforts, and Apgar scores are not used to guide decision making during a resuscitation. However, it is always appropriate to take time to dry the infant and clear the airway. Prevention of heat loss is essential; oxygen consumption is increased in cold-stressed neonates, and this will worsen the asphyxia and make resuscitation more difficult.

### Do You Begin Bag and Face Mask Ventilation or Proceed Directly to Tracheal Intubation?

#### Problems with Bag and Face Mask Ventilation

Bag and face mask ventilation is only marginally effective in resuscitating an extremely asphyxiated neonate; measured tidal volumes are only one-third of those recorded following endotracheal intubation.[2] In situations in which bag and mask ventilation is effective, it usually is due to stimulation of the infant's face; this triggers reflex inspiratory gasping. This reflex is unlikely to be elicited in an infant with severe central nervous system depression (flaccid, ashen, absent pulses, absent gag). Also, bag and face mask ventilation is inferior to ventilation through an endotracheal tube in establishing an adequate functional residual capacity (FRC) within the lungs of a newborn infant.[2] A normal infant can generate up to 40 to 50 $cmH_2O$ of negative intrathoracic pressure with its initial breaths; such pressures contribute greatly to the rapid establishment of an adequate FRC and also the clearing of lung water from the airways and alveoli. It is difficult to achieve such pressures with a bag and face mask.

Another concern with attempting bag and face mask ventilation in an asphyxiated infant is that it is possible to distend the stomach and thus impair ventilation due to restricted diaphragmatic movement. One study of this issue in asphyxiated newborns found that a mean inflation pressure of 54 $cmH_2O$ was required to inflate the esophagus. However, there was a wide intrapatient variation, and in one infant air entered the esophagus at only 24 $cmH_2O$.[3] This confirms what most anesthesiologists know from experience: high ventilatory pressures when using a bag and face mask may put more air into the stomach than the lung, particularly in the case of partial or total airway obstruction or severe lung disease resulting in poor pulmonary compliance.

## Functional Residual Capacity and Tracheal Intubation

The importance of FRC is that it represents a reservoir of oxygen within the alveoli such that during both inspiration and expiration, blood flowing through the lungs is able to be oxygenated. In the absence of an FRC, the loss of lung volume during expiration results in blood traversing the lung at a time when there are no open alveoli. Very low lung volumes are also associated with high pulmonary vascular resistance. The net result of all these factors is increased right-to-left shunting (intrapulmonary, intracardiac, and at the level of the great vessels) and worsened hypoxemia.

The best way to establish an FRC in an asphyxiated infant is to intubate the trachea with an appropriate-size tube and deliver a sustained positive pressure breath, slowly increasing the inflation pressure to a peak of 30 $cmH_2O$ over 5 seconds.[4] Subsequent tidal breaths should be at a rate of 30 to 40/min at a pressure of 15 to 20 $cmH_2O$. However, if this pressure is insufficient to expand the thorax, higher pressures may be necessary. Higher inflation pressures increase the risk of a pneumothorax, and this is a complication that should be anticipated in newborns with noncompliant lungs (i.e., extremely premature infants).

> The infant's trachea is intubated and ventilation is initiated as recommended above. The infant remains flaccid and the person palpating the umbilical cord is unable to feel a pulse. *Elapsed time: 1 minute.*

## What Should You Do Now?

It is essential that correct placement of the endotracheal tube be confirmed. It is most reassuring to visualize the tube passing between the vocal cords, but it is also essential to observe chest movement and listen over the thorax and abdomen. However, using breath sounds to verify tube placement is notoriously unreliable in infants, particularly asphyxiated infants who have not initiated spontaneous respirations and whose lungs may not be fully expanded.

Increasingly, capnography is being used to both verify endotracheal tube placement and evaluate cardiorespiratory performance during cardiopulmonary resuscitation (CPR).[5] The presence of a $CO_2$ waveform indicates that some degree of both ventilation and perfusion are occurring. If a repetitive $CO_2$ pattern is present, it excludes esophageal placement. While the presence of $CO_2$ may initially be detected following esophageal intubation due to diffusion of $CO_2$ from acidotic tissues into the stomach cavity, the $CO_2$ tracing will not be sustained with repetitious inflation and deflation of the stomach. If the $CO_2$ trace is absent or very low, *this does not necessarily indicate failure to intubate the trachea,* as this can occur whenever there is no blood flow to the lungs. Thus, in an asphyxiated newborn whose lungs are not yet inflated and in whom much of the blood flow from the right heart bypasses the pulmonary bed by traversing the ductus arteriosus (pulmonary artery to descending aorta), capnography may not be reliable as a method of verifying tracheal positioning of the tube immediately following presumed tracheal intubation. However, if a $CO_2$ trace is present, it validates tracheal or bronchial positioning and can serve as a guide to the efficacy of cardiac output during CPR. This concept is discussed more fully in Case 2.

There are two basic types of capnography sample systems: one involves a flow-through cuvette with an in-line sensor, and the other involves an aspiration system with a tiny-lumen tube connected to a remote analyzer. Both methods have been found to be reliable in newborns.[6]

> An in-line capnograph is placed in the newborn's breathing circuit. There is no $CO_2$ waveform. The chest moves symmetrically with ventilation, and, with the use of a laryngoscope, the tube can be seen passing through the vocal cords.

As discussed above, capnography (when indicating no expired $CO_2$) is not a reliable marker for tracheal positioning in this setting due to the absence of pulmonary blood flow, but nevertheless may be very useful as the resuscitation proceeds. Alternative modalities are required for verification of tube placement, and have been employed.

## What Action Is Now Called For?

In the case of a flaccid and ashen infant, chest compressions should be begun as soon as the trachea is intubated and ventilation begun. It is important to stress that there is no justification for ventilating the lungs with anything less than 100 percent oxygen in the setting of CPR, and issues regarding possible retinal toxicity are of no consequence in a pulseless neonate.

The AHA recommends that in neonates, after 15 to 30 sec of ventilation with 100 percent oxygen, chest compressions be begun if the heart rate is less than 60 bpm (Table 11-1). However, in the case of an infant in extremis, there is no need to wait to observe the potential benefits of ventilation before beginning chest compressions.

> Manual chest compressions at a rate of 120 per minute are begun, depressing the sternum approximately 2 cm each time. There is no improvement in the newborn's clinical condition. The pediatrician has still not arrived, but two nurses from the neonatal intensive care unit are assisting you. *Elapsed time: 2.0 minutes.*

**Table 11-1.** Guidelines for Chest Compressions in Neonates

| Initiate chest compressions for: |
|---|
| Heart rate $< 60$ bpm |
| Heart rate $> 60$ and $< 80$ and not increasing |
| Any pulseless or nonperfusing electrocardiogram rhythm |

## What Is Your Next Move?

In the case of severely asphyxiated infants, especially those who have experienced intrapartum hemorrhage, merely providing basic CPR consisting of ventilation and manual chest compressions will often be insufficient to allow successful resuscitation. The hallmark of the PALS courses is their emphasis on "advanced" life support strategies. When basic life support measures are ineffective, advanced life support involves prompt but sophisticated assessment, diagnosis, and treatment based upon this information, followed by reassessment and evaluation of the efficacy of any intervention.

You order epinephrine and request that an umbilical catheter be placed while continuing to provide ventilation with 100 percent oxygen and manual chest compressions. A low $CO_2$ pressure is now recorded in the expired gas (peak level 2 to 4 mmHg). *Elapsed time: 2.1 minutes.*

## How Much Epinephrine Should Be Administered and by What Route?

Endotracheal intubation almost always precedes the placement of an intravascular catheter in cases of delivery room resuscitation, so that the first available route for epinephrine is usually via the trachea. However, for any drug to be effective systemically when administered intratracheally, it must reach the central circulation. This requires that the drug cross biologic membranes and be absorbed into the bloodstream. In cases of hemorrhagic shock, there will be minimal mucosal blood flow to allow absorption of drugs that are topically applied to the trachea and bronchi. Even a drug that is distributed as far distally as the respiratory bronchioles and the alveoli may be minimally absorbed due to insufficient blood flow through the pulmonary capillaries. Particularly in the case of a newborn, adequate pulmonary blood flow requires that the lungs be inflated; prior to lung inflation, the airways are filled with lung fluid and there is minimal blood flow through the lung. Even after the lungs are expanded, pulmonary vascular resistance must decrease to a level below peripheral vascular resistance before blood will cease to be shunted away from the pulmonary bed. In the case of severe shock with no blood pressure and minimal peripheral resistance, this transition from fetal physiology to normal newborn physiology as regards pulmonary–systemic pressure gradients does not occur. Most right-heart output will bypass the lung and enter the descending aorta via the ductus arteriosus. Also, in hemorrhagic shock there is a large increase in portions of the lung that are ventilated but minimally perfused (physiologic dead space); epinephrine reaching such lung units can be expected to provide delayed, if any, pharmacologic circulatory benefits. Furthermore, a portion of the administered dose will fail to reach the alveoli, instead adhering to the walls of the endotracheal tube, the trachea, and the bronchi.

It is clear that during CPR a significant portion of intratracheally administered epinephrine, in recommended doses, will not reach the central circulation in a timely manner.[6] In newborns, intratracheal epinephrine is even less likely to be effective for the reasons given above. Using current AHA recommendations for intratracheal administration of epinephrine, Orlowski et al. found that in 12 normotensive dogs, 8 had no blood pressure response to standard (0.01 mg/kg) or double (0.02 mg/kg) dosages of intratracheal epinephrine, and one normotensive dog had no blood pressure response to 0.04

mg/kg.[7] In the opinion of Orlowski and associates, the AHA recommendations for intratracheal administration of epinephrine must be seen as inadequate for the arrest state, since this dosage is not reliable even in the normal state. They cite a number of other studies that support this inadequacy and that suggest that, in animal models, an effective dose of intratracheal epinephrine is approximately *10 times* the effective intravenous dosage. However, there is increasing evidence that the recommended AHA intravenous dosage as well may be too low (see below).

In a newborn rabbit model in which the animals were normotensive, Mullett and colleagues[8] detected very low levels of epinephrine in the heart after intratracheal doses of 100 μg/kg. This study confirms the futility of using such doses in cases of shock. Because of impaired mucosal blood flow in the trachea and major bronchi during shock, it is imperative that epinephrine reach the distal airways and alveoli where there may be some blood flow. This is best achieved by using generous amounts of saline to facilitate distal drug delivery.[9] Table 11-2 provides a guide for intratracheal epinephrine dosages based upon either weight or height.

The weight of the baby is estimated to be 3 kg. Using a syringe attached to a 5.0 Fr feeding catheter passed through and beyond the endotracheal tube, 1.5 mg of epinephrine (1.5 ml of a 1:1,000 solution) is diluted in 10 ml of saline and injected into the trachea. Electrocardiogram (ECG) leads are attached and demonstrate very wide QRS complexes at a rate of 20 bpm. After almost two minutes with continued chest compressions, there is no change in heart rate and no palpable pulse. Your assistants are attempting to place a catheter in an umbilical vessel while at the same time continuing chest compression, but the motion of the baby's body is making this task extremely difficult. *Elapsed time: 4.0 minutes.*

## What Is Your Assessment of the Situation?

Failure to promptly resuscitate an asphyxiated neonate is indicative of either a failure of ventilation or circulation, or both. In attempting to differentiate among these factors, there are clinical signs that may be useful. A patient who is dusky or cyanotic most likely has impaired oxygenation; cardiac output may still be adequate to circulate desaturated blood. In such cases, all efforts should be directed toward restoration of oxygenation. In contrast, a patient exhibiting extreme pallor (ashen) must be assumed to be in a state of circulatory shock (inade-

**Table 11-2.** Length- and Weight-Based Epinephrine Dosages for Pediatric Arrest[a]

| | | *Epinephrine Dose (mg)*[b] | |
|---|---|---|---|
| *Length (cm)* | *Average Weight (kg)* | *Intravenous* | *Intratracheal* |
| 45 | 2.5 | .25–.50 | 1.25 |
| 50 | 3.2 | .30–.60 | 1.5 |
| 60 | 5.5 | .50–1.0 | 2.5 |
| 70 | 8.5 | .80–1.5 | 4.0 |
| 80 | 11 | 1.0–2.0 | 5.0 |
| 100 | 15 | 1.5–3.0 | 7.5 |
| 120 | 22 | 2.0–4.0 | 10.0 |
| 140 | 33 | 3.5–5.0 | 15.0 |

[a] Based upon dose recommendation of 100–200 μg/kg.
[b] Dosages are for full cardiac arrest. Smaller dosages may be appropriate for lesser degrees of circulatory failure.

quate perfusion), a situation that can occur with normal alveolar oxygen delivery (adequate ventilation). Thus, while it is imperative that adequate ventilation and oxygenation be verified in an ashen patient, patient survival will depend upon restoration of circulatory function. In cases of hemorrhagic shock, this requires that the heart be provided with enough blood to generate sufficient cardiac output (stroke volume × heart rate) to deliver enough oxygen to the brain and the myocardium to prevent irreversible injury. In this infant, your assessment should be that this child needs blood immediately, with no delay for any laboratory tests (i.e., hematocrit) or crossmatching of blood. While this infant's clinical presentation could be caused by a major tension pneumothorax, the history of maternal abruption, during which the fetus sustained known blood loss via the placenta, makes extreme hypovolemia secondary to hemorrhage a much more likely diagnosis. The rapid establishment of intravascular access in order to restore intravascular volume with blood is thus of paramount importance and should take precedence over other diagnostic efforts.

> Blood is ordered. It is requested that it be as fresh as possible. CPR continues with no change in the clinical status of the infant. *Note:* This should have been done as soon as the diagnosis of abruption was suspected, and the blood should have been in the delivery room and warmed by the time the baby was delivered. Precious time has been lost. *Elapsed time: 4.2 minutes.*

## How Should Vascular Access Be Established?

The AHA guidelines state that the umbilical vein is easily located and cannulated, and indeed this is the most commonly used site for initial vascular access in the newborn undergoing resuscitation in the delivery room. A 5.0 or 8.0 Fr catheter with a single end hole and radiopaque markings should be used, and inserted just deep enough to obtain blood return freely. Either the umbilical arteries or the umbilical vein may be utilized for delivery of resuscitation fluids and blood products, although the arteries are usually more technically difficult to cannulate; for the arteries, a 3.5 Fr catheter may be more appropriate. While the level at which the catheter tip is placed is of consequence for both arterial and venous catheters, this concern should not delay fluid resuscitation in cases of cardiac arrest. For example, umbilical artery catheters in which the tip remains at the level of the renal arteries in the aorta place the child at increased risk for subsequent renovascular hypertension. There is an increased risk of vascular complications with low placement (bifurcation of aorta) compared to tip placement in the thoracic (T6–T8) region (26.6 versus 16.0 percent).[10] Most complications appear to involve vasospasm that resolves with catheter removal; a small percentage involve embolic events to the toes. No difference in the incidence of intraventricular hemorrhage has been found associated with catheter position.[10] The important point is that catheter complications are usually due to clot formation on the tip and are of no consequence during emergency resuscitation involving a freshly placed catheter.

Likewise for umbilical venous catheters, thrombosis from clot formation can occur and injure the liver. Also, hypertonic drugs infused directly into the liver may cause hepatic injury. However, hypoxia and hypotension are also extremely harmful to the liver, and it is not appropriate to delay vital resuscitation fluids (crystalloid and blood and possibly vasopressors) in order to verify correct catheter tip placement. When blood return is obtained, the catheter is intravascular and, in an emergency, that is the correct position. Once the child is resuscitated, any necessary catheter repositioning can be undertaken.

> The individual attempting to cannulate the umbilical vein has yet to obtain blood return. *Elapsed time: 4.5 minutes.*

## What Do You Do Now?

This newborn, in shock with no pulses despite CPR, will die unless adequate intravascular volume and cardiac filling pressures are promptly restored. If vascular access via the umbilical vessels is not accomplished within 1 to 2 minutes from initiation of the procedure, a decision must be made immediately whether to have someone else attempt umbilical vessel cannulation (although in cases of cardiac arrest, the most skilled person in the room should already be doing this task) or to try an alternative route. One such route is the marrow space of a large bone, such as the tibia or femur.[11] The intraosseous space is a noncollapsible part of the vascular tree, and fluid or medications injected into this space are as efficacious as when injected into peripheral or central veins. Individuals who take the PALS course will learn this technique using a bone from the leg of a turkey or chicken. *Warning:* Do not hold the child's extremity in your hand during this procedure in such a way that a firmly inserted needle can pass through the child's bone, exit the soft tissue, and cause a puncture wound in your palm.

There is an additional route that every anesthesiologist should be aware of and that is well suited for the person who has intubated the infant's trachea and is still at the patient's head. This is cannulation of the superior sagittal sinus (Fig. 11-1). This is a large vein that runs directly beneath the anterior fontanelle in the space between the two cerebral hemispheres (Fig. 11-2). This technique has been in the pediatric armamentarium for decades,[12] but has not gained wide usage, probably reflecting a fear of injuring the brain. In children other than newborns or those with major head trauma, this should not be a concern; there is a large amount of space within the interhemispheric groove, with little risk of injuring neural tissue. However, in a newborn who has just come through the birth canal, there may be displacement of landmarks and overlapping sutures as the skull is compressed and distorted, and the sagittal sinus may not immediately underlie the anterior fontanelle in such cases. In the case of an infant delivered by cesarean section without prior labor, distortion of the skull bones is rarely a concern. However, regardless of the risks, *if other attempts at vascular access fail,* there should be no hesitancy about placing a cannula in the superior sagittal sinus. It

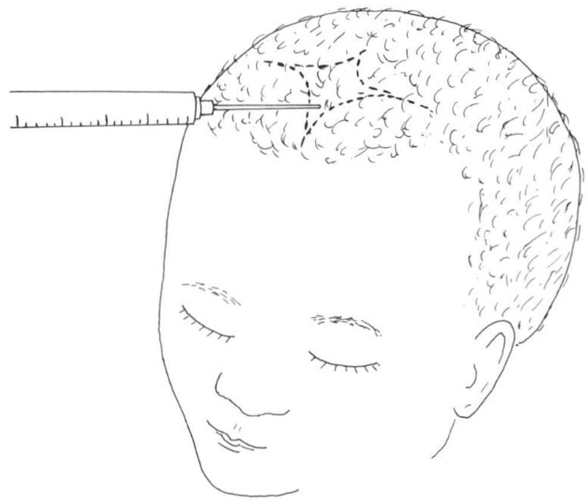

**Fig. 11-1.** Cannulation of the superior sagittal sinus. Catheter insertion is accomplished through the anterior fontanelle (broken lines) with the head in a dependent position. Needle direction is parallel to the long axis of the head. Once blood is aspirated, the plastic catheter is advanced and secured as with any other venous catheter.

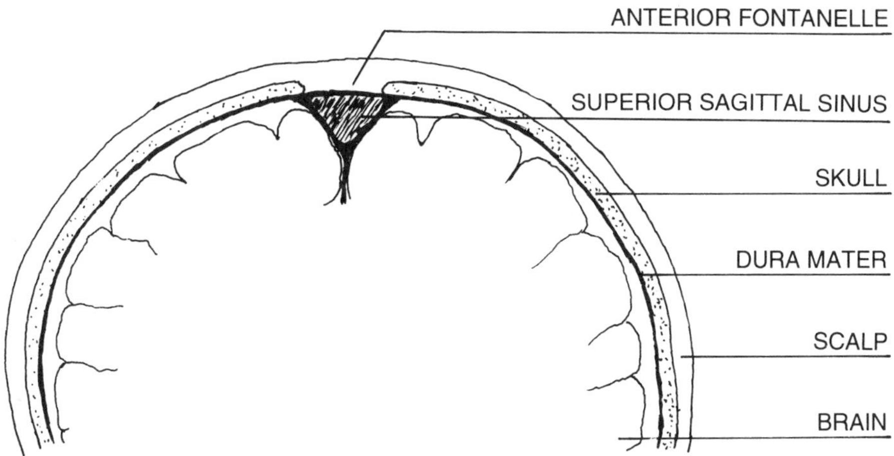


**Fig. 11-2.** Anatomic relationships of the superior sagittal sinus. A frontal section through the cranium at the level of the anterior fontanelle is illustrated. The walls of the superior sagittal sinus are formed by layers of dura mater.

is important that the infant be placed in a head-dependent position to allow distention of this vessel with venous blood.

> Before you attempt cannulation of the superior sagittal sinus, another caregiver is successful in passing a catheter into the umbilical vein. *Elapsed time: 5.0 minutes.*

## Should You Give Intravenous Epinephrine after Having Given a Large Dose Intratracheally? If So, What Dosage?

Once vascular access is established by whatever route, intravenous epinephrine should be administered immediately if the patient is still in a state of cardiac arrest. As discussed above, there is no assurance that any of the intratracheally administered drug has reached the heart or the arterial circulation, and there is no justification for reducing the intravenous dosage.

The old AHA recommendation for intravenous epinephrine in cardiac arrest was 10 to 30 μg/kg/dose every 5 minutes. New guidelines suggesting much larger dosages were expected to be issued in early 1993. Reconsideration of this issue has been prompted by reports of successful resuscitations using larger than recommended doses of epinephrine as well as the fact that there were no scientific studies to support the original AHA-recommended dose of epinephrine. At that time, the studies available to the AHA resuscitation committee indicated that a dosage of 1 mg epinephrine appeared efficacious in resuscitating dogs, and the recommendation for humans was established at 0.5 to 1 mg for adults.[13] However, the dogs in these studies weighed only 10 kg, and so the weight-based dose was 100 μg/kg. Thus, the recommended adult dosage was 7 to 10 times too small based upon the animal data used to determine the dose. Unfortunately, even though the AHA committee did not convert the dog data into a weight-based dosage recommendation for adults, they took their dosage of 0.5 to 1 mg for a 70-kg adult and converted it to a per-kilogram dosage for infants. Thus, the dosage for a 10-kg infant was set at a level that was 10 times less than the dosage required to resuscitate a dog of the same weight.

The dosage of epinephrine is important, because it is the ability of epinephrine to increase aortic diastolic blood pressure and hence increase coronary perfusion pressure and myocardial oxygen delivery that accounts for its efficacy in cardiac resuscitation, and these factors have been shown to correlate with outcome.[14] There are now a number of studies that show improved outcomes when a dosage of epinephrine in the range of 100 to 200 μg/kg is used as opposed to standard dosages of 10 to 20 μg/kg.[15–19] Use of high-dose epinephrine negates the necessity for maintaining neonatal epinephrine (1:10,000) as an emergency drug, and thus makes for a more simple dosing protocol.

The dosage of epinephrine for neonatal cardiac arrest I recommend is 100 to 200 μg/kg, which is 0.1 to 0.2 ml/kg of a standard 1:1,000 solution. Table 11-2 provides dosage guidelines for intravenous epinephrine. Using this table, a full-term 3-kg infant might get one-third of an ampule (0.3 mg) as an initial dose, and another one-third in 1 or 2 minutes if there is no initial response. This dose should be repeated every 2 to 3 minutes until spontaneous circulation returns or the resuscitation efforts are discontinued. Other causes for refractory cardiac arrest (i.e., tension pneumothorax, pericardial tamponade) should be continuously considered in a patient who is adequately volume resuscitated.

In terms of the timing of epinephrine doses, Orlowski et al.[6] have shown in dogs that during shock (but not cardiac arrest), the maximal effect upon diastolic blood pressure occurs within 40 seconds of epinephrine administration. Thus, in the case of an infant who is not in an arrest state but is hypotensive and has a delayed (> 1 minute) and minimal response to epinephrine, a low-output state (hypotensive shock) can be assumed; further resuscitative efforts should focus upon correction of the underlying problem. However, if the patient is in cardiac arrest, then cardiac output during chest compressions is likely to be very low and the time for epinephrine to reach the aorta and the peripheral vasculature and to increase vascular tone may be greatly prolonged, and the eventual effect may be greatly attenuated. Unfortunately, I am aware of no good scientific studies that have adequately addressed this issue; a dosing interval of every 2 to 3 minutes is empirical.

Epinephrine 300 μg (0.3 ml) is administered intravenously. This is immediately followed by a fluid bolus of 60 ml (20 ml/kg) of lactated Ringer's solution and 60 ml of 5 percent albumin delivered rapidly using a 60-ml syringe. There is still no palpable pulse. The heart rate has increased to 45 bpm. The QRS complexes are still very wide. The $CO_2$ trace now has a peak level of 8 mmHg. A venous blood sample is withdrawn for analysis and is noted to appear very dilute. There is no blood for transfusion in the room yet. You are informed that the courier from the blood bank is stuck in a malfunctioning elevator. The blood bank clerk asks if this is really an emergency and, if so, could you send another courier? The blood bank is seven flights below the delivery suite. *Elapsed time: 7.5 minutes.*

## What Do You Do Now?

In most cases of severe asphyxia, either crystalloid or colloid solutions are satisfactory for restoration of intravascular volume, assuming the adequacy of circulating red blood cells. However, in the case of peripartum hemorrhage in which the neonate has lost a major portion of its oxygen-carrying capacity, blood is the essential resuscitation fluid. As already stated, warmed blood should have already been in the delivery room. If there is a delay in obtaining blood for any reason in a case such as this, draw blood from the mother and transfuse this blood into the baby. If the mother's health status excludes her as a donor, blood can be obtained from medical personnel in the delivery suite. Blood should be obtained via venapuncture after site sterilization and withdrawn into a large syringe that has been wetted with heparin. At cesarean delivery, the obstetrician can easily obtain the blood from a uterine vessel.

## Is a Crossmatch Necessary?

Neonates under the age of 3 to 4 months do not mount an immunologic response to transfused cells, so a host-versus-graft reaction is not a concern. Anti-A and anti-B isohemagglutinins present in the donor serum may cause lysis of recipient red blood cells (graft-versus-host), but in the case of profound anemia this is less of a concern, and is not immediately life-threatening. Ideally, use of O-negative blood in such an emergency would be preferred if such a donor was immediately available. The use of cord blood (although it is of fetal origin) is not recommended due to the possible presence of substances that may precipitate disseminated intravascular coagulation and impair cardiovascular performance. Also, in cases of peripartum hemorrhage, the most likely scenario requiring emergency transfusion, there may not be sufficient cord blood available for neonatal resuscitation.

Sixty ml of blood is withdrawn from the mother and transfused immediately into the infant. The heart rate increases to 70 bpm and the QRS complex narrows somewhat. A faint pulse is palpable. The first blood pressure that is obtained is 20 mmHg (systolic). The expired $CO_2$ is 20 mmHg. *Elapsed time: 10 minutes.*

## Now What Do You Do?

As stated earlier, advanced life support requires continual action and reassessment until the patient is stabilized. Therefore, reassess the infant. While this should actually be going on continually, it is useful to occasionally make a conscious effort to systematically reassess the status of the patient. The hallmark of this process is to rapidly cover all the basics, since these factors are subject to change during resuscitative efforts and, if overlooked, may contribute to a failure to resuscitate. *Airway:* Is the endotracheal tube still in proper position? Is the tube kinked or obstructed with blood or secretions? *Breathing:* Are breath sounds present bilaterally? Does the chest rise with positive pressure breaths? *Circulation:* Is the pulse strong or weak? How are the skin color, capillary refill, and muscle tone? The underlying circulatory question is whether or not there is an adequate stroke volume accompanying each heart beat. The presence of a normal capnographic waveform provides verification and a rough quantification of all components of the basics—airway, breathing, and circulation.

The pulses are very weak. The child still appears very pale and is totally flaccid. There is no detectable capillary refill. The heart rate remains at 70 bpm. The venous blood sample drawn prior to transfusion had a hemoglobin concentration of 3 mg/dl, a pH of 6.8, a $PvCO_2$ of 88 mmHg and a $PvO_2$ of 22 mmHg. *Elapsed time: 11 minutes.*

## Can Chest Compressions Be Ceased Now?

The heart rate is less than 80 bpm and is not increasing (see Table 11-1). Also, the baby still appears to be in shock. Therefore, continue chest compressions and seek to determine the reason for the persistent bradycardia.

An additional dose of epinephrine of 200 μg (one-fifth of an ampule) is given IV. The heart rate increases to 90 bpm and the systolic blood pressure increases to 35 mmHg. The expired $CO_2$ is 23 mmHg. However, the clinical appearance (pale, cool, mottled extremities, flaccid) does not change.

## What Does a Large Disparity Between $CO_2$ Blood Tension and Expired Gas Tension Indicate?

Assuming correct physiologic data, a wide disparity between $CO_2$ blood tension (88 mmHg) and the expired gas tension (23 mmHg) indicates either a severe diffusion defect (extremely rare in this setting) or, much more likely, a dilution of the $CO_2$-laden gas from the lung with other gas that has no $CO_2$. This latter situation results from ventilation of lung units having impaired pulmonary blood flow, a process that results in physiologic dead space. In this case, the large gradient between venous and expired carbon dioxide is indicative of a major mismatch between ventilation and perfusion, and is corrected not by increasing ventilation (which is already relatively excessive) but by improving pulmonary blood flow. This is often difficult in newborns, and the next major breakthrough in neonatal care may involve special pulmonary artery vasodilating agents, with nitric oxide being one of the most promising.[20] At present, optimal management consists of maintaining good right-heart function (volume, possibly ionotropic agents) and trying to avoid known constrictors of the pulmonary vasculature (hypoxia and hypercarbia).

## Could the Infant Still Be Very Anemic?

Yes. The infant's normal red blood cell mass should be approximately 140 ml, based upon a weight of 3 kg, an expected blood volume of 85 ml/kg, and a normal newborn hematocrit of 55 percent. The 60 ml of maternal whole blood (expected hematocrit, 35 percent) would contain approximately 20 ml red blood cells. Thus, less than 15 percent (20/140) of the infant's red blood cell volume has been transfused. The hemoglobin value of 3 mg/dl is indicative of a hematocrit of approximately 9 percent. These calculations and the clinical examination indicate the need for additional blood, either from the blood bank or the mother. Since the infant now has maternal serum (which may contain anti-A and anti-B isohemagglutinins) as well as red blood cells, uncrossmatched blood should be O-negative and should consist only of red blood cells, rather than whole blood that may contain antibodies that could attack the just-transfused maternal red blood cells in the infant.

## Are Other Resuscitation Fluids Needed?

The fact that this child still appears to be in shock is suggestive of an ongoing extracellular fluid deficit. In adults, hemorrhagic shock is associated with an extracellular fluid deficit of 4 L. In the newborn, a similar estimate would be 200 ml (60 to 70 ml/kg). Shock is associated with movement of fluid into cells (extracellular-to-intracellular shift), and following hemorrhage and replacement of lost blood there may still be a large extracellular (intravascular and interstitial) fluid deficit. Restoration of the intravascular volume alone is not sufficient; the interstitial space needs to be repleted as well. Additional packed cells should be accompanied by crystalloid solutions.

A hemoglobin measured after the transfusion of maternal blood is 6 mg/dl. The infant receives an additional 75 ml of fresh O-negative packed red blood cells. The heart rate increases to 100 bpm and the QRS complexes continue to narrow. An umbilical artery catheter is inserted and attached to a pressure transducer. The blood pressure is 45/20 mmHg and the waveform appears grossly normal. The infant's color is somewhat pink centrally, but the extremities are still pale and cool. The infant is not moving her arms or legs spontaneously, but the tone in her extremities has improved. The end tidal $CO_2$ is 55 mmHg. *Elapsed time: 15 minutes.*

## Can You Stop Chest Compressions Now?

Since the heart rate is over 80 bpm and the infant appears clinically improved on the basis of blood pressure, expired $CO_2$, color, and tone, it is appropriate to stop chest compressions. However, the presence of a QRS complex on an ECG screen and an acceptable heart rate still does not insure adequacy of cardiac output, and it is essential to closely observe the infant to make sure that the clinical status does not deteriorate once chest compressions are stopped.

The heart rate is increasing and the clinical condition continues to improve once chest compressions are stopped. Within 4 to 5 minutes the infant begins to make spontaneous inspiratory efforts. The heart rate is 130 bpm and the blood pressure 50/30. Shortly after this, as she is being assessed by a pediatrician, the heart rate slows to 40 bpm and the infant becomes apneic. The arterial pressure decreases to 30/15 mmHg. *Elapsed time: 20 minutes.*

## What Is Going On?

Even though the infant was adequately resuscitated centrally (heart and brain), the blood supply to her muscle bed has been impaired for an extended period and anaerobic metabolism in these tissues has produced a very large lactic acid load that has not been removed by the circulation. As the infant warmed up she was able to vasodilate her peripheral circulatory bed and increase blood flow to muscle tissue; this allowed a large reservoir of lactic acid to be shifted into the central circulation. Such a massive acid load may be sufficient to precipitate severe myocardial depression, especially in a heart that may still be "stunned."

## What Action Do You Take?

You return to the ABC's (airway, breathing, circulation) and verify correct endotracheal tube placement, manually ventilate, begin chest compressions, and administer vasopressors as necessary. Once you have resuscitated the child, it will be important to keep her intubated and adequately ventilated until her extremities are well perfused, she is warm, and she has normalized her acid–base status.

An arterial blood gas sample drawn at the time of this bradycardic episode was reported as pH, 6.8; $PaCO_2$, 70; and $PaO_2$, 25, with a hemoglobin concentration of 15 mg/dl. The arterial pressure is now 40/18 mmHg without chest compressions.

## What Concerns Do These Data Raise?

Despite seemingly adequate volume resuscitation, the child is hypotensive. The normal systolic pressure should be 60 mmHg. This may indicate continued myocardial depression from the period of anoxia and hypotension or may indicate a still inadequate restoration of extracellular fluid volume coupled with an attenuation of the effects of the previously administered epinephrine. The low oxygen tension is suggestive of either low cardiac output and/or some degree of right-to-left shunting.

A repeat arterial blood gas after the infant is resuscitated is as follows: pH, 7.28; $PaCO_2$, 47; $PaO_2$, 55. The end-tidal $CO_2$ is 40 mmHg.

## Are There Continuing Concerns?

The data indicate a very large alveolar-to-arterial oxygen tension gradient. The good $CO_2$ waveform and the modest end tidal-to-arterial $CO_2$ gradient suggest that the major cause for the low oxygen tension is shunting and not low cardiac output, although both factors may be involved and are interdependent; that is, the lower the cardiac output, the greater will be the deleterious effects of a given amount of right-to-left shunting.[21] The most likely site for right-to-left shunting in this infant would be the ductus arteriosus. Although it is rarely necessary to make a precise diagnosis in the setting of a delivery room resuscitation, the ideal way to evaluate these possibilities is using echocardiography, possibly coupled with Doppler techniques.

The systolic blood pressure falls to 38 mmHg and a dopamine infusion (5 μg/kg/min) is begun. Additional 5 percent albumin and crystalloid is administered. The blood pressure increases to 55/30 mmHg.

At this dosage, dopamine has beneficial effects on cardiac output by increasing inotropy and augmenting preload as a result of a modest increase in venous tone. It also exerts beneficial dopaminergic effects on the renal vasculature. The increase in blood pressure is probably not due to any increase in afterload (arterial vasoconstriction) at this modest dose.

## What Postresuscitation Care Is Appropriate?

Infants who have sustained severe peripartum asphyxia should be admitted to a special care nursery, preferably a neonatal intensive care unit experienced in the management of such infants. Even after a successful cardiopulmonary resuscitation, there may be persistent injury to other organ systems. In the nursery, the infant will be observed for evidence of central nervous system injury, which could manifest with seizures or more subtle neurologic findings. Asphyxia can also cause injury to the kidneys (acute tubular necrosis) and to the bowel. Asphyxiated premature infants are considered to be at risk for necrotizing enterocolitis, and care will be taken before enteral feeding is begun. Babies resuscitated from shock are also considered to be at high risk for sepsis. Even though the etiology of shock in this instance was maternal hemorrhage, an appropriate sepsis workup and possible prophylactic antibacterial therapy may nonetheless be initiated.

In some cases, it may be necessary to transport a newborn to another hospital for such care, and it may take hours for a transport team to arrive. In cases of critically ill neonates (e.g., a newborn requiring a dopamine infusion to maintain blood pressure), it may be necessary for the anesthesiologist to remain actively involved until an appropriately skilled health provider can assume care. It is unlikely that an anesthesiologist who has been crucial to the successful resuscitation of a neonate who would have likely died without such cross-specialty intervention is going to leave the baby's side until the care is assumed by someone of comparable competence, as long as the primary patient, the mother, is well cared for.

Because there may be undetected but permanent sequelae following episodes of neonatal shock/asphyxia requiring cardiopulmonary resuscitation, it is important that explanations to the family be somewhat guarded. In the overwhelming relief that occurs following restoration of life to a lifeless infant, there is a natural desire to tell the parents that the baby is alive and that everything is going to be okay. Such information should come from the primary caregivers after a thorough evaluation.

## Additional Comments

Neonatal shock can occur with an essentially normal intravascular blood volume. Asphyxia and severe acidosis, as from a prolapsed umbilical cord, may cause myocardial depression and profound vasodilation. The impaired heart needs extra volume to take advantage of the Starling forces, yet venodilation results in peripheral pooling and decreased cardiac return. Diminished preload from venodilation, impaired contractility, and greatly diminished afterload from arteriolar dilation may together produce a situation of cardiovascular collapse. There may also be valvular dysfunction of the heart due to papillary muscle ischemia.

It is essential to recognize the difference between cyanosis (blue) and extreme pallor (gray). A cyanotic baby appears blue because of circulating desaturated hemoglobin. However, the critical distinction is the presence of *circulation.* Cyanosis is usually associated with a recent interruption of gas exchange (i.e., a ventilatory problem). In such cases, the primary focus must be upon identifying and correcting the cause for respiratory insufficiency before subsequent circulatory impairment results. Thus, a patent airway and not vascular access is the prime concern when confronted with a cyanotic child. In almost all such cases, restoration of oxygenation is sufficient therapy and volume resuscitation and vasopressors are unnecessary.

In contrast, when a patient is ashen, there is an inadequacy of circulating hemoglobin, which can be due to either severe anemia (hemorrhage, hemolysis) or severely impaired cardiac output (heart failure, massive pulmonary embolus, hypovolemia, drug-induced myocardial depression). When the patient is ashen, appropriate therapy includes not only establishing adequate oxygen delivery to the lungs, but restoration of circulating oxygenated hemoglobin. A simple rule is that when a baby is *blue,* think *airway/oxygen/ventilation;* when the baby is *gray,* think *airway/oxygen/ventilation/heart/intravascular volume/blood.* Thus, following tracheal intubation of an ashen infant, the failure to respond to oxygenation and positive pressure ventilation should not lead to a prolonged assessment focused on the respiratory tract. (Is the tube down a mainstem bronchus?) Rather, therapy should immediately focus on cardiocirculatory etiologies of shock.

Although the timing of the resuscitative efforts in this case is representative of many real-life situations, it still must be considered suboptimal. What was lacking was a clearly defined plan and proper advance preparation. The most essential life-sustaining element—blood—was not available when it was needed. Too much time was spent before vascular access was established and volume resuscitation begun. Ideally, this infant in profound circulatory decompensation would have been delivered, quickly dried, tracheally intubated, ventilated, and had an umbilical venous catheter placed. If this was not immediately accomplished, a catheter would have been placed in the superior sagittal sinus or a bone marrow space and the already warmed blood (ideally fresh blood with reasonably normal potassium levels) transfused. Under the best of circumstances, this could be accomplished within 2 to 3 minutes. However, such speed can only be achieved when there are skilled practitioners with a well-defined plan of action. In addition to PALS instruction, there is much to be gained from running mock "codes," particularly in areas such as the delivery suite where there is often a paucity of personnel with critical care training and experience.

## CASE 2: RESUSCITATION IN THE EMERGENCY ROOM

You arrive in the emergency department as the rescue squad carries in a 15-month-old who has been struck by a motor vehicle, speed unknown. The history provided by the rescue squad is as follows:

> At the scene the child was found unconscious but breathing spontaneously; the blood pressure was 90/55 mmHg and the heart rate was 150 bpm; his eyes were closed, but he responded to a pinch by withdrawing his arm. En route to the hospital the blood pressure decreased to 50/30 mmHg and the heart rate increased to 180 bpm. Attempts to place an intravenous catheter during transport were unsuccessful. Oxygen was administered using a face mask and a breathing bag. *Transport time: 15 minutes.*

A pediatric critical care specialist is present in the emergency department to direct the resuscitation.

### What Do You Do First?

The first step in such situations is always assessment. Take a few seconds to obtain a global view of the patient as the child is transferred to the resuscitation table. This phase is also referred to as the primary survey, and can proceed even as resuscitative measures are begun.

> The male child is on a backboard; his neck is stabilized with two sandbags and tape across the forehead. His skin color is ashen, and he is cool to the touch. There are no spontaneous respirations and no palpable pulses. There is no evidence of capillary refill in the fingertips. The abdomen is tense and distended. The child is somewhat obese, but both thighs appear grossly enlarged, and the right upper leg is abnormally angulated. There are multiple abrasions and contusions of the face, scalp, thorax, abdomen, and extremities. There is a deep laceration of the scalp but it is not bleeding. The portable ECG displays very wide QRS complexes; the rate is now 20 bpm. No blood pressure is obtainable. Chest compressions are begun. *Elapsed time: 30 seconds.*

### After Assessment, What Is Your First Priority?

Your primary responsibility is to ensure a patent airway. In the case of an unconscious trauma patient with unknown gastric contents, the airway should be secured and protected with an endotracheal tube. The use of cricoid pressure during such a procedure, as well as during bag and face mask ventilation, is controversial in the setting of possible cervical spine trauma. The risk of applying cricoid pressure is movement of the bony structures of the neck and possible spinal cord injury; however, the risk of not applying cricoid pressure is possible aspiration pneumonitis should gastric contents be regurgitated.

There is no chest wall movement with manual ventilation delivered by bag and face mask. A pulse oximeter is applied to a finger but no oxygen saturation data is reported by the machine. Vascular access in both antecubital fossae is being attempted. *Elapsed time: 1 minute.*

## What Do You Do Now?

The clinical evidence suggests that you have failed to secure an airway. There are several management options. Since the most likely etiology for a failure to ventilate in such situations is upper airway obstruction caused by soft tissue (or occasionally a foreign body), attempts can be made to relieve the obstruction. Alternatively, you may attempt immediate tracheal intubation via direct laryngoscopy. Regardless of which option is selected, it is essential to begin thinking about what you might do if the first two approaches are unsuccessful.

In terms of relieving airway obstruction, conventional maneuvers such as extension of the head on the neck are not appropriate in someone with a potential unstable cervical spine. An oral airway may or may not be helpful. If it is too small, it may be occluded by the soft tissue at the base of the tongue; if it is too large, it may force the epiglottis down and occlude the laryngeal inlet. Radiographic studies have demonstrated that the soft palate, rather than the tongue, is often the source of upper airway obstruction in supine, unconscious patients.[22] Obstruction of this nature is best relieved by a nasopharyngeal airway. However, in the setting of major head trauma with possible basilar skull fracture, there is always some degree of concern about the potential for brain injury resulting from a rigid catheter or tube penetrating the brain through a bony disruption in the nasopharynx. This problem can be circumvented by using a soft rubber catheter as a guide (essentially a soft stylet) and verifying that the rubber catheter has entered the oropharynx (either visually or manually) before the tube or nasal airway is advanced over the soft rubber guide. Use of such a guide also decreases the risk of tissue trauma and bleeding as the tube is advanced. Pediatric nasal trumpets may not be readily available in an emergency room, so endotracheal tubes may be substituted.

If you elect to proceed with tracheal intubation, you must recognize that the situation is complicated by the fact that the patient is extremely hypotensive, has a possible cervical spine injury, and has a presumed closed head injury. Thus, drugs that would help protect the brain from sharp increases in intracranial pressure (ICP) would likely have severe effects upon circulatory function. Management in this case is a matter of judgment, recognizing that anoxia is the greatest immediate threat to the brain and must be promptly corrected, if possible. In the case of this unconscious child undergoing cardiopulmonary resuscitation, we would opt for an intubation using no medications. Cerebral hypotension poses a much greater threat to this patient than does the potential for cerebral hypertension following tracheal intubation. It is important that an assistant stabilize the head to prevent excessive head or neck motion during laryngoscopy; axial traction is not advisable. External manipulation of the larynx to improve the laryngoscopic view may cause displacement of cervical fractures, and must be done with great caution.

If an airway cannot be established rapidly by either of the approaches outlined above, be prepared to proceed with an alternative approach, usually translaryngeal entry via a cricothyrotomy or a needle with a high-pressure oxygen delivery system. Both cricothyrotomies and tracheostomies are technically more difficult in young children.

## What Size Endotracheal Tube Is Appropriate?

Table 11-3 gives endotracheal tube sizes based upon weight and length. A weight is not available for this child, but he is measured and found to be 75 cm long. Thus, a 4.0-mm tube is chosen.

With the infant's head immobilized, direct laryngoscopy is performed. A large lumen suction device is immediately at hand in the event gastric contents or blood is encountered. The tip of the epiglottis is visible, but not the arytenoid cartilages or the vocal cords. The tracheal tube is advanced beneath the epiglottis. Chest compressions are interrupted and the chest wall is observed for movement with positive pressure ventilation. The right side of the chest moves considerably more than the left. A capnograph (correct function had been verified immediately prior to use by breathing through the sample tube and observing a normal waveform) is attached to the breathing circuit. A normal capnographic tracing is not obtained when repetitive positive pressure is delivered through the tube; rather, there is a waveform with a peak level of only 4 to 5 mmHg. *Elapsed time: 1.5 minutes.*

## Does the Capnogram Indicate an Esophageal Intubation?

Capnography is now considered by many to be the gold standard for the confirmation of tracheal intubation. However, it can detect only that $CO_2$ that is delivered to the lungs, and in the case of low cardiac output states, this may be minimal or, in the case of cardiac arrest, absent.

Chest compressions are resumed and the capnograph waveform displays a peak of 8 mmHg (normal range, 35 to 40 mmHg). There has been no change in the clinical status of the patient. *Elapsed time: 2 minutes.*

A repetitive $CO_2$ waveform cannot be

**Table 11-3.** Recommended Size and Depth of Endotracheal Tubes Relative to Age and Length

| *Age* | *Length (cm)* | *Endotracheal Tube (internal diameter in mm)* | *Tube Depth (cm)*[a] |
|---|---|---|---|
| Premature infants | < 45 | 2.5–3.0 | 7 |
| Normal newborns | 50 | 3.0–3.5 | 9 |
| 1 year | 75 | 3.5–4.0 | 11 |
| 2 years | 87 | 4.0–4.5 | 12 |
| 4 years | 102 | 4.5–5.0 | 14 |
| 6 years | 117 | 5.0–5.5 | 15 |
| 12 years | 150 | 6.0–6.5 | 18 |

[a] Measured from alveolar ridge or teeth.

obtained from the esophagus. The presence of $CO_2$ may initially be detected following unintended esophageal intubation, since high tissue levels of carbon dioxide (in an extremely acidotic patient) will readily diffuse into the stomach. However, with repetitious inflation and deflation of the stomach, this $CO_2$ will promptly disappear. On the other hand, *failure to see a $CO_2$ waveform does not exclude correct tracheal intubation,* as this can occur whenever there is no blood flow to the lungs (e.g., following cardiac arrest or a massive pulmonary embolus).

Capnographic determinations in the setting of cardiac arrest are usually low, and have been correlated with outcome of CPR.[5] Capnography readings in such a setting have no relation to tissue $CO_2$ levels because of severe ventilation–perfusion inequalities that exist in the lungs.[23]

There is now a small, single-use commercial device (Easy Cap, from Nellcor Corp.) for the colorimetric detection of end-tidal $CO_2$ in settings in which capnography is not available. This technology has been verified in pediatric patients,[24] and promises to be of value for field use.

If capnography is not available, or if there is no waveform, then verification during direct laryngoscopy of the tube passing between the vocal cords is the next best approach to assuring tracheal intubation. When, as in this case, the laryngoscopic view is limited and vigorous maneuvers involving the neck carry a risk for spinal cord injury, clinical assessment using a stethoscope over both lungs and the abdomen may have to suffice. One clinical pearl that may be useful is that if the tube is in the esophagus and vigorous suction is applied to the tube, it will collapse the soft tissue of the esophagus and no gas will come out.[25] This is not the case if the tube is in the trachea. One caveat for this test is that it is possible to distend to esophagus with air during vigorous positive pressure mask ventilation, in which case it may be possible to suction air from the esophagus. However, prior ventilation through a tube deliberately placed in the esophagus has been shown to have no effect on the accuracy of this technique.[24] However, prior decompression of the stomach and the esophagus using a large-bore suction catheter will eliminate any concern for this as well as decrease the volume of gastric contents.

> The end-tidal $CO_2$ level of 8 mmHg is sustained during repetitious positive pressure breaths. Breath sounds are heard bilaterally, but the left hemithorax moves only minimally compared with the right side. *Elapsed time: 2.3 minutes.*

## What Can Account for Bilateral Breath Sounds in the Presence of Asymmetrical Hemothorax Movement?

The limitations of human hearing coupled with the transmission of sounds within the thorax of an infant or small child make auscultation notoriously unreliable for detecting asymmetrical lung ventilation in cases of endobronchial intubation or pneumothorax. The presence of abnormalities on auscultation is highly significant; the absence of abnormalities on auscultation may be reported in cases where there are life-threatening derangements of ventilation. The major differential diagnosis in this child includes endobronchial intubation, tension pneumothorax, and hemothorax. Rare etiologies in this setting would be unilateral pulmonary aspiration (blood, gastric contents) or bronchial disruption. Intra-abdominal trauma and diaphragmatic injuries can also produce asymmetries of chest wall excursion and possibly differences in auscultatory findings.

A soft large-lumen tube is passed transorally into the stomach and suction applied; the distended abdomen decreases somewhat, but still feels firm. Chest excursion is not affected. The endotracheal tube is noted to be taped at a depth of 11 cm, measured at the lips. The child is measured and found to be 75 cm long. The child's clinical condition is unchanged following tracheal intubation and ventilation with 100 percent oxygen. *Elapsed time: 3.0 minutes.*

## How Can Endobronchial Intubation and Tension Pneumothorax Be Differentiated?

Radiographic examination is probably the most reliable diagnostic technique. However, examination of the markings on the endotracheal tube should reveal whether or not the tube is obviously in too deep. A useful guide to tube depth, using the alveolar ridge as a reference, is presented in Table 11-3, along with suggested endotracheal tube sizes based on both age and body length. The latter is readily measured even during resuscitation procedures and can be used as a guide for both proper equipment size and drug dosages, since weight is often not available and may be difficult to estimate.[26] For those who prefer to use a formula, the following is a close approximation based upon the data in Table 11-3.

Tube depth from alveolar ridge

= body length/10 + 3 cm

This child's length of 75 cm indicates that a tube depth of 11 cm from the alveolar ridge is appropriate, so no tube repositioning is warranted.

While a chest radiograph would certainly be helpful in the diagnosis, any delay in initiating treatment is unacceptable in a case such as this. This child has a presumed tension pneumothorax, and the proper management is the insertion of a plastic catheter over a needle (e.g., Jelco, Angiocath) into the pleural space at the second intercostal space in the midclavicular line, followed by prompt evacuation of air (or possibly blood) using a large (60-ml) syringe and a stopcock.

A 20-g intravenous catheter is inserted into the pleural space on the left. Aspiration produces 200 ml of air. Afterward, chest wall motion appears symmetrical and breath sounds appear to be equal. The heart rate increases to 50 bpm, but the QRS complexes remain wide and the rhythm is very irregular. The child is still ashen with cold extremities, and no pulses are palpable. Chest compressions produce a peak $CO_2$ level of 12 mmHg. Attempts at vascular access have not been successful. Epinephrine (5 mg) is administered intratracheally after diluting 5 ampules of epinephrine 1:1,000 in 10 ml of saline (dose derived from Table 11-2). Within 30 seconds, the heart rate increases to 90 bpm and the rhythm becomes even more irregular. There are still no palpable pulses. The end-tidal $CO_2$ level decreases to 8 mmHg. *Elapsed time: 5 minutes.*

## Why Did the Expired $CO_2$ Decrease When the Heart Rate Increased?

This result is frequently seen when epinephrine is administered during CPR, and may be due to vasoconstrictive effects upon the pulmonary vasculature.[27,28] There is evidence that epinephrine may actually decrease overall cardiac output during CPR, but selectively increases coronary and cerebral perfusion.

## How Is the Epinephrine Dosage Determined?

As discussed in the previous case, intratracheal epinephrine is unreliable in the setting of shock or cardiac arrest due to the impairment of tracheal mucosal blood flow under such circumstances.[6,8] Thus, the dose is purely empirical, based upon the assumption that an intravenous dose of 100 to 200 μg/kg would be called for, and that a large portion of an intratracheal dose will never reach the central circulation. Table 11-2 gives recommended epinephrine dosages for both intratracheal and intravenous administration.

## What Do You Do Now?

Having taken care of the first two components of life support (airway patency and ventilation with oxygen), it is imperative that circulatory function be restored. Prompt diagnosis and treatment of the tension pneumothorax were essential first steps. The absence of pulses with QRS complexes, the low levels of $CO_2$ on the capnograph, and the ashen appearance of the child are all consistent with a persistent low cardiac output state. Volume resuscitation is obviously a critical priority.

> Blood is ordered from the blood bank. Multiple attempts at vascular access have been unsuccessful. The pediatric resident in the emergency department has taken a PALS course, and is preparing to insert a bone marrow needle into the child's tibial plateau. *Elapsed time: 6 minutes.*

## Is Attempting Vascular Access via the Tibia the Most Appropriate Course of Action?

This child has obvious bilateral femoral fractures as well as likely intra-abdominal trauma. There is no assurance that fluids administered into a leg vessel or bone marrow will reach the central circulation. Even a catheter placed in the femoral vein above the level of the fracture may still be downstream from a major vascular disruption or from an obstructing hematoma.

Access to the jugular vessels in the neck is limited by the need to maintain neck immobility and the presence of a cervical restraining device. A subclavian approach to the central circulation requires the interruption of chest compressions. If the child is severely hypovolemic, this interruption may be of little consequence since chest compressions are so ineffective. Successful placement of a subclavian venous catheter requires a certain degree of operator skill and, when a child is in hemorrhagic shock, may be time consuming even in the hands of experts.

An optional route for vascular access is the marrow space of the humerus. This technique has been discussed previously, although the upper arm is rarely considered as an access site. However, the widest aspect of the proximal humerus, just beneath the capsule of the shoulder joint, is an accessible site. While concerns have been raised about potential long-term bone injury from damage to the growth plate in children, this complication does not appear to be a significant problem.[11]

An alternative approach in emergencies such as this in young children is placement of a catheter in the superior sagittal sinus (see Figs. 11-1 and 11-2). The anterior fontanelle normally closes sometime between 9 and 15 months of age, and may or may not be patent in this particular child. The only required preparation is placement of the child in a head-dependent position; no special operator skill or expertise is required. In the case of massive cerebral edema, the superior sagittal sinus may be obliterated. In the case of a midline shift of the brain due to a large subdural hematoma, location of the sinus may be problematic. Otherwise, this is a route that may be available in young children in the event other routes are unsuccessful, and is a route that is readily accessible to the anesthesiologist at the head of the table once the airway is secure. In the setting of traumatic brain injury, this is a site that should be attempted only when more conventional approaches have failed and the life of the patient is at risk, as in this case.

> A 14-g catheter is placed in the left subclavian vein (the side with the evacuated hemithorax) with the child in steep Trendelenburg (head-down) position. Blood is withdrawn for laboratory studies. Epinephrine (0.5 mg) is administered intravenously along with a bolus (300 ml) of lactated Ringer's solution and 250 ml of 5 percent albumin (the patient's weight is estimated to be 12 kg, even though Table 11-2 would predict an average weight of 10 kg for a child 75 cm in length; this is a fat baby). The heart rate increases to 160 bpm; the rhythm is irregular due to multiple ectopic beats. No pulses are palpable. The expired $CO_2$ without chest compressions is now 14 mmHg. A spun hematocrit on blood drawn through the subclavian catheter before the fluid resuscitation is reported as 20 percent. The pH of the central venous blood sample is 6.9; $PvCO_2$, 90 mmHg; $PvO_2$, 25 mmHg; base deficit, 15 mEq/L; serum potassium, 3.2 mEq/L; ionized calcium, 3.2 mg/dl (normal range, 4.2 to 5.0 mg/dl). *Elapsed time: 11 minutes.*

The dose of epinephrine (slightly more than 40 μg/kg) is based upon information previously discussed, with modification for the child's clinical condition. This child is not in cardiac arrest, but has a poorly perfusing rhythm. He has already received and partially responded to an intratracheal dose of epinephrine. Subsequent dosages must be based upon a clinical assessment of the patient and not a preset formula. It is still good to remember that we have had years of experience using doses of epinephrine that, in retrospect, were much too small. We have yet to determine how much epinephrine is too much. Do not err on the side of giving too little.[29]

## Should the Child Be Left in the Trendelenburg Position?

Do not leave the infant in the Trendelenburg position. During shock, the Trendelenburg position is associated not with an increase in cardiac output, but rather with a decrease.[30,31] This is because during shock, there is a redistribution of a limited blood volume to the most vital of structures, with the brain being the preferential beneficiary. Thus, in the head-down position, the increased portion of cardiac output delivered to the brain becomes venous blood that is lower than the level of the heart, and hence cardiac return is impaired and is not offset by increased return from the lower half of the body, from which blood has already been shunted away. These events are even more pronounced in small children, as compared with adults, due to the size of the head relative to the rest of the body. These hemodynamic events do not apply to a patient with severe cerebral hypertension; the increased intracranial pressure prevents increases in arterial flow to the brain as well as venous pooling, regardless of gravitational effects.

## Is the Hematocrit Value Consistent with the Patient's Profound Shock?

In cases of hemorrhage, time is required for extravascular (interstitial and intracellular) fluid to be translocated to the intravascular compartment (bloodstream) in an attempt to support circulation. In cases of rapid exsanguination, the small volume of blood left in the vascular system may still have a relatively normal hemoglobin concentration.

A repeat hematocrit spun after the infusion of lactated Ringer's solution and albumin was 11 percent. A repeat central venous blood gas is reported as follows: pH, 6.9; $PvCO_2$, 70 mmHg; $PvO_2$, 26 mmHg; base deficit, 17 mEq/L; serum potassium, 3.3 mEq/L; ionized calcium, 3.1 mg/dl. Two 18-gauge intravenous catheters are placed, one in each antecubital fossa. An arterial catheter is placed in the left femoral artery. The peak arterial blood pressure is 25 mmHg both with and without CPR. The end-tidal $CO_2$ is 14 mmHg and is not affected by chest compressions. The heart rate is 150 bpm. The central venous pressure (CVP) is measured through the subclavian catheter and is 8 mmHg. Chest compressions are suspended. Radiographs of the chest and cervical spine are taken. *Elapsed time: 14 minutes.*

## What Is the Significance of These Data?

These data indicate that your patient is extremely anemic and has a profound mixed (metabolic and respiratory) acidosis. Also, in spite of vigorous ventilation and proper CPR technique, there is mismatching of ventilation and perfusion, presumably due to poor pulmonary blood flow; otherwise, the expired $CO_2$ levels would be higher than the current capnograph reading of 14 mmHg. This is very disconcerting, since you had expected the fluid resuscitation to improve this.

The hypotension with and without CPR is most suggestive of decreased preload (hypovolemia, impaired venous return). However, the relatively normal CVP should call into question the diagnosis of decreased preload.

## Should the Patient Receive Sodium Bicarbonate Until the Cause of the Hypotension Is Determined?

At this point, presumably because of ventilation–perfusion mismatching in the lung, the patient is already hypercarbic. The administration of sodium bicarbonate would worsen the metabolic component of the acidosis, as carbonic acid would be created but not removed by the lung as expired carbon dioxide. While bicarbonate may increase the systemic pH, it has very little effect on intracellular pH, and has been shown to actually worsen myocardial energy metabolism.[32] This may account for the fact that a number of investigators have found that bicarbonate administration during severe metabolic acidosis results in myocardial depression and a worsening of cardiac output; this issue has been reviewed recently by Arieff.[33] While the role of bicarbonate therapy in the treatment of metabolic acidosis is controversial, what is not debated is the futility of using this drug when ventilation is inadequate. This case represents such a situation.

A rapid transfusion of type O packed red blood cells is begun. After the infusion of one unit (approximately 280 ml), the systolic blood pressure is 30 mmHg. The central venous pressure increases to 12 mmHg. The QRS complexes narrow somewhat, but the S-T segments and the T wave morphology are grossly abnormal, with severely depressed S-T segments and inverted T waves that are much larger than the QRS complexes. There are still irregular beats (10 to 15 per minute). The heart rate is 140 bpm. Because of the persistent hypotension, an additional dose of epinephrine (0.1 mg) is given intravenously. The heart rate immediately increases to 190 bpm, the irregularity worsens, and a brief period of a very rapid rhythm is followed by ventricular fibrillation. The end-tidal $CO_2$ trace is flat. *Elapsed time: 18 minutes.*

## What Action Do You Take?

As in all arrest situations, it is essential to take care of the ABC's of resuscitation and to then move on to advanced levels of diagnosis and treatment.

You immediately resume chest compressions (noting the return of the expired $CO_2$ trace with a peak level of 12 mmHg), administer calcium chloride (125 mg IV) and lidocaine (25 mg IV), and order the power on the defibrillator set to 25 J (approximately 2 J/kg). *Elapsed time: 19 minutes.*

The success of direct current countershock will depend upon correction of the underlying problem. The differential diagnosis of treatable conditions at this stage of the resuscitation includes (1) hyperkalemia due to rapid infusion of banked blood with elevated potassium levels and (2) myocardial irritability resulting from a cardiac contusion and exacerbated in the presence of severe tissue acidosis and the administration of exogenous catecholamines. If the main problem is hyperkalemia, calcium is the drug of choice for this condition; if myocardial irritability is the cause for the fibrillation, lidocaine will help stabilize the membranes of myocardial conductive tissue and decrease the likelihood of malignant arrhythmias once a perfusing rhythm is restored.

You administer direct current countershock and the patient promptly converts to sinus tachycardia at a rate of 165 bpm. There is less ectopy than had been present previously. The blood pressure is 35 mmHg. Fluid resuscitation with lactated Ringer's solution and albumin continues. The CVP is 15 mmHg. The hematocrit is now 19 percent. Arterial blood gas data: pH, 7.1; $PaCO_2$, 60 mmHg; $PaO_2$, 40 mmHg; base deficit, 10 mEq/L. End-tidal $CO_2$ on the capnograph is 15 mmHg. *Elapsed time: 21 minutes.*

## Why Did This Child Fibrillate?

The cause of fibrillation is unclear from the information available. The packed red blood cells were 2 weeks old. A serum potassium level drawn after the episode of fibrillation was reported as 6.2 mEq/L. This level would normally be associated with ECG changes (peaked T waves, widening of the QRS complex), and such changes were present in this case. While ventricular fibrillation or asystole usually occurs at higher serum levels (8 to 10 mEq/L), values similar to the ones in this case have been associated with cardiac arrest in pediatric patients in the setting of rapid transfusion during major hemorrhage.[34] In all these cases the hyperkalemia was acute in onset rather than chronic. Hyperkalemia associated with rapid transfusion of banked blood is discussed extensively in Case 3.

On the other hand, epinephrine in the presence of hypercarbia is highly arrhythmogenic, particularly in an injured heart. The well-known arrhythmogenic properties of epinephrine have led some investigators to suggest the use of other vasoconstrictors such as norepinephrine, phenylephrine, and methoxamine, all of which tend to be less likely to induce ventricular arrhythmias than epinephrine, yet appear to be equally effective as vasoconstrictors.[35–37] It is currently believed that the beneficial effects of epinephrine during cardiac arrest result from stimulation of $\alpha_1$- and $\alpha_2$-receptors on blood vessels. This causes an increase in aortic pressure and hence improved coronary perfusion.[38] In this somewhat special case in which there is a high likelihood of a myocardial contusion (as evidenced by ECG changes and persistent ventricular ectopy), a good case can be made for using an alternative and less arrhythmogenic vasopressor.

As to the etiology of the ventricular fibrillation, it most likely represents a combination of factors, including hyperkalemia, myocardial irritability, hypercarbia, epinephrine, and possibly ischemia due to hypotension and/or myocardial injury.

## What Is the Major Concern at This Point?

The child is still hypoxic and hypotensive, despite the administration of crystalloid, colloid, blood, epinephrine and calcium. For the past 10 minutes, this child has had a poorly perfusing cardiac rhythm that has yet to be corrected or even properly addressed.

> **Fresh packed red blood cells are obtained from the blood bank, and an additional 280 ml is administered rapidly. The CVP increases to 24 mmHg. The arterial blood pressure remains at 35 mmHg. A chest tube has been placed in the left hemithorax and connected to an underwater suction device. *Elapsed time: 25 minutes.***

## What Could Account for the Persistent Hypotension?

Low cardiac output and hypotension coupled with high central venous pressures are highly suggestive of pericardial tamponade. The myocardial irritability (ventricular ectopy) and ischemic changes on the ECG are also consistent with injury to the heart.

> The chest radiograph taken earlier shows a heart that appears normal in size and position. There is evidence of a small pneumothorax on the left side. The tracheal tube is above the carina. There are no rib fractures. The left clavicle is fractured and displaced. The chest tube appears to be in proper position. Chest compressions are interrupted as, using a subzyphoid approach, a 20-gauge needle attached to a syringe is advanced cephalad toward the heart until blood is aspirated; 15 ml of blood is removed. Immediately, the end-tidal $CO_2$ increases to 30 mmHg and the blood pressure increases to 60/40 mmHg. The irregular rhythm and the S-T segment changes are unchanged. The CVP decreases to 5 mmHg. For the first time, the pulse oximeter begins to function, and the oxygen saturation is 83 percent. The head wound begins to bleed. Blood replacement is resumed. A pig-tailed catheter is advanced over a wire and left in place in the pericardium. *Elapsed time: 30 minutes.*

Because a child's chest wall is compliant, it is not uncommon to have significant organ injury (myocardial and pulmonary contusions) in the presence of minimal evidence of soft tissue or bony trauma. It takes only a small amount of pericardial blood to cause a major impairment in cardiac output. If there is any question about whether the blood aspirated during attempted pericardiocentesis is from the pericardium or not, it can be observed for clotting in a clear tube. Pericardial blood will not clot due to the presence of endogenous fibrinolytic compounds. However, in many cases the clinical response will confirm the relief of pericardial tamponade.

## Should This Child Now Be Rushed to the Operating Room for Chest Exploration?

Most pericardial bleeding following trauma is from venous tears, and these tend to seal off without surgical intervention. Pericardial tamponade from an arterial site is usually a lethal lesion. The presence of a soft catheter in the pericardial space will allow for monitoring of any continual bleeding, as well as for relief of any reaccumulation of blood. With the restoration of a reasonable cardiac output, it is now time to perform a secondary survey, which includes reassessing all the basics plus directing attention to less life-threatening concerns.

A thorough physical examination is performed. There is no blood or spinal fluid in the ear canals. Probing of the deep scalp laceration reveals a bony defect, indicating a possible penetrating injury to the brain. Both pupils are dilated and respond minimally to light. The child moves his arms in response to painful stimuli, but does not open his eyes spontaneously. A gag reflex is present. While neck stability is maintained, the back is examined; it appears uninjured. The pelvis is unstable, but there are no bony fragments palpated on a rectal examination. The prostate gland cannot be felt. The rectal sphincter tone is normal. Abdominal and lower extremity radiographs confirm the presence of bilateral displaced femoral fractures and pelvic fractures. *Elapsed time: 35 minutes.*

## What Management Is Now Indicated?

The child has evidence for a severe closed head injury, and brain protection is now a prime concern. While the use of epinephrine can account for dilated pupils, this child is unconscious, minimally responsive, and has a deep scalp laceration. Evaluation and treatment of brain injury become paramount once basic cardiovascular function is reestablished.

The patient is vigorously ventilated, and a repeat arterial blood gas indicates a $PaCO_2$ of 24 mmHg (simultaneous capnography reading is 19 mmHg) and a $PaO_2$ of 185 mmHg on 100 percent oxygen. The pH is now 7.4. A mannitol infusion is begun. *Elapsed time: 40 minutes.*

Hyperventilation is one of the most readily available methods for lowering ICP. As already discussed, hyperventilation is possible only when there is adequate blood flow to the lungs. Before the relief of the pericardial tamponade, it would have been impossible to induce hypocarbia in this child. The administration of mannitol is also a standard method for lowering ICP by removing brain water via an osmotic gradient.

## Why Is the pH Normal while the $PaCO_2$ Is Abnormally (but Intentionally) Low?

There is still a metabolic acidosis present that has not totally resolved with the restoration of an adequate cardiac output. The base deficit associated with the most recent arterial blood gas data was 10 mEq/L. This corresponds to a plasma bicarbonate level of 14.5 mEq/L (normal range, 24 to 26 mEq/L). However, as the citrate in the banked blood is metabolized by the liver, the bicarbonate level will increase, as bicarbonate is the major metabolic by-product of citrate metabolism. Intracellular pH is well maintained during metabolic acidosis, and further therapy is unwarranted.

## Is a Urinary Catheter Contraindicated in Pelvic Trauma?

While pelvic trauma may be associated with a partial disruption of the urethra in adults, this is not usual in children; thus, a catheter should be inserted to help in the fluid management of this child, particularly after the administration of an osmotic diuretic such as mannitol.

## Is Peritoneal Lavage Indicated, Given the Tense Abdomen?

The detection of blood in the peritoneal cavity by lavage does little to identify the site of bleeding. Abdominal computed tomography (CT) is now considered the method of choice for evaluation of possible intra-abdominal injuries following trauma. The use of contrast media also allows for assessment of renal function and urinary system integrity.

## Should This Child Be Taken to the Operating Room Rather than the CT Scanner?

While the delay for CT scanning imposes some risks, the benefit of having a much more precise assessment of the degree of cerebral and thoracoabdominal injuries allows for better surgical and medical management. As long as hemodynamic stability can be maintained, the imaging information is usually worth the risk.

The child is transported to a radiology suite for CT scanning of the head, chest, and abdomen. *Elapsed time: 55 minutes.*

## What Are the Primary Concerns at This Point?

The child has ongoing blood loss from the multiple fracture sites and possibly from intra-abdominal sites as well. He is at risk of hypothermia from exposure and low ambient temperatures in the radiology suites. Care must be taken to warm all fluids and to continue hemodynamic monitoring and appropriate fluid therapy. In essence, this represents a continuing resuscitation, a process most anesthesiologists have experienced in the operating room when there are massive ongoing fluid losses. The unfamiliarity of the radiology setting should not serve as a deterrent to good medical care; institutions that provide pediatric trauma care should develop systems for management of patients requiring ongoing volume resuscitation during diagnostic studies.

## Comments

There are some anatomic differences in children that should be kept in mind when dealing with major trauma, since these differences increase the likelihood of multisystem injury.

### Head

In children, the head represents a proportionately larger part of the total body compared to adults, thus increasing the risk for head injury when a violent impact occurs. Because of the disproportionate distribution of weight to the head in young children, the center of gravity is shifted cranially. During rapid decelerations, this makes it more likely that the head will function as the leading structure (battering ram) as the child is projected toward a dashboard or a windshield. The unfused cranial bones of young children (< 1 year) provide for a more compressible protective covering for the brain, increasing the chance of brain injury following head trauma. Children are also more prone to develop reactive cerebral edema following head injury. Fortunately, the brain in children is still somewhat plastic, and children are better able to recover than adults with similar degrees of injury.

### Cervical Spine

Cervical spine injuries are uncommon in children, due to greater flexibility of the bony structures and a shorter neck length compared to adults. However, when cervical spine injuries do occur, the shorter neck of an infant or small child increases the likelihood of injury in the atlanto-occipital, C1, and C2 regions, as opposed to lower cervical levels (C4 and C5) in the older child and adults. Also, because of greater flexibility, cord injury without cervical spine fracture may occur in children. Thus, the absence of radiographic findings does not preclude the possibility of an unstable cervical spine and, particularly in a child with a history of weakness or paresthesia (even transient) following head and neck trauma, a spinal cord injury should be presumed until proven otherwise, possibly with CT or magnetic resonance imaging (MRI) studies. As with adults, cervical spine injury must be presumed in most cases of traumatic head injury (falls, automobile-related injuries) and managed initially with head and neck stabilization and immobilization.

### Rib Cage

Because the rib cage in young children is so supple and the overlying muscle and fat are thinner than in adults, blunt injury communicates more force to underlying organs. This increases the risk for myocardial and pulmonary contusions and rupture of abdominal viscera when compared to adults sustaining similarly severe impact. Chest wall compliance also results in a lower incidence of rib fractures in children. The abdominal organs of children are less enclosed by the rib cage, so that the liver and spleen are more exposed and less protected than in adults.

## Additional Comments

This case illustrates the usefulness of capnography in assessing cardiac output during cardiac arrest. In this case, it confirmed the persistence of a low cardiac output state in spite of seemingly appropriate resuscitative measures, and facilitated the diagnosis of pericardial tamponade. It may also be helpful in documenting endotracheal tube placement. I believe that the absence of some device to detect expired carbon dioxide can lead to delays in definitive resuscitative care, since time must be spent trying to verify endotracheal tube positioning in a child in cervical traction. Most experienced pediatric practitioners have encountered children in the emergency department who have been transported in a state of cardiac arrest, with ongoing CPR, only to find that the breathing tube was in the esophagus rather than the trachea, making the resuscitative efforts futile. Capnography is now considered essential for the optimum care of children in the operating room. I believe that the same level of care needs to be extended to other locations where critically ill or injured children requiring endotracheal intubation are likely to be encountered.

If, in this case, you had taken time to transduce the subclavian catheter and measure the CVP when it was first inserted, it is unlikely a high CVP (despite pericardial tamponade) would have been present due to profound hypovolemia. However, once vigorous volume replacement occurred, there was a continual increase in CVP without a parallel improvement in blood pressure or cardiac output (as estimated from capnography). This information, which was not properly appreciated at the earliest possible moment, is highly suggestive of severe myocardial dysfunction. In this case, the most likely etiologies would be pericardial tamponade or severe myocardial contusion, possibly with valvular disruption. In some institutions, echocardiographic examination in the resuscitation suite would have enabled rapid identification of the impaired cardiac filling due to tamponade and to exclude valvular injury.

During transport the child was hypotensive, had a rapid heart rate, and sustained major blood loss. His condition upon arrival may have been improved had vascular access and volume resuscitation been initiated during transport. However, the success rate of intravenous cannulation in infants and small children by nonanesthesiologists in the field is poor. There are now several reports that document a high rate of success when intraosseous infusions are utilized following a brief training period.[39–43] Intraosseous needle placement is clearly a technique that every anesthetist and provider of prehospital emergency care should be prepared to utilize in injured children.

Although this discussion has proceeded rather slowly, in a real situation this child's life would depend upon an extremely rapid restoration of circulating oxygenated blood. This requires correction of the tension pneumothorax, recognition and treatment of the hemopericardium, and rapid blood replacement, thus necessitating vascular access. Only individuals with a high degree of commitment, training, and skill are likely to be able to accomplish these tasks quickly enough.

## CASE 3: RESUSCITATION IN THE OPERATING ROOM

A 6-month-old 7-kg male is undergoing an emergency laparotomy for severe upper gastrointestinal bleeding. The abdomen is open, but the surgeon has not yet identified the bleeding site. The abdomen is filled with bright red blood, some of which has clotted. Vascular access includes three peripheral venous catheters (20-gauge) and an arterial catheter that is being transduced for blood pressure monitoring. Packed red blood cells are being administered rapidly through two catheters using an in-line manually activated blood pump. The infant has already received 3 adult units of packed cells (280 ml each) over a 3-hour period from the time of admission and during a selective aortogram in the radiology suite. Through the other intravenous catheter, fresh frozen plasma is being rapidly administered, to be followed by platelets. The blood pressure is 80/45 and the heart rate is 170 bpm. Additional monitoring includes pulse oximetry ($SaO_2$, 99 percent) and capnography (end-tidal $CO_2$, 30 mmHg). A nasogastric tube on continuous suction is delivering bright red blood to a wall canister at a rate of approximately 50 ml/min. The most recent laboratory data was obtained on blood drawn approximately 10 minutes earlier and is as follows: hematocrit, 20 percent; serum potassium, 4.6 mEq/L; and ionized calcium, 3.4 mg/dl (normal range, 4.2 to 5.0 mg/dl). Arterial blood gas data: pH, 7.32; $PaCO_2$, 38 mmHg; $PaO_2$, 168 mmHg; base deficit, 7 mEq/L.

The blood pressure decreases to 50/30. The arterial waveform, which previously had a brisk upstroke, now appears damped. The heart rate decreases to 120 bpm. In addition to slowing of the rate, the ECG trace indicates a modest increase in the height of the T waves. The rate of blood delivery to the wall canister appears unchanged. Observation of the surgical field reveals that extreme traction is being applied to the right upper quadrant.

## What Is Your First Response?

The first response to hypotension during exsanguinating hemorrhage is to increase the rate of volume replacement, if possible. This should be done immediately, as this infant's survival depends upon your ability to keep up with ongoing blood losses until the surgeon obtains control of the bleeding site. At the same time, the surgeon should be informed of the hypotension in order to participate in the assessment of the etiology.

The rate of blood replacement is increased, and the fresh frozen plasma infusion is accelerated. The surgeon informs you that the hypotensive episode was not preceded by an increase in the hemorrhaging, and she is able to release the traction on the liver. The blood pressure decreases further to 40/20 and the heart rate decreases to 80 bpm. There is a noticeable widening of the space between the QRS complexes and the T waves (Q-T interval).

## What Do You Do Now?

Unfortunately, the life-saving properties of banked blood and its constituents (platelets, clotting factors) coexist with potential life-threatening properties, particularly when rapid transfusion is required. The ability of the heart to maintain an effective circulatory pump can be impaired by citrate-induced hypocalcemia, such that the administration of even more blood to treat hypotension may only worsen the degree of hypotension. Citrate binds calcium, and will decrease the level of ionized calcium. The previous laboratory value confirmed a low ionized calcium level, and the arterial waveform changes are consistent with a further decrease in the level of this ion. Even though present in this case, the absence of obvious Q-T prolongation on the ECG does not exclude a diagnosis of hypocalcemia.

Calcium chloride (70 mg) is administered; the blood pressure increases to 85/40, and the arterial waveform displays a sharper upstroke. The heart rate increases to 150 bpm. The Q-T interval narrows with administration of calcium.

The likelihood of citrate toxicity is a function of both the rate of citrate administration and the capacity of the liver to metabolize citrate. The concentration of citrate is approximately *five times* higher in fresh frozen plasma (436 mg/dl) than in packed cells (87 mg/dl). The citrate concentration of banked whole blood is intermediate at 280 mg/dl. The rapid infusion of fresh frozen plasma and other blood products may exceed the ability of the liver to metabolize citrate, particularly if surgical traction in the abdomen compromises hepatic blood flow or cardiac output by impeding venous return to the heart from the lower half of the body. Because of its high citrate load, fresh frozen plasma is not an optimum agent for volume expansion during hemorrhage in children. If a colloid solution is desired, there are alternatives, such as albumin concentrate, that present a much lower potential for citrate toxicity and do not carry the risk of transfusion-related diseases.

While citrate-induced hypocalcemia is usually self-correcting as long as there is adequate cardiac output, the severe hypotension and the continuing need for rapid administration of citrate-containing blood component therapy in this case justifies prompt treatment with calcium chloride at a dose of 10 mg/kg via a central line, if present. Calcium can cause severe tissue damage if it extravasates.

An alternative explanation for sudden hypotension and bradycardia could be vena caval obstruction caused by surgical traction. The response of the heart to a sudden decrease in venous return is slowing, the so-called right atrial reflex: temporarily, venous baroreceptors predominate over arterial baroreceptors, and the response of the right heart to decreased filling is to slow its rate in order to allow more time for passive filling.[44] This reflex may be masked in the current setting by the high level of sympathetic nervous system tone resulting from light anesthesia. Insisting that the surgeon relax traction during a critical time in the procedure in order to correct this problem may only delay getting control of the bleeding site; thus, it is important to rapidly exclude other causes of hypotension and bradycardia before interrupting the progress of surgery.

> As vigorous blood volume replacement continues, the blood pressure gradually decreases to 70/35 mmHg and the heart rate decreases to 110 bpm. The pulse oximeter indicates a decrease in oxygen saturation from 98 to 85 percent. Suddenly the heart rate decreases to 40 to 50 bpm and the blood pressure decreases to 40/25 mmHg. Peaked T waves and a widened QRS complex are seen on the ECG; progressive slowing of the heart rate is rapidly followed by asystole.

## What Actions Do You Take to Counteract Cardiac Arrest?

When the presence of cardiac arrest is established, it is imperative that airway patency and ventilation be verified and cardiac compressions be initiated immediately. In most operating room situations, a member of the surgery team is in the best position to do the latter. If any inhalational anesthetic agent is being administered (it is not in this case) it should be discontinued and 100 percent oxygen delivered.

> Chest compressions are initiated, and the $CO_2$ waveform on the capnograph indicates an end-tidal concentration of 15 mmHg. No signal is obtained by the pulse oximeter. The chest moves with manual inflations of the breathing bag and the surgeon can see the diaphragm, through the open incision, moving normally with ventilation.

This evidence, obtained in a matter of seconds, should shift your focus from problems with ventilation to problems with perfusion, especially in the setting of massive hemorrhage. Move immediately from airway and breathing considerations to evaluation and support of circulatory function.

## What Information Does the Capnograph Provide at This Point?

The capnograph confirms that the breathing tube is somewhere in the airway (critically important information during a cardiac arrest) and that CPR is at least adequate enough to deliver some blood to the lungs. In addition, it focuses the differential diagnosis on pump problems (the heart) rather than obstructive problems such as a massive pulmonary embolus. Since chest compressions in this case generate reasonable pulmonary blood flow (as documented by $CO_2$ delivery), adequate pulmonary artery patency as well as alveolar-to-atmospheric airway patency is established.

> Chest compressions generate a systolic blood pressure of 45 mmHg. The ECG tracing is flat. The pulse oximeter is still in a search mode.

## What Measures Do You Take Now?

The T-wave changes noted on the ECG just before asystole were highly suggestive of hyperkalemia, and the drug of choice for the emergent treatment of life-threatening hyperkalemia is calcium chloride administered intravenously.

Calcium chloride (70 mg IV) is administered. In addition, epinephrine (500 μg IV) is also given. Within one minute, the patient's rhythm reverts to a sinus tachycardia (180 bpm). The blood pressure increases to 170/90. The end-tidal $CO_2$ reading is 55 mmHg. Chest compressions are stopped. The pulse oximeter indicates an oxygen saturation of 95 percent.

## Why Was the End-Tidal $CO_2$ Abnormally Low During Cardiopulmonary Resuscitation?

Chest compressions may not generate sufficient pulmonary artery pressures or blood flow to deliver blood to all areas of the lung. This results in ventilation–perfusion inequalities of a dead space nature. That is, there are alveoli that are ventilated but not perfused. This results in delivered gas returning to the trachea having not participated in gas exchange, so that it has given up no oxygen and received no carbon dioxide. This gas mixes with carbon dioxide–laden gas coming from alveoli that are perfused. The mixing of these two gases produces a mixture that will have a carbon dioxide concentration that must be lower than that in the venous blood and the tissues. Thus, in shock or cardiac arrest states, an end-tidal $CO_2$ waveform may have no correlation with the acid–base status of the patient, and a patient with a $PaCO_2$ in excess of 100 mmHg may have a capnograph with an end-tidal $CO_2$ of less than 20 mmHg.

During cardiopulmonary resuscitation, there is a $CO_2$ gradient from the tissues to the central circulation, due to the response of the body to shock. Blood flow is shunted away from nonessential organs such as skin and muscle, and preferentially delivered to the heart and brain. Thus, as nonperfused tissues convert to anaerobic metabolism and produce excess $CO_2$ and lactate, there is insufficient tissue blood flow to remove these metabolic byproducts, and tissue levels rise. The blood that does perfuse these tissues returns to the central circulation with a very high $CO_2$ content and a low pH. This small volume of blood perfuses a highly ventilated lung, and arterial blood gases, as well as capnography, may indicate low levels of $CO_2$ at a time of high tissue acidosis. Thus, there are major acid–base differences between arterial and venous blood during CPR, and this difference is due to ventilation–perfusion abnormalities arising in the lung due to low cardiac output and poor pulmonary perfusion.[45]

## Why Did the Pulse Oximeter Not Respond During CPR?

The pulse oximeter will often fail during chest compressions because of movement artifact and the irregularity of the pulse waveform. The oximeter requires several successive pulses that meet certain predetermined criteria for uniformity before saturation and heart rate data are released to the front screen for display.[46] Thus, even with CPR adequate for cerebral perfusion, the signal may not be "clean" enough for the oximeter to work. Also, peripheral vasoconstriction, a condition often present during cardiac arrest, impairs the functioning of pulse oximeters.

## How Did You Decide Upon the Epinephrine Dosage?

The arrest was witnessed, and the drug was administered immediately thereafter. The $CO_2$ waveform indicated some cardiac output. The dosage given was 70 μg/kg, slightly less than the recommended dosages in Table 11-2. It is important to stress that these recommendations are only guidelines and cannot substitute for clinical assessment. The dosage administered was based upon clinical judgment, not a cookbook.

The surgeon informs you that she has isolated and controlled the bleeding site, an aneurysm of the right gastroepiploic artery. The laboratory informs you that a serum potassium drawn just before the arrest was 6.7 mg/dl, that the pH was 7.1 mEq/L, the $PaCO_2$ was 71 mmHg (simultaneous end-tidal $CO_2$ was 25 mmHg), and the $PaO_2$ was 42 mmHg. A blood sample drawn shortly after restoration of spontaneous cardiac activity was reported as follows: potassium, 7.7 mEq/L; pH, 7.38; $PaCO_2$, 31 mmHg; $PaO_2$, 128 mmHg; and Hct, 30 percent.

The laboratory data confirm the diagnosis of hyperkalemia. Note that even though the serum potassium is still at a toxic level after the restoration of sinus rhythm, the calcium therapy has facilitated restoration of membrane potentials to a range that allows for normal cardiac electrical activity.

## What Other Therapies Are Available to Acutely Lower Extracellular Potassium?

There are other therapies that lower elevated potassium levels, but all are slower and/or less efficacious than calcium administration. β-agonists such as isoproteranol and ritodrine shift potassium intracellularly. Although epinephrine also has β-2 properties, this particular catecholamine may in fact transiently increase serum potassium levels, at least in the arterial circulation.[47] This is significant, since it is the potassium concentration of the arterial blood supply to the coronary circulation which is of critical concern. Studies that have measured venous plasma levels have found that doses of epinephrine in the dose range used for cardiac resuscitation decreases potassium levels by a modest amount (~ 20 percent).[48] The combination of glucose and insulin is also useful in shifting potassium from the extra- to the intracellular space, as is the use of bicarbonate. Although cumbersome in the operating room setting, hemodialysis is another modality for treating life-threatening hyperkalemia.

The patient is given glucose (3.5 gm IV) and regular insulin (1.5 U IV). Blood analysis in the operating room 5 minutes later using a Chem-Strip (Boekringer Mannheim) test kit and glucometer indicates a glucose level of over 400 mg/dl. A repeat dose of insulin (1.5 U) is given and a follow-up arterial blood analysis minutes later shows the following: glucose, 310 mg/dl; pH, 7.21; $PaCO_2$, 54 mmHg; $PaO_2$, 160 mmHg; base deficit, 7 mEq/L; potassium, 6.6 mEq/L. Additional increments of insulin are given and followed with Chem-Strip glucose measurements to avoid hypoglycemia.

As demonstrated, dextrose and insulin can be used to decrease serum potassium levels by an amount similar to that seen with β-agonist therapy. β-agonists tend to lower the blood pressure due to vasodilation, and hence are not the optimal agent for a patient in shock.

## What Level of Potassium Can Be Expected in Banked Blood?

The level of potassium in banked blood is a function of the age of the blood. Potassium concentrations may be as high as 40 mEq/L in stored whole blood and 120 mEq/L in stored red blood cells. However, the amount of plasma present in packed cells is only a fraction of that present in a unit of whole blood, so that the total potassium load per equal volume of red blood cells is actually less with packed cells.

The packed red blood cells that you were administering were diluted in Plasma-lyte at roughly a 50:50 ratio. A blood sample drawn from this mixture had a potassium level of 18 mEq/L and a hematocrit of 39 percent.

## If Continued Rapid Blood Administration Is Needed, What Strategies Could Decrease the Risk of Hyperkalemia and Cardiac Arrest?

If fresh whole blood is available, it is preferable for a number of reasons, including (1) decreased risk of hyperkalemia associated with stored blood and (2) the platelets and clotting factors it provides.

Another alternative, when only banked blood is available, is to process the red blood cells through a cell-saver device that will essentially wash away the extracellular fluid that contains the high concentration of potassium ($K^+$). In many institutions the blood bank can perform this function. The main drawback is the time required.

All strategies that maintain cardiac output also decrease the risk of hyperkalemia, since this allows for delivery of blood to as much of the body's intracellular space as possible. The main mechanism by which the body buffers abrupt increases in serum potassium is to shift $K^+$ ions into cells. A large reservoir for potassium consists of the cells of the skin (the largest organ of the body), the skeletal muscle, and the gut. During shock, blood flow is shunted away from the these areas. This decreases the volume of the sink for excess $K^+$ ions and also effectively centralizes the blood volume, so that a given amount of exogenous potassium circulates in a small volume, producing a higher concentration. Thus, when administering large volumes of banked blood rapidly, it becomes crucial to maintain blood flow to skin, muscle, and gut. This requires sufficient intravascular volume, adequate pump function, and the avoidance of hypothermia. Because maintaining cardiac output during massive transfusion is so essential, empiric calcium therapy is warranted to avoid hypocalcemia and myocardial depression; this therapy also provides some protection against the adverse consequences of hyperkalemia should it occur.

## What Can Be Done to Avoid Hypothermia?

The ambient temperature of the room should be kept as warm as possible, irrespective of the comfort level of the surgical staff. A warming blanket should be in place beneath the patient, and all areas outside the surgical field should be covered. Warming lights can be used.

All fluids and blood should be warmed and infused at as near body temperature as possible. In emergency situations, I have used a microwave oven to warm blood products, testing frequently to make sure overheating is avoided and mixing to avoid uneven heating. A number of in-line commercial warming devices are available, some incorporating microwave energy,[49] as are very expensive rapid-infusion machines that are used during such procedures as liver transplantation.

A final strategy that can be used during laparotomy is to irrigate the abdominal cavity with warm saline. This can increase core body temperature by several degrees over a period of 5 to 10 minutes. While this approach is not practical during rapid intra-abdominal hemorrhage, it can be utilized once the bleeding is controlled.

The aneurysm is repaired and the wound is closed without further complications. The child is transported to a pediatric intensive care unit. The first arterial blood gas is as follows: pH, 7.50; $PaCO_2$, 40; $PaO_2$, 180; base excess, 5 mEq/L.

## What Accounts for the Change from Acidosis to Metabolic Alkalosis?

The large amount of citrate that was administered in the banked blood and the fresh frozen plasma has now been metabolized by the liver with the resultant production of excessive amounts of bicarbonate. Had sodium bicarbonate been used in an attempt to treat the mixed acidosis that was present intraoperatively, the subsequent alkalosis would have been even worse.

## Comments

In all cases of exsanguinating hemorrhage in children, rapid blood replacement requires sufficient vascular access and strategies for avoiding the deleterious effects of hyperkalemia, hypocalcemia, and hypothermia. The use of fresh blood or washed cells can minimize problems with potassium. Because the child will sustain major evaporative, convective, and radiant heat loss from a large abdominal wound with profuse bleeding, it is imperative that efforts be made to minimize the degree of hypothermia through such measures as using warming pads, wrapping all parts of the body outside the surgical field, using warming lights, and infusing all fluids at a temperature of approximately 37°C. Hypocalcemia due to citrate toxicity can best be managed by maintaining cardiac output and hence hepatic blood flow to the extent possible to allow metabolism of the citrate as well as administration of calcium based on the hemodynamic condition of the patient.

## Additional Concerns

The appropriate resuscitation fluid during massive hemorrhage is blood. Exclusive use of either lactated Ringer's or a mixture of hypertonic saline and dextran in the setting of uncontrolled bleeding has been associated with increased hemorrhage and worsened outcomes in animal studies.[50] This is an area of inquiry that needs further clarification, since initial fluid management in many patients in hemorrhagic shock remains rapid infusion of a crystalloid solution.

There is a growing body of evidence that suggests that even modest hyperglycemia during global cerebral ischemia may lead to worsened neurologic outcomes.[51,52] It is theorized that the glucose substrate increases the amount of anaerobic metabolism that occurs in the absence of oxygen and leads to intraneuronal lactic acidosis; normally, intracellular pH is well maintained despite marked systemic acidosis.[32] The availability of inexpensive and reliable technology for measuring serum glucose levels within 2 minutes (Chem-Strip) should end the practice of administering prophylactic dextrose to unconscious patients who fail to respond to usual resuscitative measures.

Another drug that has almost no emergency utility for the anesthesiologist is naloxone. The only use for this drug is in reversal of narcotic-induced respiratory depression. In a patient whose airway is

**Table 11-4.** Drugs and Dosages for Pediatric Resuscitation

| *Agent* | *Initial Dose (mg/kg)* | *Indication* |
|---|---|---|
| Epinephrine | 0.1–0.2 | Cardiac arrest |
| Calcium chloride | 10–20 | Severe hypotension secondary to hypocalcemia; hyperkalemia |
| Lidocaine hydrochloride | 1–2 | Ventricular ectopy |
| Phenylephrine | 0.5–1 | Cardiac arrest |
| Norepinephrine | 0.15 | Cardiac arrest |
| Atropine sulfate | 0.02 | Anticholinergic poisoning |

properly managed and whose respirations are supported, this is not a life-threatening concern. Likewise, atropine for the treatment of hypoxia-induced bradycardias is of no benefit. The agent of choice for this condition is oxygen.

Resuscitation from cardiac arrest is an area of ongoing research, and many questions remain unanswered. For example, it is not at all clear that epinephrine is indeed the best adrenergic agent in this situation. Now that more appropriate dosing is being utilized in many protocols, it may be possible to identify which of the various pressors does in fact lead to the best clinical outcomes. For a review of this issue, the reader is referred to the article by Brown and Werman.[53] A guide to the recommended dosages for these agents, plus other select drugs of use in some cases of cardiac arrest, is given in Table 11-4.

## REFERENCES


1. Chameides L (ed): Textbook of Neonatal Resuscitation. American Heart Association, Dallas, 1990
2. Milner AD, Vyas H, Hopkin IE: Efficacy of facemask resuscitation at birth. Br Med J 289:1563, 1984
3. Vyas H, Milner AD, Hopkin IE: Face mask resuscitation: does it lead to gastric distension? Arch Dis Child 58:373, 1983
4. Vyas H, Milner AD, Hopkin IE, Boon AW: Physiologic responses to prolonged and slow-rise inflation in the resuscitation of the asphyxiated newborn infant. J Pediatr 99:635, 1981
5. Callaham M, Barton C: Prediction of outcome of cardiopulmonary resuscitation from end-tidal carbon dioxide concentration. Crit Care Med 18:358, 1990
6. Bagwell JM, Heavener JE: End-tidal carbon dioxide pressure in neonates and infants measured by aspiration and flow-through capnography. J Clin Monit 7:285, 1991
7. Orlowski JP, Gallagher JM, Porembka DT: Endotracheal epinephrine is unreliable. Resuscitation 19:103, 1990
8. Mullett CJ, Kong JQ, Romano JT, Polak MJ: Age-related changes in pulmonary venous epinephrine concentration, and pulmonary vascular response after intratracheal epinephrine. Pediatr Res 31:458, 1992
9. Redding JS, Asuncion JS, Pearson JW: Effective routes of drug administration during cardiac arrest. Analg Anesth 46:253, 1967
10. Umbilical Artery Trial Study Group: Relationship of intraventricular hemorrhage or death with the level of umbilical catheter placement: a randomized clinical trial. Pediatrics 90:881, 1992
11. Fisher DH: Intraosseous infusions. N Engl J Med 327:1579, 1990
12. Hughes WT, Buescher ES: Collection of blood specimens. p. 71. In Pediatric Procedures. 2nd Ed. WB Saunders, Philadelphia, 1980

13. Redding JS, Pearson JW: Evaluation of drugs for cardiac resuscitation. Anesthesiology 24:203, 1963
14. Neimann JT, Criley JP, Rosborough JP et al: Predictive indices of successful cardiac resuscitation after prolonged arrest and experimental CPR. Ann Emerg Med 14:521, 1985
15. Hebert P, Weitzman BN, Stiell IG, Stark RM: Epinephrine in cardiopulmonary resuscitation. J Emerg Med 9:487, 1991
16. Goetting MG, Parasis NA: High dose epinephrine in refractory pediatric cardiac arrest. Crit Care Med 17:1258, 1989
17. Goetting MG, Parasis NA: High-dose epinephrine improves outcome from pediatric cardiac arrest. Ann Emerg Med 20: 22, 1991
18. Barton C, Callaham M: High-dose epinephrine improves the return of spontaneous circulation rates in human victims of cardiac arrest. Ann Emerg Med 20:722, 1991
19. Lindner KH, Ahnefeld FW, Prengel AW: Comparison of standard and high-dose adrenaline in the resuscitation of asystole and electromechanical dissociation. Acta Anaesthesiol Scand 35:253, 1991
20. Rich GF, Roos CM, Anderson SM et al: Inhaled nitric oxide: dose response and the effects of hemoglobin in the isolated rat lung. J Appl Physiol (in press)
21. Pontoppidan H, Geffin B, Lowenstein E: Acute respiratory failure in the adult. N Engl J Med 287:690, 1972
22. Nandi PR, Charlesworth CH, Taylor SJ et al: The effect of general anesthesia on the pharynx. Brit J Anaesth 66:157, 1991
23. Angelos MG, DeBehnke DJ, Leasure JE: Arterial blood gases during cardiac arrest: markers of blood flow in a canine model. Resuscitation 23:101, 1992
24. Kelly JS, Wilhoit RD, Brown RE, James R: Efficacy of the FEF colorimetric end-tidal carbon dioxide detector in children. Anesth Analg 75:45, 1992
25. Foutch RG, Magelssen MD, MacMillan JG: The esophageal detector device: a rapid and accurate method for assessing tracheal versus esophageal intubation in a porcine model. Ann Emerg Med 21: 1073, 1992
26. Luten RC, Wears RL, Broselow J et al: Length-based endotracheal tube and emergency equipment in pediatrics. Ann Emerg Med 21:900, 1992
27. Gonzales ER, Ornato JP, Garnett AR et al: Dose-dependent vasopressor response to epinephrine during CPR in human beings. Ann Emerg Med 18:920, 1989
28. Callaham M, Barton C, Matthay M: Effect of epinephrine on the ability of end-tidal carbon dioxide readings to predict initial resuscitation from cardiac arrest. Crit Care Med 20:337, 1992
29. Callaham M: Epinephrine doses in cardiac arrest: is it time to outgrow the orthodoxy of ACLS? Editorial. Ann Emerg Med 18:1011, 1989
30. Taylor J, Weil MH: Failure of the Trendelenburg position to improve circulation during clinical shock. Surg Gynecol Obstet 124:1005, 1967
31. Sibbald WJ, Paterson AM, Holliday RL, Baskerville J: The Trendelenburg position: hemodynamic effects in hypotensive and normotensive patients. Crit Care Med 7:218, 1979
32. Zahler R, Barrett E, Mujamdar S et al: Lactic acidosis: effect of treatment on intracellular pH and energetics in the living rat heart. Am J Physiol 262:H1572, 1992
33. Arieff AI: Indications for the use of bicarbonate in patients with metabolic acidosis. Br J Anaesth 67:165, 1991
34. Brown KA, Bissonnette B, McIntyre B: Hyperkalemia during rapid blood transfusion and hypovolemia cardiac arrest in children. Can J Anaesth 37:747, 1990
35. Lindner KH, Ahnefeld FW, Schuermann W, Bowdler IM: Epinephrine and norepinephrine in cardiopulmonary resuscitation. Effects on myocardial oxygen delivery and consumption. Chest 97:1458, 1990
36. Midei MG, Sugiura S, Maughan WL et al: Preservation of ventricular function by treatment of ventricular fibrillation with phenylephrine. Am J Coll Cardiol 16:489, 1990
37. Hoekstra JW, Ligten PV, Neumar R et al: Effect of high dose norepinephrine versus epinephrine on cerebral and myocardial blood flow during CPR. Resuscitation 19: 227, 1990

38. Otto CW, Yakatis RW, Blitt CD: Mechanism of action of epinephrine in resuscitation from asphyxial arrest. Crit Care Med 9:321, 1981
39. Brunette DD, Fischer R: Intravascular access in pediatric cardiac arrest. Am J Emerg Med 6:557, 1988
40. Glaeser PW, Losek JD, Nelson DB et al: Pediatric intraosseous infusions: impact on vascular access time. Am J Emerg Med 6:330, 1988
41. Fuchs S, LaCovey D, Paris P: A prehospital model of intraosseous infusion. Ann Emerg Med 20:371, 1991
42. Seigler RS, Tecklenburg FW, Shealy R: Prehospital intraosseous infusion by emergency medical services personnel: a prospective study. Pediatrics 84:173, 1989
43. Miner WF, Corneli HM, Bolte RG et al: Prehospital use of intraosseous infusion by paramedics. Pediatr Emerg Care 5:5, 1989
44. Baron JF, Decaux-Jacolot A, Edouard A et al: Influence of venous return on baroreflex control of heart rate during lumbar epidural anesthesia in humans. Anesthesiology 64:188, 1986
45. Weil MH, Rackow EC, Trevino R et al: Difference in acid–base state between venous and arterial blood during cardiopulmonary resuscitation. N Engl J Med 315: 153, 1986
46. Woods AM, Lawson D: Valsalva maneuver in obstetrics: the influence of peripheral circulatory changes on function of the pulse oximeter. Anesth Analg 73:765, 1991
47. Lindner KH, Ahnefeld FW, Bowdler IM: The effect of epinephrine on hemodynamics, acid–base status and potassium during spontaneous circulation and cardiopulmonary resuscitation. Resuscitation 16:251, 1988
48. Follett DV, Loeb RG, Haskins SC, Patz JD: Effects of epinephrine and ritodrine in dogs with acute hyperkalemia. Anesth Analg 70:400, 1990
49. Holzman S, Connolly RJ, Schwaitzberg SD: The effect of in-line microwave energy on blood: a potential modality for blood warming. J Trauma 33:89, 1992
50. Bickell WH, Bruttig SP, Millnamow GA et al: Use of hypertonic saline/dextran versus lactated Ringer's solution as a resuscitation fluid after uncontrolled aortic hemorrhage in anesthetized swine. Ann Emerg Med 21:1077, 1992
51. Nakakimura K, Fleischer JE, Drummond JC et al: Glucose administration before cardiac arrest worsens neurologic outcome in cats. Anesthesiology 72:1005, 1990
52. Robertson CS, Goodman JC, Narayan RK et al: The effect of glucose administration on carbohydrate metabolism after head injury. J Neurosurg 74:43, 1991
53. Brown CG, Werman HA: Adrenergic agonists during cardiopulmonary resuscitation. Resuscitation 19:1, 1990

# Appendix

# Antibiotics:

| *Type* | *Indications* | *Resistance* | *Generic Name* |
|---|---|---|---|
| Chloramphenicol | Gram-positive aerobes, anaerobes, *Rickettsia, Chlamydia* | | Chloramphenicol |
| Vancomycin | Gram-positive *Staphylococcus aureus, Staphylococcus epidermidis, Streptococcus pneumoniae,* Enterococcus | Gram-negative | Vancomycin |
| Macrocide | Gram-positive cocci, *Legionella, Mycoplasma, Chlamydia, Bordetella pertussis* | Gram-negative | Erythromycin |
| Monobactam | Gram-negative aerobes | Gram-positive, gram-negative anaerobes | Aztreonam |
| Carbepenem | Gram positive plus gram-negative<br>Wide spectrum | | Imipenem |
| Aminoglycosides | Gram-negative | Anaerobic<br>Gram-positive | Gentamicin<br>Tobramycin<br>Amikacin |
| Clindamycin | Gram-positive cocci, anaerobes | Gram-negative | Clindamycin |
| Trimethoprim-sulfamethoxazole (TMP-SMX) | Gram-negative *Staphylococcus aureus, Pneumocystis carinii* | *Serratia marcescens*<br>*Pseudomonas*<br>Group A beta-hemolytic streptococcus (GABHS) | TMP-SMX |
| Metronidazole | Obligate anaerobes | | Metronidazole |

## β-Lactams

| *Trade Name* | *Dosage* | *Adverse Reactions* | *Anesthetic Considerations* |
|---|---|---|---|
| Chloromycetin | 15–25 mg/kg q6h | Reversible anemia; rare aplastic anemia; left ventricle dysfunction | May cause peripheral neuropathy |
| Vancocin, Vancoled, Vancomycin | 10–15 mg/kg q6h | Dose-related renal and ototoxicity; hypersensitivity; Redman syndrome | Enhance the neuromuscular blocking effect of vecuronium and other nondepolarizing relaxants; cardiac arrest has occurred following rapid administration during anesthesia—must be given slowly over 60 min; delay induction of anesthesia if patient has recently had large dose by rapid intravenous injection |
| Ilisone, Erythromycin, Pediazole, Ilotycin | 5 mg/kg q6h | Hepatic metabolism and drug interactions; gastrointestinal irritation with oral therapy | Prolonged effect of alfentanil has been reported following erythromycin administration |
| Azactam | 20–40 mg/kg q6h | Hypersensitivity reactions; increased serum creatinine | Patient may have cross allergy to penicillins and cephalosporins; causes pain and thrombophlebitis at injection site; may cause hypotension, confusion, and seizures; thrombocytopenia may occur |
| Primaxin | 15–25 mg/kg q6h | Nephrotoxicity; hypersensitivity reactions | May cause hypotension and seizures; use with caution in patients with history of seizures |
| Gentamycin, Garamycin<br>Nebcin<br>Amikin | 2–2.5 mg/kg q8h<br>2–2.5 mg/kg q8h<br>7.5 mg/kg q12h | Dose-related renal toxicity and ototoxicity; neuromuscular blockade | Augments the depolarizing block of succinylcholine and potentiates the non-depolarizing blocking agents |
| Cleosin<br>Clindamycin | 5–10 mg/kg q6h | Hypersensitivity; hepatotoxicity; colitis | Acts as cardiac depressant (avoid rapid injection); may potentiate neuromuscular blocking drugs |
| Bactrim<br>Septra | TMP: 4 mg/kg q12h<br>SMX 20 mg/kg q12h | Nausea and vomiting; Stevens-Johnson syndrome | May cause confusion depression, ataxia, and seizures |
| Flagyl | 10 mg/kg q6h | Peripheral neuropathy; seizures | May cause peripheral neuropathy, headaches, dizziness, confusion, and seizures |

## Antibiotics:

| *Type* | *Indications* | *Resistance* | *Generic Name* |
|---|---|---|---|
| First-generation | Gram-positive cocci<br>Most staphylococci<br>*Escherichia coli*<br>*Proteus mirabilis* | Penicillinase<br>*Haemophilus influenzae*<br>Clostridia<br>Enterococcus | Cefazolin<br>Cephapirin<br>Cephradine<br>Cephalexin<br>Cefadroxil<br>Cefaclor |
| Second-generation | Same as for first-generation, with enhanced effect against anaerobes | Same as for first-generation | Cefoxitin |
| | Gram-positive cocci<br>*Staphylococcus, Haemophilus influenzae*<br>*Neisseria, Escherichia coli*<br>*Klebsiella Salmonella* | Enterococcus | Cefuroxime |
| Third-generation | Fewer gram-positive<br>More gram-negative<br>*Haemophilus influenzae* | Variable *Pseudomonas* resistance, plus *Staphylococcus* | Cefotaxime<br>Ceftriaxone<br>Cefoperazone<br>Ceftazidime<br>Cefixime |

## Antibiotics:

| *Type* | *Indications* | *Resistance* | *Generic Name* |
|---|---|---|---|
| Penicillin | Gram-positive organisms<br>Group A beta-hemolytic streptococci<br>*Neisseria meningitidis*<br>Oral anaerobes<br>Clostridium<br>Syphilis<br>Lyme disease<br>Rat bite fever | *Staphylococcus* species<br>Gram-negative organisms<br>Some *Streptococcus pneumoniae* | Penicillin G |
| | | | Penicillin V |
| | | | Procaine penicillin G |

## Cephalosporins

| *Trade Name* | *Dosage* | *Adverse Reactions* | *Anesthetic Considerations* |
|---|---|---|---|
| Ancef Cefazolin, Kefzol | 20–30 mg/kg q8h | Pseudomembraneous entercolitis; immunologic-based reactions; rash; urticaria | Cross sensitivity with penicillins; may cause transient elevation of liver enzymes; use caution in patients with impaired renal function |
| Cefadyl | 10–20 mg/kg q6h | | |
| Cephradine, Velosef | 6–25 mg/kg q6h | | |
| Biocef, Keflex | 25 mg/kg q6h | | |
| Duricef, Ultracef | 15 mg/kg bid | | |
| Ceclor | 10–15 mg/kg tid | | |
| Mefloxin | 20–40 mg/kg q6h | Same as for first-generation; fever | As for first-generation; gastrointestinal bleeding, headache, and dizziness |
| Kefurox, Zinacef | 12–25 mg/kg q6h | | |
| Claforam (intramuscular) | 40–50 mg/kg q6h | Pseudomembraneous enterocolitis; immunologic-based reactions | Cross sensitivity with penicillins; may cause transient elevation of liver enzymes; use caution in patients with impaired renal function; gastrointestinal bleeding, headache, and dizziness |
| Rocephin (intramuscular) | 40 mg/kg q12h | | |
| Cefobid | 30–60 mg/kg q8h | | |
| Ceptaz, Taziaf, Taxidime | 50–70 mg/kg q8h | | |
| Suprax | 8 mg/kg/d | | |

## Penicillins[a]

| *Trade Name* | *Dosage* | *Adverse Reactions* | *Anesthetic Considerations* |
|---|---|---|---|
| Bicillin, Wycillin | 25–100,000 U/kg/d | Immunologic-based reaction; rash, anaphylaxis, vasculitis, serum sickness, Stevens-Johnson syndrome, fever | May cause convulsions, confusion, drowsiness, myoclonus; thrombophlebitis may occur |
| Oral Pen Vee K, Betapen | 30,000 U/kg q8h | | As for penicillin G |
| IM | 25–100,000 U/kg/d | | As for penicillin G; may cause myocardial depression and conduction disturbances |

(*Continues*)

## Antibiotics:

| Type | Indications | Resistance | Generic Name |
|---|---|---|---|
| | | | Benzathine penicillin G |
| Antistaphylococcal penicillin | *Staphylococus aureus* | Up to one-third of all *Staphylococcus aureus* | Methicillin |
| | | | Nafcillin |
| | | | Oxacillin |
| | | | Cloxacillin |
| | | | Dicloxacillin |
| Aminopenicillins | Same as penicillin<br>*Haemophilus influenzae*<br>Enterococcus | Penicillinase<br>*Haemophilus influenzae*<br>*Staphylococcus* species | Ampicillin |
| | *Listeria monocytogenes*<br>*Streptococcus pneumoniae*<br>Some enterobacteria | *Escherichia coli*<br>*Shigella*<br>*Salmonella* | Amoxicillin<br>Bacampicillin<br>Cyclacillin |
| Broad-spectrum penicillins | Gram-positive except *Staphylococcus*<br>Enterococcus<br>*Bacteroides fragilis*<br>*Pseudomonas aeruginosa*<br>Gram-negative anaerobic<br>*Klebsiella*<br>*Serratia* | *Staphylococcus*<br>Penicillinase<br>*Haemophilus influenzae* | Carbenicillin<br>Ticarcillin<br>Piperacillin<br>Mezlocillin |

[a] It should be remembered that all antibiotics have the possibility of producing either an anaphylactic

## Penicillins[a] (*Continued*)

| *Trade Name* | *Dosage* | *Adverse Reactions* | *Anesthetic Considerations* |
|---|---|---|---|
| Bicillin | 25–100,000 U/kg/d | | As for penicillin G; use with caution if patient has impaired renal function, myocardial depression, or seizure disorder |
| Staphcillin | 25–75 mg/kg q6h | As for penicillin G | |
| Nafcil, Unipen | 25–50 mg/kg q6h | | Irritant solution: avoid extravasation; causes pain and thrombophlebitis; use caution in patients with renal and hepatic impairment |
| Prostaphlin | 25–75 mg/kg q6h | As for penicillin G | May cause nausea and vomiting; occasional hepatotoxicity |
| Tegopen | 12–25 mg/kg q6h | As for penicillin G | |
| Dynapen | 6 mg/kg q6h | As for penicillin G | May cause elevated liver enzymes, leukopenia and thrombocytopenia, fever, and serum sickness-like reaction |
| Polycillin, Ampicillin | 15–20 mg/kg tid | Rash, anaphylaxis, vasculitis, serum sickness, Stevens-Johnson syndrome, fever | May cause nausea and vomiting; Decrease dosage if creatinine clearance is diminished |
| Polymox | 25 mg/kg q12h | | |
| Spectrobid | 25 mg/kg q12h | | Decrease dosage is renal function in impaired |
| Cyclanpen-W | 25 mg/kg q8h | | |
| Geocillin | 30 mg/kg qid | Rash, fever, eosinophila, exfoliative dermatitis, hemolytic anemia, neutropenia, interstitial nephritis | May cause bleeding diathesis; inhibits platelet aggregation, hypernatremia, hypokalemia, and metabolic alkalosis; seizures and hepatitis may occur |
| Ticar | 70 mg/kg q6h | | |
| Pipracil | 70 mg/kg q6h | | Prolongs bleeding time; may cause seizures, hypokalemia, and elevated liver enzymes |
| Meglin | 70 mg/kg q6h | | |

or an anaphylactoid reaction.

## Antiviral Drugs

| Generic Name | Trade Name | Dosage | Adverse Reactions | Anesthetic Considerations |
|---|---|---|---|---|
| Zidovudine (AZT) | Retrovir | 30 mg/kg/d | Anemia; granulocytopenia | Lorazepam, acetaminophen, cimetidine, or indomethacin may increase toxicity of AZT; confusion, dizziness, tremor, or seizures may occur |
| Acyclovir | Zovirax | 30 mg/kg/d | Nausea and vomiting | |

## Anticonvulsants

| Generic Name | Trade Name | Dosage | Adverse Reactions | Anesthetic Considerations |
|---|---|---|---|---|
| Phenytoin | Dilantin | 4–8 mg/kg/d | Blood dyscrasias | May increase requirements for nondepolarizing relaxants; also increases requirements for fentanyl; may cause hypotension, bradycardia, and cardiovascular collapse; give loading dose slowly—not to exceed 1 mg/kg/min; may cause peripheral neuropathy |
| Mephenytoin | Mesantoin | 3–6 mg/kg/d | Blood dyscrasias | |
| Phenobarbital | Phenobarbital | 3–6 mg/kg/d | Drowsiness | |
| Primidone | Mysoline | 10–25 mg/d | Ataxia, vertigo | |
| Carbamazepine | Tegretol | 20–30 mg/kg/d | Dizziness, vomiting | |
| Valproic acid | Depakene | 15–60 mg/kg/d | Hepatotoxicity | |

## Chemotherapeutic

| Class | Type | Generic Name | Trade Name |
|---|---|---|---|
| **Natural products** | Vinca alkaloids | Vinblastine | Velban, Velbe, Velsar |
| | | Vincristine | Vincrex, Oncovin, Vincasar |
| | Epipodophyllotoxins | Etoposide | VePesid, VP-16 |
| | | Teniposide | VM-26 |
| | Antibiotics | Dactinomycin (actinomycin D) | Cosmegen |
| | | Daunorubicin (daunomycin, rubidomycin) | Cerubidine |
| | | Doxorubicin | Adriamycin, Rubex |

## Bronchodilators

| Generic Name | Trade Name | Dosage | Adverse Reactions | Anesthetic Considerations |
|---|---|---|---|---|
| Theophylline | Theophyl, Choledyl | 7 mg/kg oral/d | Nausea and vomiting | Severe arrhythmias may occur with halothane |
| Aminophylline | Slo-Phyllin, Theodur | | | |
| Albuterol | Proventil, Ventolin | 0.15 mg/kg tid | Tachycardia, tremor | May cause spurious readings from mass spectrometer respiratory gas monitors |
| Metaproterenol | Alupent, Metapril | 0.5 mg/kg tid | Tachycardia, tremor | |
| Terbutaline | Brethaire | 0.075 mg/kg tid | Tachycardia, tremor | May decrease the time of onset and duration of succinylcholine block |
| Isoproterenol | Isuprel | Aerosol | Tachycardia, tremor | |
| Isoetharine | Bronkosol | Aerosol | Tachycardia, tremor | |

## Agents[a]

| Dosage | Adverse Reactions | Anesthetic Considerations |
|---|---|---|
| 2.5–7.5 mg/m$^2$ BSA[b] | Neurotoxicity | May cause peripheral neuropathy; conduction anesthesia contraindicated |
| 10–30 μg/kg one a week | Cardiotoxicity; neurotoxicity | Neurotoxic effects, seizures, central nervous system depression |
| Not established | | None described |
| 5 mg/kg twice a week | Myelosuppression | None described |
| 10–15 mcg/kg/d for 5 days | Cardiotoxicity | Severe cardiac depression may occur with halothane; avoid myocardial depressants |
| 25 mg/m$^2$ BSA | Cardiotoxicity | Cardiotoxic effects may be markedly potentiated by halothane; avoid myocardial depressants |
| 30 mg/m$^2$ BSA on 3 successive days for 4 weeks | Cardiotoxicity | Cardiotoxic effects may be markedly potentiated by halothane; avoid myocardial depressants |

(*Continues*)

## Chemotherapeutic

| *Class* | *Type* | *Generic Name* | *Trade Name* |
|---|---|---|---|
| | | Bleomycin | Blenoxane |
| | | Plicamycin (mithramycin) | Mithracin |
| | | Mitomycin (mitomycin C) | Mutamycin |
| | Enzymes | L-asparaginase | Kidrolase, Elspar |
| **Miscellaneous agents** | Platinum coordination complexes | Cisplatin (cis-DDEP), carboplatin | Abiplatin, Platinol |
| | Methyl hydrazine derivatives | Procarbazine (N-methylhydrazine, MIH) | Matulane, Natulan |
| | Adrenocortical suppressants | Amsacrine | Amsidyl |
| | Antifungal | Ketoconazole | Nizoral |
| **Alkylating agents** | Nitrogen mustards | Mechlorethamine ($HN^2$) | Mustargen |
| | | Cyclophosphamide | Cytoxan, Neosar, Procytox |
| | | Ifosfamide<br>Melphalan (L-sarcolysin)<br>Chlorambucil | IFEX<br>Alkeran<br>Leukeran |
| | Ethylenimines and methylmelamines | Hexamethyl-melamine<br>Thiotepal | |
| | Alkyl sulfonates | Busulfan | Myleran |
| | Nitrosoureas | Carmustine (BCNU)<br>Lomustine (CCNU)<br>Streptozocin (streptozotocin) | BiCNU<br>CeeNU<br>Zanosar |
| | Triazenes | Dacarbazine (DTIC [dimethyltriazenoimid-azolecarboxamine]) | DTIC-Dome |
| **Antimetabolites** | Folic acid analogs | Methotrexate (amethopterin) | Rheumatrex, Methotrexate |
| | Pyrimidine analogs | Fluorouracil (5-FU) | Adrucil, 5-FU |
| | | Floxuridine (FUdR)<br>Cytarabine (cytosine arabinoside) | FUDR<br>Cytosar |
| | Purine analogs and related inhibitors | Mercaptopurine (6-mercaptopurine; 6-MP) | 6 MP, Purinethol |

[a] All drugs used in tumor therapy may cause myelosupression, with anemia, leukopenia, and thrombocy
if intravenous extravasation occurs.

[b] BSA, body surface area.

## Agents (*Continued*)

| *Dosage* | *Adverse Reactions* | *Anesthetic Considerations* |
|---|---|---|
| 15 U/m$^2$ BSA for 4–5 days | Pulmonary toxicity | Excess oxygen increases pulmonary damage; avoid fluid overload |
| 25–30 μg/kg/d | Cardiotoxicity | May cause coagulopathy, hepatorenal failure |
| 10–20 mg/m$^2$ BSA | Cardiotoxicity; pulmonary toxicity | Pulmonary fibrosis may be present |
| 6,000 U/m$^2$ BSA 3 times a week | Neurotoxicity | May cause coagulopathy, lethargy and somnolence; coma may occur |
| 20 mg/m$^2$ BSA for 5 days | Cardiotoxicity; neurotoxicity; nephrotoxicity | |
| 50 mg/d (variable dosages) | Pulmonary toxicity; neurotoxicity | Central nervous system depressant drugs potentiated; use with caution; inhibits monoamine oxidase inhibitors |
| 0–200 mg/m$^2$ | Cardiotoxicity; myelosuppression | |
| 5–10 mg/kg/d | Hepatotoxicity | |
| Variable | Bone marrow depression | |
| 1.2 gm/m$^2$ BSA for 5 days | Cardiotoxicity; pulmonary toxicity; neurotoxicity; nephrotoxicity | Inhibition of plasma cholinesterase to prolong block with succinylcholine |
| 250 μg/kg/d | Pulmonary toxicity | |
| .10–.20 ml/kg/d (up to a total dose of 8–12 mg/kg/body weight) | Pulmonary toxicity | |
| 60–120 μg/kg/d | Pulmonary toxicity; neurotoxicity | Reduce plasma cholinesterase to prolong succinylcholine effect |
| 40 mg/m$^2$ BSA/d for 5 days | Pulmonary toxicity | |
| Variable | Pulmonary toxicity | |
| 500 mg/m$^2$ BSA/d for 5 days | Nephrotoxicity | |
| 2–4.5 mg/kg/d | Bone marrow depression | |
| 20–40 mg/m$^2$ BSA once a week | Pulmonary toxicity; neurotoxicity; nephrotoxicity | |
| 7–12 mg/kg/d | Cardiotoxicity; neurotoxicity | |
| 100–600 μg/kg | | |
| 3 mg/kg/d for 5–10 days | Pulmonary toxicity | |
| 2.5 mg/kg/d | Pulmonary toxicity; neurotoxicity | |

topenia. They also cause stomatitis and enterocolitis. Many are neurotoxic. Severe tissue burns will result

## Immunosuppressive Agents

| *Generic Name* | *Trade Name* | *Dosage* | *Adverse Reactions* | *Anesthetic Considerations* |
|---|---|---|---|---|
| Cyclosporine | Sandimmine | Variable | Nephrotoxicity | Cyclosporine absorption after oral administration is decreased by isoflurane anesthesia |
| Azathioprine | Imuran | 1–3 mg/kg/d | Infection | |
| Methotrexate | Folex Mexate | 2–5 mg/kg/d | Leukopenia, nausea | |
| Corticosteroids | Multiple | Variable | Hypertension, infection | |

## Antihypertensive Agents

| *Type* | *Generic Name* | *Trade Name* | *Dosage* | *Adverse Reactions* | *Anesthetic Considerations* |
|---|---|---|---|---|---|
| α-blockers | Prazosin | Minipress | 0.4 mg/kg/d | Hypotension; bradycardia | May potentiate the dissociative effects of ketamine |
| β-blockers | Atenolol<br>Propranolol<br>Metoprolol | Tenormin<br>Inderal<br>Lopressor | 2 mg/kg/d<br>4–6 mg/kg/d<br>6 mg/kg/d | Bronchospasm; cardiac output | May potentiate the myocardial depressant effects of volatile anesthetic agents; prevent fasciculations with succinylcholine; neostigmine or other anticholinesterases may cause serious bradycardia |
| α- and β-blockers | Labetalol | Trandate | 10–12 mg/kg/d | Hypotension; rash | |
| Central adrenergic agonists | Clonidine<br>Methyldopa<br>Guanabenz | Catapres<br>Aldoment<br>Wytensin | 30 μg/kg/d<br>40 mg/kg/d<br>1 mg/kg/d | Sedation; hypotension | May prolong effects of local anesthetics; Decrease postoperative shivering, postoperative oxygen uptake, cardiovascular responses to intubation, and heart rate response to atropine; may supplement depressants and analgesics |
| Direct vaso-dilators | Hydralazine<br>Minoxidil | Apresolin<br>Loniten | 8 mg/kg/d<br>1–2 mg/kg/d | Tachycardia; renin release | May cause peripheral neuritis, weakness; indomethacin interacts to reduce effort |

*(Continues)*

## Antihypertensive Agents (*Continued*)

| *Type* | *Generic Name* | *Trade Name* | *Dosage* | *Adverse Reactions* | *Anesthetic Considerations* |
|---|---|---|---|---|---|
| Angiotensin-converting enzyme inhibitors | Captopril<br>Enalapril<br>Lisinopril | Capoten<br>Vasotec<br>Zestril | 5 mg/kg/d<br>1 mg/kg/d<br>0.1–0.8 mg/kg bid | Neutropenia; renal damage | Severe hypotension may occur with volume depletion; indomethacin reduces antihypertensive effect of captopril |
| Calcium channel blockers | Nifedipine<br>Verapamil<br>Diltiazem | Procardia<br>Calan<br>Cardizem | 1 mg/kg/d<br>7.0 mg/kg/d<br>3.5 mg/kg/d | Atrioventricular conduction disturbance; reduced heart rate; hypotension | Peak blood levels may be higher if drug is administered during halothane anesthesia; potentiate effects of nondepolarizing relaxants |
| Diuretics | Hydrochlorothiazide<br>Furosemide<br>Triamterene<br>Spironolactone | Hydrodiuril<br>Lasix<br>Dyazide<br>Aldactone | 5 mg/kg/d<br>5 mg/kg/d<br>6 mg/kg/d<br>3 mg/kg/d | Hypokalemia; hyperkalemia | Hyperkalemia predisposes to succinylcholine-induced arrhythmias; furosemide may prolong the effect of D-tubocurarine; hypokalemia may prolong the action and delay reversal of effects of muscle relaxants |
| Digitalis | Digoxin | Lanoxin | Premature infant (<1,250 g): 6 μg/kg/d<br>Premature infant (>1,250 g): 8 μg/kg/d<br>Newborn: 10 μg/kg/d<br>7 months–2 years: 16 μg/kg/d<br>2–5 years: 14 μg/kg/d<br>5–10 years: 9 μg/kg/d<br>>10 years: 4 μg/kg/d | Nausea and vomiting arrhythmias | Digoxin may increase bupivacaine toxicity; indomethacin increases digoxin plasma level |

# Index

Page numbers followed by *f* indicate figures; those followed by *t* indicate tables.